Advances in Computer Vision and Pattern Recognition

For further volumes:
www.springer.com/series/4205

Klaus D. Toennies

Guide to Medical Image Analysis

Methods and Algorithms

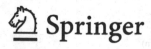

Springer

Prof. Klaus D. Toennies
Computer Science Department, ISG
Otto-von-Guericke-Universität Magdeburg
Magdeburg
Germany

Series Editors
Prof. Sameer Singh
Research School of Informatics
Loughborough University
Loughborough
UK

Dr. Sing Bing Kang
Microsoft Research
Microsoft Corporation
Redmond, WA
USA

ISSN 2191-6586   e-ISSN 2191-6594
Advances in Computer Vision and Pattern Recognition
ISBN 978-1-4471-6096-0   ISBN 978-1-4471-2751-2 (eBook)
DOI 10.1007/978-1-4471-2751-2
Springer London Dordrecht Heidelberg New York

British Library Cataloguing in Publication Data
A catalogue record for this book is available from the British Library

Printed on acid-free paper

Springer is part of Springer Science+Business Media (www.springer.com)

Preface

Hans Castorp, in Thomas Mann's Magic Mountain, keeps an x ray of his lover as it seems to him the most intimate image of her to possess. Professionals will think differently of medical images, but the fascination with the ability to see the unsccable is similar. And, of course, it is no longer just the x ray. Today, it is not sparseness, but the wealth and diversity of the many different methods of generating images of the human body that make the understanding of the depicted content difficult. At any point in time in the last 20 years, at least one or two ways of acquiring a new kind of image have been in the pipeline from research to development and application. Currently, optical coherence tomography and magnetoencephalography (MEG) are among those somewhere between development and first clinical application. At the same time, established techniques such as computed tomography (CT) or magnetic resonance imaging (MRI) reach new heights with respect to the depicted content, image quality, or speed of acquisition, opening them to new fields in the medical sciences.

Images are not self-explanatory, however. Their interpretation requires professional skill that has to grow with the number of different imaging techniques. The many case reports and scientific articles about the use of images in diagnosis and therapy bears witness to this. Since the appearance of digital images in the 1970s, information technologies have had a part in this. The task of computer science has been and still is the quantification of information in the images by supporting the detection and delineation of structures from an image or from the fusion of information from different image sources. While certainly not having the elaborate skills of a trained professional, automatic or semi-automatic analysis algorithms have the advantage of repeatedly performing tasks of image analysis with constant quality, hence relieving the human operator from the tedious and fatiguing parts of the interpretation task.

By the standards of computer science, computer-based image analysis is an old research field, with the first applications in the 1960s. Images in general are such a fascinating subject because the data elements contain so little information while the whole image captures such a wide range of semantics. Just take a picture from your last vacation and look for information in it. It is not just Uncle Harry, but also the beauty of the background, the weather and time of day, the geographical location, and many other kinds of information that can be gained from a collection of pixels of which the only information is intensity, hue, and saturation. Consequently, a variety of methods have been developed to integrate the necessary knowledge in an interpretation algorithm for arriving at this kind of semantics.

Although medical images differ from photography in many aspects, similar techniques of image analysis can be applied to extract meaning from medical images. Moreover, the profit from applying image analysis in a medical application is immediately visible as it saves times or increases the reliability of an interpretation task needed to carry out a necessary medical procedure. It requires, however, that the method is selected adequately, applied correctly, and validated sufficiently.

This book originates from lectures about the processing and analysis of medical images for students in Computer Science and Computational Visualistics who want to specialize in Medical Imaging. The topics discussed in the lectures have been rearranged to provide a single comprehensive view on the subject. The book is structured according to potential applications in medical image analysis. It is a different perspective if compared to image analysis, where usually a bottom-up sequence from pixel information to image content is preferred. Wherever it was possible to follow the traditional structure, this has been done. However, if the methodological perspective conflicted with the view from an application perspective, the latter was chosen. The most notable difference is in the treatment of classification and clustering techniques that appears twice since different methods are suitable for segmentation in low-dimensional feature space compared to classification in high-dimensional feature space.

The book is intended for medical professionals who want to get acquainted with image analysis techniques, for professionals in medical imaging technology, and for computer scientists and electrical engineers who want to specialize in the medical applications. A medical professional may want to skip the second chapter, as he or she will be more intimately acquainted with medical images than the introduction in this chapter can provide. It may be necessary to acquire some additional background knowledge in image or signal processing. However, only the most basic material was omitted (e.g., the definition of the Fourier transform, convolution, etc.), information about which is freely available on the Internet. An engineer, on the other hand, may want to get more insight into the clinical workflow, in which analysis algorithms are integrated. The topic is presented briefly in this book, but a much better understanding is gained from collaboration with medical professionals. A beautiful algorithmic solution can be virtually useless if the constraints from the application are not adhered to.

As it was developed from course material, the book is intended for use in lectures on the processing and analysis of medical images. There are several possibilities to use subsets of the book for single courses, which can be combined. Three of the possibilities that I have tried myself are listed below (Cx refers to the chapter number).

- Medical Image Generation and Processing (Bachelor course supplemented with exercises to use Matlab or another toolbox for carrying out image processing tasks):
  - C2: Imaging techniques in detail (4 lectures),
  - C3: DICOM (1 lecture),

- C4: Image enhancement (2 lectures),
- C5: Feature generation (1 lecture),
- C6: Basic segmentation techniques (2 lectures),
- C12: Classification (1 lecture),
- C13: Validation (1 lecture).
- Introduction to Medical Image Processing and Analysis (Bachelor course supplemented with a student's project to solve a moderately challenging image analysis task; requires background on imaging techniques):
  - C2: Review of major digital imaging techniques: x ray, CT, MRI, ultrasound, nuclear imaging (1 lecture),
  - C3: Information systems in hospitals (1 lecture),
  - C4: Image enhancement (1 lecture),
  - C6: Basic segmentation techniques (2 lectures),
  - C7: Segmentation as a classification task (1 lecture),
  - C8–C9: Introduction to graph cuts, active contours, and level sets (2 lectures),
  - C10: Rigid and nonrigid registration (2 lectures),
  - C11: Active Shape Model (1 lecture),
  - C13: Validation (1 lecture).
- Advanced Image Analysis (Master course supplemented with a seminar on hot topics in this field):
  - C7: Segmentation by using Markov random fields (1 lecture),
  - C8: Segmentation as operation on graphs (3 lectures),
  - C9: Active contours, active surfaces, level sets (4 lectures),
  - C11: Object detection with shape (4 lectures).

Most subjects are presented so that they can also be read on a cursory level, omitting derivations and details. This is intentional to allow a reader to understand the dependencies of a subject on other subjects without having to go into detail in each one of them. It should also help to teach medical image analysis on the level of a Bachelor's course.

Medical image analysis is a rewarding field for investigating, developing, and applying methods of image processing, computer vision, and pattern recognition. I hope that this book gives the reader a sense of the breadth of this area and its many challenges while providing him or her with the basic tools to take the challenge.

Magdeburg, Germany   Klaus D. Toennies

Acknowledgements

There are many who contributed to this book who I wish to thank. First and foremost, there is the Unknown Student. Many of the students who took part in the lectures on which this book is based took a real interest in the subject, even though image processing and image analysis requires more background in mathematics than many students care to know. Their interest in understanding this subject certainly helped to clarify much of the argumentation.

Then there are the PostDocs, PhD and Master students who contributed with their research work to this book. The work of Stefan Al-Zubi, Steven Bergner, Lars Dornheim, Karin Engel, Clemens Hentschke, Regina Pohle, Karsten Rink, and Sebastian Schäfer produced important contributions in several fields of medical image analysis that have been included in the book. I also wish to thank Stefanie Quade for proofreading a first version of this book, which certainly improved the readability.

Finally, I wish to thank Abdelmalek Benattayallah, Anna Celler, Tyler Hughes, Sergey Shcherbinin, MeVis Medical Solutions, the National Eye Institute, Siemens Sector Healthcare, and Planilux who provided several of the of the pictures that illustrate the imaging techniques and analysis methods.

Contents

1   The Analysis of Medical Images   1
   1.1   Image Analysis in the Clinical Workflow   5
   1.2   Using Tools   8
   1.3   An Example: Multiple Sclerosis Lesion Segmentation in Brain
       MRI   13
   1.4   Concluding Remarks   18
   1.5   Exercises   18
   References   19

2   Digital Image Acquisition   21
   2.1   X-Ray Imaging   24
       2.1.1   Generation, Attenuation, and Detection of X Rays   24
       2.1.2   X-Ray Imaging   29
       2.1.3   Fluoroscopy and Angiography   32
       2.1.4   Mammography   34
       2.1.5   Image Reconstruction for Computed Tomography   35
       2.1.6   Contrast Enhancement in X-Ray Computed Tomography .   43
       2.1.7   Image Analysis on X-Ray Generated Images   44
   2.2   Magnetic Resonance Imaging   44
       2.2.1   Magnetic Resonance   45
       2.2.2   MR Imaging   48
       2.2.3   Some MR Sequences   51
       2.2.4   Artefacts in MR Imaging   53
       2.2.5   MR Angiography   54
       2.2.6   BOLD Imaging   56
       2.2.7   Perfusion Imaging   57
       2.2.8   Diffusion Imaging   58
       2.2.9   Image Analysis on Magnetic Resonance Images   60
   2.3   Ultrasound   60
       2.3.1   Ultrasound Imaging   61
       2.3.2   Image Analysis on Ultrasound Images   63
   2.4   Nuclear Imaging   64
       2.4.1   Scintigraphy   65
       2.4.2   Reconstruction Techniques for Tomography in Nuclear
           Imaging   66

2.4.3   Single Photon Emission Computed Tomography (SPECT)   71
2.4.4   Positron Emission Tomography (PET)   72
2.4.5   Image Analysis on Nuclear Images   73
2.5   Other Imaging Techniques   74
2.5.1   Photography   74
2.5.2   Light Microscopy   75
2.5.3   EEG and MEG   76
2.6   Concluding Remarks   77
2.7   Exercises   78
References   80

3   **Image Storage and Transfer**   83
3.1   Information Systems in a Hospital   84
3.2   The DICOM Standard   91
3.3   Establishing DICOM Connectivity   96
3.4   The DICOM File Format   98
3.5   Technical Properties of Medical Images   100
3.6   Displays and Workstations   101
3.7   Compression of Medical Images   106
3.8   Concluding Remarks   107
3.9   Exercises   108
References   108

4   **Image Enhancement**   111
4.1   Measures of Image Quality   112
4.1.1   Spatial and Contrast Resolution   112
4.1.2   Definition of Contrast   113
4.1.3   The Modulation Transfer Function   117
4.1.4   Signal-to-Noise Ratio (SNR)   117
4.2   Image Enhancement Techniques   119
4.2.1   Contrast Enhancement   119
4.2.2   Resolution Enhancement   120
4.2.3   Edge Enhancement   123
4.3   Noise Reduction   127
4.3.1   Noise Reduction by Linear Filtering   128
4.3.2   Edge-Preserving Smoothing: Median Filtering   131
4.3.3   Edge-Preserving Smoothing: Diffusion Filtering   133
4.3.4   Edge-Preserving Smoothing: Bayesian Image Restoration   138
4.4   Concluding Remarks   144
4.5   Exercises   144
References   145

5   **Feature Detection**   147
5.1   Edge Tracking   148
5.2   Hough Transform   152
5.3   Corners   154
5.4   Blobs   157

        5.5   SIFT and SURF Features 159
        5.6   MSER Features 161
        5.7   Key-Point-Independent Features 162
        5.8   Saliency and Gist 165
        5.9   Bag of Features 165
        5.10   Concluding Remarks 166
        5.11   Exercises 166
        References 167

6   Segmentation: Principles and Basic Techniques 171
        6.1   Segmentation Strategies 172
        6.2   Data Knowledge 175
                6.2.1   Homogeneity of Intensity 177
                6.2.2   Homogeneity of Texture 179
        6.3   Domain Knowledge About the Objects 182
                6.3.1   Representing Domain Knowledge 183
                6.3.2   Variability of Model Attributes 184
                6.3.3   The Use of Interaction 185
        6.4   Interactive Segmentation 188
        6.5   Thresholding 190
        6.6   Homogeneity-Based Segmentation 195
        6.7   The Watershed Transform: Computing Zero-Crossings 197
        6.8   Seeded Regions 199
        6.9   Live Wire 203
        6.10   Concluding Remarks 206
        6.11   Exercises 206
        References 208

7   Segmentation in Feature Space 211
        7.1   Segmentation by Classification in Feature Space 212
                7.1.1   Computing the Likelihood Function 214
                7.1.2   Multidimensional Feature Vectors 217
                7.1.3   Computing the A Priori Probability 219
                7.1.4   Extension to More than Two Classes 221
        7.2   Clustering in Feature Space 221
                7.2.1   Partitional Clustering and k-Means Clustering 222
                7.2.2   Mean-Shift Clustering 225
                7.2.3   Kohonen's Self-organizing Maps 228
        7.3   Concluding Remarks 231
        7.4   Exercises 231
        References 232

8   Segmentation as a Graph Problem 235
        8.1   Graph Cuts 236
                8.1.1   Graph Cuts for Computing a Segmentation 236
                8.1.2   Graph Cuts to Approximate a Bayesian Segmentation . . 242

          8.1.3   Adding Constraints 247
          8.1.4   Normalized Graph Cuts 247
    8.2   Segmentation as a Path Problem 250
          8.2.1   Fuzzy Connectedness 250
          8.2.2   The Image Foresting Transform 252
          8.2.3   Random Walks 254
    8.3   Concluding Remarks 257
    8.4   Exercises 257
    References 258

9 **Active Contours and Active Surfaces** 261
    9.1   Explicit Active Contours and Surfaces 262
          9.1.1   Deriving the Model 263
          9.1.2   The Use of Additional Constraints 266
          9.1.3   T-snakes and T-surfaces 268
    9.2   The Level Set Model 270
          9.2.1   Level Sets 272
          9.2.2   Level Sets and Wave Propagation 273
          9.2.3   Schemes for Computing Level Set Evolution 277
          9.2.4   Computing Stationary Level Set Evolution 281
          9.2.5   Computing Dynamic Level Set Evolution 284
          9.2.6   Segmentation and Speed Functions 285
          9.2.7   Geodesic Active Contours 288
          9.2.8   Level Sets and the Mumford–Shah Functional 290
          9.2.9   Topologically Constrained Level Sets 294
    9.3   Concluding Remarks 295
    9.4   Exercises 295
    References 296

10 **Registration and Normalization** 299
    10.1   Feature Space and Correspondence Criterion 301
    10.2   Rigid Registration 312
    10.3   Registration of Projection Images to 3D Data 319
    10.4   Search Space and Optimization in Nonrigid Registration . . . 322
    10.5   Normalization 325
    10.6   Concluding Remarks 328
    10.7   Exercises 328
    References 329

11 **Detection and Segmentation by Shape and Appearance** 333
    11.1   Shape Models 335
    11.2   Simple Models 338
          11.2.1   Template matching 338
          11.2.2   Hough Transform 340
    11.3   Implicit Models 341
    11.4   The Medial Axis Representation 343

	11.4.1 Computation of the Medial Axis Transform	344
	11.4.2 Shape Representation by Medial Axes	345
11.5	Active Shape and Active Appearance Models	347
	11.5.1 Creating an ASM	348
	11.5.2 Using ASMs for Segmentation	351
	11.5.3 The Active Appearance Model	352
11.6	Physically Based Shape Models	353
	11.6.1 Mass Spring Models	354
	11.6.2 Finite Element Models	360
11.7	Shape Priors	371
11.8	Concluding Remarks	374
11.9	Exercises	374
	References	376

12 Classification and Clustering 379
12.1	Features and Feature Space	380
	12.1.1 Linear Decorrelation of Features	380
	12.1.2 Linear Discriminant Analysis	382
	12.1.3 Independent Component Analysis	384
12.2	Bayesian Classifier	386
12.3	Classification Based on Distance to Training Samples	387
12.4	Decision Boundaries	390
	12.4.1 Adaptive Decision Boundaries	391
	12.4.2 The Multilayer Perceptron	393
	12.4.3 Support Vector Machines	398
12.5	Classification by Association	401
12.6	Clustering Techniques	403
	12.6.1 Agglomerative Clustering	404
	12.6.2 Fuzzy c-Means Clustering	405
12.7	Bagging and Boosting	407
12.8	Multiple Instance Learning	409
12.9	Concluding Remarks	410
12.10	Exercises	410
	References	411

13 Validation 413
13.1	Measures of Quality	415
	13.1.1 Quality for a Delineation Task	416
	13.1.2 Quality for a Detection Task	420
	13.1.3 Quality for a Registration Task	422
13.2	The Ground Truth	424
	13.2.1 Ground Truth from Real Data	425
	13.2.2 Ground Truth from Phantoms	427
13.3	Representativeness of Data	433
	13.3.1 Separation Between Training and Test Data	433
	13.3.2 Identification of Sources of Variation and Outlier Detection	434

          13.3.3 Robustness with Respect to Parameter Variation 435
    13.4 Significance of Results 436
    13.5 Concluding Remarks 439
    13.6 Exercises 439
    References 440

14 Appendix 443
    14.1 Optimization of Markov Random Fields 443
          14.1.1 Markov Random Fields 443
          14.1.2 Simulated Annealing 445
          14.1.3 Mean Field Annealing 447
          14.1.4 Iterative Conditional Modes 448
    14.2 Variational Calculus 449
    14.3 Principal Component Analysis 451
          14.3.1 Computing the PCA 452
          14.3.2 Robust PCA 454
    References 456

Index 459

List of Abbreviations

AAM   active appearance model
AC   anterior commissura
ACR   American College of Radiology
AdaBoost   adaptive boosting
AE   application entity (DICOM)
ANSI   American National Standards Institute
ART   algebraic reconstruction technique
ASM   active shape model
AVM   arteriovenous malformation

Bagging   bootstrap aggregating
BOLD   blood oxygen level dependency

CAT   computed axial tomography (=CT)
CCA   connected component analysis
CRT   cathode ray tube
CSF   cerebrospinal fluid
CT   computed tomography
CTA   CT angiography

DICOM   digital communication in medicine
DIMSE   DICOM message service element
DoG   difference of Gaussians
DRR   digitally reconstructed radiograph
DSA   digital subtraction angiography
DSM   deformable shape model
DTI   diffusion tensor imaging

EEG   electroencephalogram
EM   expectation maximization
EPI   echoplanar imaging
eV   electron volt (unit)

FBP   filtered backprojection
FEM   finite element model

FID	free induction decay
fMRI	functional MRI
FOM	figure of merit
FOV	field of view
GLCM	gray-level co-occurrence matrix
GM	gray matter
GVF	gradient vector flow
HIS	hospital information system
HL7	health level 7
HOM	hit-or-miss operator
HU	Hounsfield unit
ICA	independent component analysis
ICM	iterative conditional modes
ICP	iterative closest point
IFT	image foresting transform
IOD	information object description (DICOM)
ISO	International Standards Organization
ITK	Insight Toolkit
keV	kilo electron volt (unit)
kNN	k-nearest-neighborhood
LDA	linear discriminant analysis
LoG	Laplacian-of-Gaussian
LOR	line of response
lpmm	line pairs per millimeter
m-rep	medial axis representation
MAP-EM	maximum a posteriori-expectation maximization
MEG	magnetoencephalogram
MIL	multiple instance learning
MIP	maximum intensity projection
MLEM	maximum likelihood expectation maximization (reconstruction)
MRA	MR angiography
MRF	Markov random field
MRI	magnetic resonance imaging
MSER	maximally stable extremal regions
MTF	modulation transfer function
MTT	mean transit time
mWST	marker-based watershed transform
NEMA	National Electrical Manufacturers Association

OpenCV	open source computer vision
OSEM	ordered set expectation maximization
OSI	open systems interconnect
OSL	one-step-late (algorithm)
PACS	picture archiving and communication system
PC	posterior commissura
PCA	principal component analysis
PDM	point distribution model
PET	positron emission tomography
PSF	point spread function
PVE	partial volume effect
QoF	quality of fit
R	röntgen (unit)
rad	radiation absorbed dose (unit)
RAG	region adjacency graph
RARE	rapid enhancement with relaxation enhancement
rCBF	relative cerebral blood volume
rCBV	relative cerebral blood volume
RIS	radiology information system
rms	root mean square
ROC	receiver operator characteristic
ROI	region of interest
SCP	service class provider (DICOM)
SCU	service class user (DICOM)
SIFT	scale-invariant feature transform
SNR	signal-to-noise ratio
SOP	service object pair (DICOM)
SPECT	single photon emission tomography
SPM	statistical parametric mapping
STAPLE	simultaneous truth and performance level estimation
SURF	speeded-up robust features
SUSAN	smallest univalue segment assimilating nucleus
SVM	support vector machine
T	Tesla (unit)
TE	echo time (MRI)
TI	inversion time (MRI)
TR	repetition time (MRI)
TFT	thin film transistor
UID	unique identifier

US   ultrasound

WST   watershed transform
WM   white matter

The Analysis of Medical Images

1

Abstract

Medical images are different from other pictures in that they depict distributions of various physical features measured from the human body. They show attributes that are otherwise inaccessible. Furthermore, the analysis of such images is guided by very specific expectations, which gave rise to acquiring the images in the first place. This has consequences on the kind of analysis and on the requirements for algorithms that carry out some or all of the analysis. Image analysis as part of the clinical workflow will be discussed in this chapter as well as the types of tools that exist to support the development and carrying out of such an analysis. We will conclude with an example for the solution of an analysis task to illustrate important aspects for the development of methods for analyzing medical images.

Concepts, notions and definitions introduced in this chapter

> Introduction to basic development strategies
> Common analysis tasks: delineation, object detection, and classification
> Image analysis for clinical studies, diagnosis support, treatment planning, and computer-assisted therapy
> Tool types: viewers, workstation software, and development tools

Why is there a need for a book on medical image analysis when there are plenty of good texts on image analysis around? Medical images differ from photography in many ways. Consider the picture in Fig. 1.1 and the potential questions and problems related to its analysis. The first question that comes to mind would probably be to detect certain objects (e.g., persons). Common problems that have to be solved are to recover the three-dimensional (3D) information (i.e., missing depth information and the true shape) to separate illumination effects from object appearance, to deal with partially hidden objects, and to track objects over time.

K.D. Toennies, *Guide to Medical Image Analysis*,
Advances in Computer Vision and Pattern Recognition,
DOI 10.1007/978-1-4471-2751-2_1, © Springer-Verlag London Limited 2012

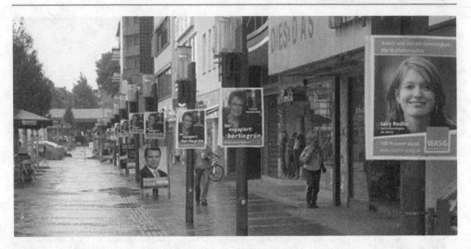

Fig. 1.1 Analysis questions for a photograph are often based on a detection or tracking task (such as detecting real persons in the image). Problems relate to reducing effects from the opacity of most depicted objects and to the reconstruction of depth information (real persons are different from those on the picture because they are 3D, and—if a sequence of images is present—because they can move)

Medical images are different. Consider the image in Fig. 1.2. The appearance of the depicted object is not caused by light reflection, but from the absorption of x rays. The object is transparent with respect to the depicted physical attribute. Although the detection of some structure may be the goal of the analysis, the exact delineation of the object and its substructures may be the first task. The variation of the object shape and appearance may be characteristic for some evaluation and needs to be captured. Furthermore, this is not the only way to gain insight into the human body. Different imaging techniques produce mappings of several physical attributes in various ways that may be subjects of inspection (compare Fig. 1.2 with Fig. 1.3). Comparing this information with reality is difficult, however, since few if any noninvasive methods exist to verify the information gained from the pictures. Hence, the focus on analysis methods for medical images is different if compared to the analysis of many other images. Delineation, restoration, enhancement, and registration for fusing images from different sources are comparably more important than classification, reconstruction of 3D information, and tracking (although it does not mean that the last three topics are irrelevant for medical image analysis). This shift in focus is reflected in our book and leads to the following structure.

- Medical images, their storage, and use will be discussed in Chaps. 2 and 3.
- Enhancement techniques and feature computation will be the subject of Chaps. 4 and 5.
- Delineation of object boundaries, finding objects and registering information from different sources will make up the majority of the book. It will be presented in Chaps. 6 to 12.

Fig. 1.2 Detail of one of the first radiographs showing the wrist and part of the hand. The image projects a physical entity that is transparent with respect to the detection technique. Bone structures are clearly visible

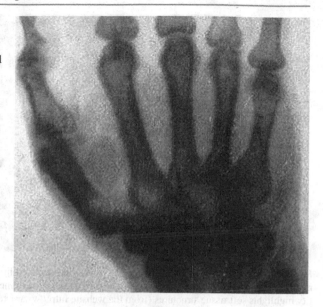

- A separate chapter, Chap. 13, will be devoted to the validation of an analysis procedure since this is particularly difficult for methods developed for medical images.

Computer-assisted analysis of medical images is meant to support an expert (the radiologist, the surgeon, etc.) in some decision task. It is possible to associate analysis tasks to the kind of decision in which the expert shall be supported (see Fig. 1.4).

- *Delineation* of an object requires solving a segmentation task.
- *Detection* of an object requires solving a classification task.
- Comparison of the object appearance from pictures at different times or from different modalities requires solving a *registration* task.

Although the characterization above is helpful in deciding where to look for solutions, practical applications usually involve aspects from not just one of the fields. Hence, before deciding on the kind of methodology that is needed, it is important to understand the technical questions associated with the practical application. Several aspects need to be discussed.

- Analysis in the *clinical work flow*: How does the analysis fit into the clinical routine within which it has been requested?
- *Strategies* to develop an analysis tool: How can it be assured that an efficient and effective solution has been chosen?
- Acquisition of necessary *a priori information*: What kind of information is necessary to solve the analysis task and how can it be acquired?
- Setup of an *evaluation scenario*: How can the quality of the analysis method be tested?
- *Tools* to support an analysis task: How can tools be used to spend as little effort as necessary to solve the analysis task?

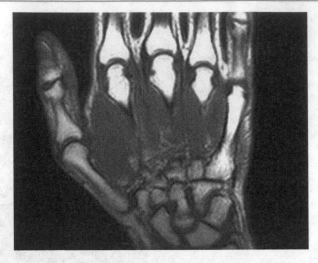

Fig. 1.3 Detail of a slice to a similar region as the one depicted in Fig. 1.2 by a magnetic resonance image (MRI). The acquisition technique produces a 3D volume and the imaged physical entity highlights soft tissue structures (from the website http://www.exeter.ac.uk/~ab233/, with kind
permission of Dr. Abdelmalek Benattayallah)

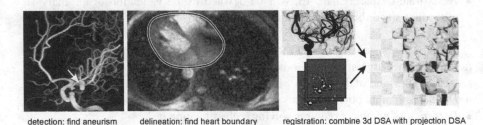

detection: find aneurism   delineation: find heart boundary   registration: combine 3d DSA with projection DSA

Fig. 1.4 Different tasks in medical image analysis require different methodology and validation
techniques

It is easy to forget about these more general questions when being confronted
with some analysis problem because

- each analysis task is different from most other analysis tasks (different organ or
  pathology to be analyzed, different imaging system, imaging parameters, imaging
  equipment);
- when being asked, finding a solution fast is usually the main motivation and other
  aspects such as fitting the solution into the workflow appear to be of lesser importance;
- the development of a method usually takes place well separated from the regular
  practice in which the method is supposed to be used;
- it is more fun to experiment with some new method or to apply a methodology
  with which the developer has experience rather than truly looking for the most
  appropriate solution.

Nonetheless, the final result needs to be an effective and ideally efficient solution. The following sections will present strategies for developing a method in the clinical environment, for deciding on the type of methodology, and for deciding on an evaluation scenario.

Digital medical images and computer-assisted methods for their interpretation have been around for quite some time. Several books exist that treat the subject. Books on specific aspects of medical image analysis will be referenced in the respective chapters. Books on medical image analysis in general are the following.

- *The Handbook of Medical Imaging and Analysis* (Bankman 2008) is an edited book containing almost 60 articles of active researchers in the field on all relevant aspects of the topic. It is a well structured text of more than 1000 pages.
- *The Handbook of Biomedical Image Analysis* (Suri et al. 2005) is another, even more extensive book on the subjects of the analysis of medical images, although—compared to Bankman (2008)—the text is slightly outdated.
- *Principles and Advanced Methods in Medical Imaging and Image Analysis* (Dhawan et al. 2008) is a reference covering a broad spectrum of topics that is particularly strong in image generation techniques.
- *Medical Image Analysis* (Dhawan 2011) is strong on the physics, generation, and information content of modern imaging modalities.

There is still a need for another text since the subject is either treated with focus on the generation of images rather than on their analysis, or the treatment requires a very good background to appreciate the information. The book at hand will introduce the subject and present an overview and detailed look at the many dependencies between different strategies for the computer-assisted interpretation of medical images.

1.1   Image Analysis in the Clinical Workflow

A newly developed method or a newly adapted method for carrying out some analysis (e.g., for determining the tumor boundary and tumor volume in brain MRI) will most likely not be implemented on the computer that is used to generate or to evaluate the images. The reason for this is that this piece of software will often not be certified as part of the equipment to be used in a clinical routine. Hence, the method will be separate from other analysis devices while still is intended to be used within some medical procedure. This has to be accounted for when developing a method. The developer will not only have to create the method, but also needs to provide an environment in which the method can be applied. The type of environment depends on the problem that has to be solved. At least four different scenarios can be differentiated (see Table 1.1).

- For a *clinical study*, images are analyzed outside a clinical routine task to understand or confirm findings based on images. In this case, images that are part of the study are often copied to some workstation where the study is taking place. The image analysis method is then implemented on this workstation and the results from analysis are kept here as well. The transfer of data to this workstation has to be organized and bookkeeping must enable a later checking of results.

Table 1.1 Different scenarios for computer-assisted image analysis have very different requirements

	Clinical study	Computer aided diagnosis	Treatment planning	Computer assisted surgery
No. of cases	Large	Small	Small	Small
Time-constraints	Low	Medium	Medium	High
Location	Anywhere	Office, Reading room	Office, ward	Operating room
Interaction	Not acceptable	Acceptable	Acceptable	Acceptable
Archival requirements	High	High	Medium	Medium

- For *diagnosis support* (computer-aided detection, computer-aided diagnosis), single cases that may consist of several studies containing images are analyzed on a medical workstation. The transfer of images to this workstation is often done by other software, but access to the images, which may be organized by the export module of the image acquisition system, has to be part of the analysis method. Diagnosis support systems often involve interaction since the user has to accept or reject the analysis result anyway. If interaction is used to supply the method with additional information by the data expert, it has to be ensured that it is intuitive and efficient and that contradictions between the results from the analysis and any overwriting actions by the user are clear.
- Analysis in *treatment planning* precedes treatment. It may be carried out in a radiology department or at a surgery department, depending on who is doing the treatment planning. Methods have to take the time into account that is acceptable for doing this task (which may be critical in some cases). Furthermore, the results from treatment planning are the input for the treatment. This input may happen by the medical expert taking numerical results from planning and using it for some kind of parameterization. The generated results should be well documented and measures should be enacted that help to avoid mistakes during the transfer from results to parameterization. The input into some treatment module may also happen automatically (after the acceptance of the result by the expert). The interface for the transfer has then to be specified as well.
- Image analysis for *computer-assisted surgery* is time-critical. Since noncertified software is usually not allowed on the imaging system, fast transfer to the system on which the analysis method is implemented has to be organized. Furthermore, the time constraints have to be known and kept by the method. With programmable graphic cards, time constraints are often adhered to by implementing some or all of the analysis method on the graphics hardware. Any constraints from the use of the system in an operating theater have to be considered and adhered to.

Any constraints, such as speed requirements, and additional methods, such as access to the data, should be included in the specification of the method to be developed. While this is a standard software engineering routine, it is sometimes neglected in practice.

An important part of the description is the definition of the problem to be solved and the underlying assumptions for a solution. This is not to be underestimated. A lot of domain knowledge exists about the appearance of structures of interest in medical images. Nevertheless, anatomical variation, artefacts from image generation, and changes of appearance due to different imaging techniques make it unlikely that the conditions to extract information from the image for some specific analysis task can be proven to be sufficient.

Arriving at a problem description is a result of a discussion between a data expert (the radiologist, surgeon, or physician) and the methodology expert (the computer scientist or engineer). An experienced radiologist will certainly have the knowledge to come to a well-founded decision based on the images presented to him or her. However, a radiologist is seldom forced to formalize this decision in some general way a priori (i.e., before looking at some evidence from the images). Hence, generating the domain knowledge for a computer-assisted method will be more difficult than making decisions based on a set of images. Furthermore, the different scientific background of the data expert and the methodology expert will make it difficult for either side to decide on the validity, representativeness, and exhaustiveness of any fact conveyed from one side to the other. Experience helps, of course, but there is still room for misunderstandings.

Reviewing the underlying assumptions for an analysis method later helps to identify sources of error. Such a description should contain the following information.

- Description of the images on which the analysis is performed (i.e., kind of images, technical parameters, etc.).
- Description of the patient group on which the analysis is performed.
- All image features that are used for the analysis method, including any assumptions about the reliability of the features.
- All a priori information that is used as domain knowledge to perform the analysis.

Any change of method to correct errors found on test data will have to result in changes of this description as well.

The description also helps to set up an evaluation scenario. Evaluation ensures that the information generated by the analysis method really reflects an underlying truth. Since the truth is usually not known, evaluation has to abstract from specific cases and has to provide some kind of "generic truth." This can be of two different types. Either the method is evaluated with respect to some other method of which the performance and quality has been proven, or the method is evaluated with respect to the assumptions made a priori. The former is the simpler way to test a method, as it shifts the responsibility of defining truth to the method against which our new method is tested. For the latter, two aspects have to be tested. The first is whether the analysis result is as expected when the assumptions from the domain knowledge hold. The second is whether the assumptions hold. This evaluation has the advantage of not relying on some gold standard, which may be difficult to come by. However, it is usually difficult to show that the domain knowledge sufficiently describes the problem. Hence, the topic of validation requires a careful look and it will be discussed in detail in the final chapter of this book.

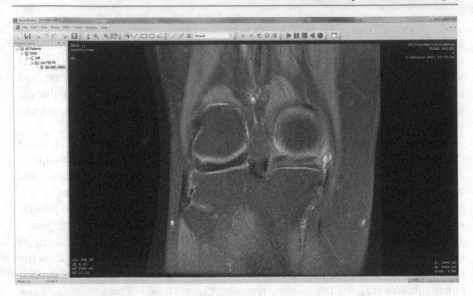

Fig. 1.5 The free MicroDicom viewer (www.microdicom.com) allows viewing DICOM images and simple operations such as annotations and some filtering operations

1.2   Using Tools

Fortunately, developing an analysis method does not mean that everything has to be created from scratch. Different types of software greatly support speedy development:

- viewer software;
- analysis software;
- rapid prototyping software;
- software libraries.

An extensive list of free software (either open source software or at least free to use for academic and/or educational purposes) to view, export, analyze, and transfer images is found at http://www.idoimaging.com.

Viewer software has been primarily developed to look at the data, but usually contains some methods for analyzing the data as well. Although it is not thought to be extended, it facilitates the development of a new analysis method by providing quick access to the image data (see Fig. 1.5 for an example of a free DICOM viewer). Commercial software can be quite comfortable and if it is found that a combination of existing methods solves the problem, development stops here. But even if it is just a way of accessing and looking at the image data, it helps to get a first impression on the kind of data, to organize a small data base on which the development of an analysis method is based, and to discuss the problem and possible solutions with the data expert.

Analysis software is different from viewer software in that it is intended to provide the user with a set of parameterizable analysis modules that perform different steps of image analysis ranging from image enhancement methods to segmentation,

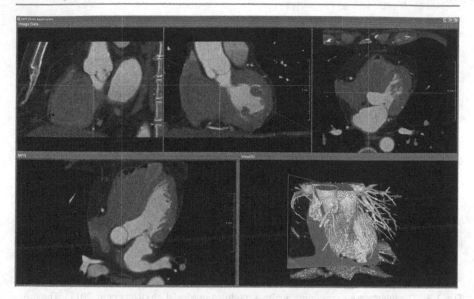

Fig. 1.6 Example of the user interface for an analysis module implemented under MeVisLab (with kind permission of MeVis Medical Solutions AG, Bremen, Germany)

registration, or classification tools. An example for such analysis software is MeVis-Lab, which exists in a commercial and a noncommercial version (www.mevis.de, see Fig. 1.6).

MeVisLab provides the user with a set of implemented, parameterizable modules that produce output from the data. Different modules can be combined using a graphic interface that allows the user to connect the output of one module with the input of another module (see Fig. 1.7). It is, for instance, possible to create a processing chain, where the data are first enhanced by removing artefacts and noise using suitable filters, and then separated into different regions by a segmentation technique of which one segment is then selected and analyzed (e.g., by measuring its volume). This kind of modularization provides much more flexibility than the usual workstation analysis software. It does, of course, require some knowledge about the implemented modules to use them in an appropriate fashion.

One step further is to use a rapid prototyping programming language such as Matlab or IDL. These are interpreter languages that are geared toward rapidly processing arrays. It makes them particularly suitable to be used for working with two dimensional (2D) and 3D image arrays.

It is possible to write programs in both languages that can be executed later (see Figs. 1.8 and 1.9 for a view at the program development interfaces of the two prototyping languages). A wealth of methods for signal and image processing makes it easy to program even more complex methods. The possibility to use the methods in interpreter mode allows for experimenting with different methods for finding a solution for some image analysis problem. For efficient use, the user should be familiar with the basic vocabulary of image processing and image analysis.

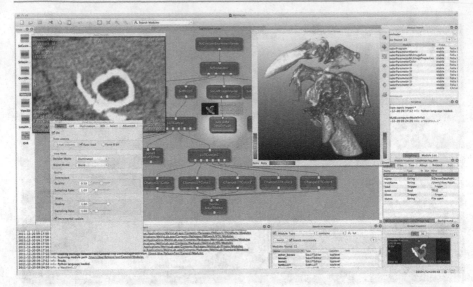

Fig. 1.7 The interface for generating analysis modules in MevisLab (Ritter et al. 2011). The programmer can combine existing modules, e.g., for filtering, segmentation, and visualization, in a way that is suitable to solve some specific problem using an intuitive graphical user interface (with kind permission of MeVis Medical Solutions AG, Bremen, Germany)

Since routines for the input of images (filters for the most common formats including DICOM) and for display are provided by IDL and Matlab, they are also excellent tools to discuss potential methods and their contribution to analysis. Without having to go into detail the developer can simply show what is happing.

There is the danger that the simple way to construct analysis modules results in *ad hoc* developments. They may be difficult to justify later except for the fact that they worked on the data provided. Still, if prototyping languages are so useful, why should they not be used for software development? If software development consists of combining modules for which Matlab or IDL have been optimized, there is little to say against such a decision except for the fact that both environments are commercial products and require licenses for the development and runtime environment.

If substantial program development is necessary, other reasons may speak against using Matlab or IDL. Both environments allow object-oriented programming, but they do not enforce it (simply because this would interfere with the nonobject-oriented fashion of the interpreter mode). It requires a disciplined development of software that is meant to be extended and used by others. Furthermore, both environments optimize the computation of matrix operations. Computation may become slow if software development requires nonmatrix operations. In such a case, the performance suffers from translating the implemented program into the underlying environment (which in both cases is C). It usually pays to implement directly into C/C++ or any other suitable language using the techniques and strategies for efficient computation.

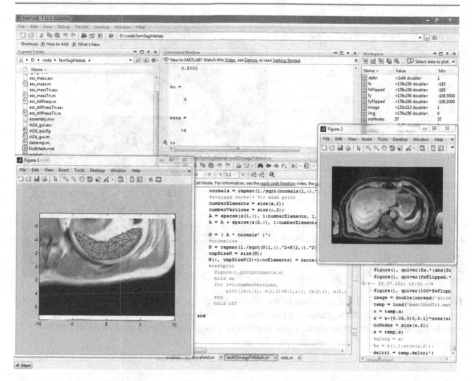

Fig. 1.8 The Matlab interface is similar to the programming environment for some programming language. The main differences are that Matlab can be used in interpreter modes and that it has toolboxes for many methods in image analysis, pattern recognition, and classification

If a method is to be implemented completely without the help of some specific programming environment, various libraries aid the developer. For analysis tasks in medical imaging, two environments are mainly of interest: OpenCV and ITK.

OpenCV began as a way to promote Intel's chips by providing an extensive and fast image processing library for Windows and Intel chips. The restriction no longer applies. OpenCV is intended to support general image processing and computer vision tasks. The input is assumed to consist of one or several 2D images. The analysis can be almost anything in the field of computer vision including, e.g., image enhancement, segmentation, stereovision, tracking, multiscale image analysis, and classification. The software has been published under the BSD license, which means that it may be used for commercial or academic purposes. With respect to medical image analysis its main disadvantage is that the processing of 3D or four-dimensional (4D) scenes is not supported.

This is different for ITK (Insight Toolkit), which focuses on the segmentation and registration of medical images. It is an open source project as well. Being meant to support medical image analysis, it also contains plenty of auxiliary methods for accessing and enhancing images. Furthermore, registration methods not included in OpenCV for rigid and nonrigid registration are part of the software. Segmentation,

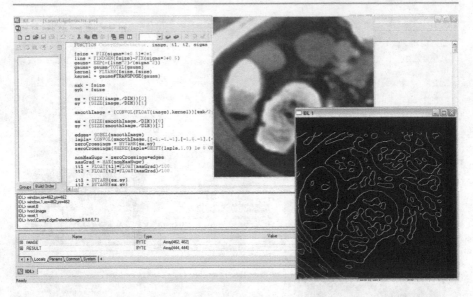

Fig. 1.9 The IDL interface is similar to the Matlab interface. Windows for program development, interactive evaluation of programs and functions, status of system variables, and generated output enable the development of methods while inspecting results from the current chain of processes

which plays a much bigger role in medical imaging compared to the analysis of other images, is extensively covered by including state-of-the-art methods.

ITK is written in C++, and the use of classes and methods is fairly simple. Being an open source project, new contributions are invited, provided that guidelines for software development within the ITK community are followed. As with OpenCV, the efficient use of ITK requires some background knowledge about the methods implemented, if only for deciding whether, e.g., the implemented level set framework can be used for a segmentation solution for which you have worked out a level set formulation. Information about OpenCV and ITK can be accessed by their respective websites (http://opencv.willowgarage.com/wiki/ and http://www.itk.org/) with Wiki and user groups. Being open source projects with voluntary supporters, it is usually expected that the questioner spent some time on research work before asking the community. A question such as "How can I use ITK for solving my (very specific) registration problem?" might receive an answer such as "We suggest reading some literature about registration first."

As with the prototyping languages, the open source libraries may be all that is needed to solve an analysis problem. But even if not, they will provide for quick access to methods that can be tested with respect to their capability for solving the problem. They also may provide state-of-the-art methods for data access, preprocessing, and postprocessing. If the solution of image analysis problems is a recurring task, it should well justify the effort to understand and efficiently use these toolkits.

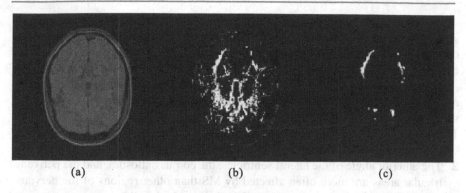

(a)   (b)   (c)

Fig. 1.10 · White matter lesions can be recognized in MR images as their signal differs from the surrounding tissue. However, this information alone is insufficient as it can be seen by comparing a simple intensity-based segmentation (**b**) of an MRI slice (**a**) with the result of a segmentation by a human expert (**c**)

1.3 An Example: Multiple Sclerosis Lesion Segmentation in Brain MRI

So far the discussion has been rather abstract. We conclude this chapter with a presentation of an example. We selected a rather complex segmentation task (see Fig. 1.10) for finding multiple sclerosis lesions to exemplify the range of models and decisions in performing the analysis. The description is based on the two publications (Al-Zubi et al. 2002) and (Admasu et al. 2003).

Multiple sclerosis (MS) is a disease of the central nervous system where the myelin shield of axons is receding. Estimating the extent and distribution of MS lesions supports understanding the development of the disease and estimating the influence of treatment. MS lesions can be detected in magnetic resonance images using spin echo imaging. The method produces registered proton density (ρ), T_1, and T_2 images (see the next chapter for details on this imaging technique), all of which are going to be used in the segmentation process.

The choice of an appropriate analysis technique was guided by the goal of replacing the manual delineation of MS lesions by some automatic procedure. Lesion detection is an active research field and the presentation of the method below by no means should indicate that this is the only or even the best way to do the segmentation. It was chosen because the author of the book contributed to the result and can comment on the various decisions and point out problems that are usually not stated in a publication.

Selecting, adapting, or developing an analysis algorithm follows the standard practice of scientific work. Information about data and possible a priori information is gathered, a representation is selected in which this information can be described and which can be used during segmentation. Then the method is implemented and tested.

Since the goal is to separate MS lesions from the background, it points to the segmentation of foreground segments. Their characteristics describe the properties of MS lesions. The properties of other structures need to be captured only to the extent of enabling the separation of lesions from the background.

Discussions with physicians, MR physicists, and the study of the related literature resulted in the following description of the appearance of MS lesions in T_2-weighted spin echo images.

1. 90–95% of all lesions occur in white matter. White matter segmentation can be used for imposing a location constraint on the lesion search.
2. The anterior angle of the lateral ventricles, the corpus callosum, and the periventricular areas are more often affected by MS than other regions of the nervous system. Identifying those regions will further restrict localization.
3. There is considerable size variation for lesions, but their shape is roughly ellipsoidal. It points to the use of shape constraints as part of the a priori knowledge.
4. MS lesions tend to appear in groups. This will require the introduction of a priori knowledge about neighboring segments.
5. The intensity of an MS lesion varies from being bright in its center to being lower at its boundaries. The intensity range is brighter than white matter intensity, but overlaps with intensity for the cerebrospinal fluid (CSF). The data-driven criterion will thus be some homogeneity constraint on intensity, but it is clear that data-driven segmentation alone will be insufficient.
6. Shading in the MR images affects the brightness of the white matter as well as of the MS lesions. Thus, the above-mentioned homogeneity criterion will be more efficient in separating lesions, if shading is considered.

It was possible to accumulate such an extensive list of attributes because of the high interest of the research community in the topic. There will be other cases where the medical partner who requested an analysis solution may be the only source of information. It will still be possible to generate a good description as the partner is an expert and trained to develop such assumptions. He or she will also be able to point to medical literature where such information can be found (even if it has not been used for generating computer-assisted solutions).

The way of describing the attributes typically involves expressions like "tends to" or "intensity varies" indicating a rather fuzzy knowledge about the permissible ranges for attribute values. Even mentioning numbers such as "90–95% of all lesions" may refer to a single study with other studies coming up with different numbers.

The research in medical science is often conducted empirically with observations leading to hypotheses. This is no problem in general. Much of the scientific research—especially if it involves complex dependencies that do not easily point to simple underlying facts—is empirical. However, for making this information useful as a priori knowledge it has to be treated as factual. The transition from empirical evidence to known facts may be a source of failure of an analysis method because the underlying model assumptions turn out to be false.

Considering possible model knowledge, a number of consequences arose regarding a successful segmentation strategy for the problem.

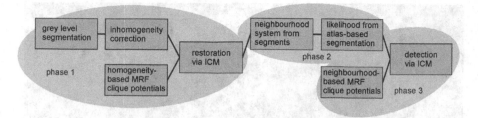

Fig. 1.11 The overall structure of the algorithm with the three different analysis phases

- Segmentation will need to include a strong model component to account for the ambiguities between the appearance of CSF and MS lesions.
- Model constraints regarding the shape and the location of lesions will need to be stated probabilistically or in some fuzzy manner (at least in some informal fashion).
- The first location constraint (condition 1 above) requires white matter segmentation. The application of the second constraint (condition 2) further requires some representation of relative positions.
- Constraint 4 requires the definition of the neighborhood among segments.

The fuzziness of the described lesion properties led us to use a Bayesian Markov random field (MRF) for representation (MRFs will be described in Sect. 14.1). An MRF allows a probabilistic description of known neighborhood dependencies, which is just what we need to describe constraints 1, 2, and 4.

Segmentation takes place in three stages (see Fig. 1.11). At the first stage, white matter and lesions are segmented based on their intensities. A classifier for separating white matter is trained which determines the expected values and variances of a multivariate Gaussian distribution for ρ, T_1, and T_2. Intensity variation due to magnetic field inhomogeneities is estimated based on segmented white matter regions (which are assumed to have constant intensity). Segmentation is repeated (see Fig. 1.12a). The subsequent MRF-based restoration reduces noise in the result since the a priori knowledge about the neighborhood states that adjacent pixels belong, more likely, to the same kind of object rather than to different objects. Finding the most probable segmentation given the MRF formulation resulted in a first estimate of potential MS lesions (see Fig. 1.12b).

The white matter segmentation of the first stage is used to find neighboring structures by atlas matching (see Fig. 1.12c). The segmentation of gray matter is difficult but necessary. We needed to differentiate between white matter bordering gray matter or the CSF of the ventricles to apply the second localization condition. The spatial continuity of the gray matter and CSF regions is exploited when assuming that the elastic registration of patient images with an anatomical atlas gives a sufficient approximation of the different structures. Lesions segmented in the previous step are reassessed using the deformed atlas as a priori information.

The shape constraint of lesions is used as a final confirmation. Because of the fuzzy a priori knowledge, thresholds in the two previous stages for segment membership were set in a way so as to not exclude potential lesion sites. The final step

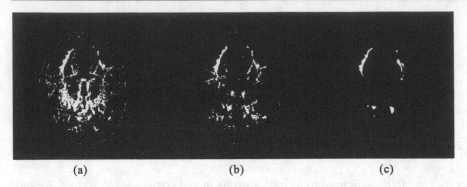

(a)   (b)   (c)

Fig. 1.12 In the first two stages, the initial segmentation (**a**) is first postprocessed using a local homogeneity constraint arriving at (**b**). Then atlas matching is used to remove lesions at unlikely locations arriving at (**c**)

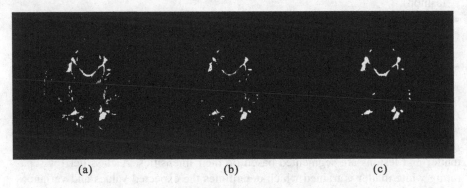

(a)   (b)   (c)

Fig. 1.13 In the final step, the result from atlas matching in (**a**) is postprocessed by defining a shape-based MRF. The result in (**b**) compares favorably with the expert segmentation in (**c**)

treats the labels of lesion segments as random variables being either a lesion or gray matter. Criteria are the deviation from the ellipsoidal shape and the distance of a segment from the ventricles. An (abstract) neighborhood system is defined. Segments in this neighborhood are assumed to have the same label, as lesions tend to appear in groups (condition 4). Labeling optimizes this MRF (see Fig. 1.13).

The stages described above accumulate the constraints derived from attributes that characterize the lesions. Selecting a sequential order was necessitated by the nature of some of the attributes (e.g., groups of lesions can only be identified when potential lesions are already segmented, the neighborhood of white matter to other tissues requires white matter segmentation first, etc.). Using a common representation for neighborhood relations at the pixel and the segment level was intentional as it enabled an easy reconsideration of segment labeling in subsequent steps.

The resulting structure of the analysis methods accumulates and evaluates semantics gradually in several steps that introduce different kinds of domain knowledge. This is typical for many automatic analysis methods, as it allows keeping the fuzziness of knowledge through many steps of the decision process. If it enables correcting erroneous decisions, it also contributes to the robustness of the method. While this is generally desired, it may hide the use of incomplete, incorrect, or inadequate domain knowledge. Evaluation should account for this by validating the expected results of the intermediate steps as well.

The modular structure of the method may also be a problem from the viewpoint of a developer. A large part of the solution lies in the proper combination of the modules. Reusing modules for a different problem solution requires the expertise of a developer since the purpose of single modules within the overall problem solution is rather abstract. This may be unwanted in a clinical environment where clinical and radiological expertise is available, but not the expertise of an engineer for image analysis solutions.

Using the methodology described above is by no means the only way to encode the prior knowledge about lesion attributes. This is proved by the numerous publications on MS lesion detection using different knowledge representations and segmentation strategies. Selecting a specific method is often influenced by reasons such as existing experience with specific types of representation or segmentation techniques, existing software, or other preferences by the developer. If the justification for some technique is conclusive nonetheless, it may not influence the effectiveness of a method. The effectiveness may only be affected when the existing prior knowledge was used incompletely or inaccurately despite the conclusiveness of the argument.

Reviewing our own decisions above, several points come to mind.

- The sequential order of removing lesions does not enable the reconsideration of the segments excluded from being lesions at later stages.
- Assuming Gaussianity for the probability distributions in the framework is an approximation that may not always be true.
- Repeated MRF optimization in the first two stages may be redundant because it uses rather similar kinds of a priori knowledge.
- Using the Bayesian framework was influenced by the type of expertise in our group at that time.

In a later revision (Admasu et al. 2003), the sequential order of the removal of lesions was replaced by a sequence of two steps, which explicitly addressed two different aspects of the prior knowledge. At a data-driven first step, segments were created by adaptive intensity region growing using the concept of fuzzy connectedness of Udupa and Samarasekera (1996). It created CSF, gray matter (GM), and white matter (WM) regions. The uncertainty of the homogeneity criterion in the data-driven step was not modeled by Gaussian distributions but by introducing interaction to indicate seed points for growing, fuzzily connected GM, WM, and CSF regions.

Regions that are enclosed by GM, WM, or CSF and that are not found by the method are labeled as potential lesion sites. The method does involve interaction, but it is robust to input errors and not very costly. Only a few seed points have to be selected for each of the connected components of GM, WM, or CSF. If any of those components are missed they will be erroneously classified as a potential lesion site, but this will be remedied in the next step. The advantage of using interaction is to avoid the specification of absolute homogeneity criteria.

The features of potential lesion sites were then fed to a trained backpropagation network. Shape and location features described a potential lesion site. The beauty of using a neural network was that it essentially creates an approximation of a decision boundary in feature space. The decision boundary describes locations in feature space where the probability of a segment being a lesion equals that of a segment not being a lesion. Other properties of the two probability distributions are not needed and are not approximated. This results in a good estimate of the decision boundary even if only relatively few samples are present. Although the relative spatial relation among lesions was not considered—an important step of the previous approach—success was in the range of the previous method and computation speed was much faster.

What can be learned from the simplification? Sometimes it pays to consider limited interaction for supplying a priori knowledge. Reconsidering the limitations of the use of model knowledge, even if the performance is very satisfactory, may lead to a more efficient computation without sacrificing quality. After all, developing a solution for a complex problem and experimenting with the results usually produces a lot of insight into the importance of applied domain knowledge and its representation. It should be noted that redesigning a method may again slant the view of the developer toward methods supporting a chosen strategy.

1.4   Concluding Remarks

Analysis in medical imaging differs from other image analysis tasks. The various medical images carry very different information and many of the analysis tasks are related to the individual quantification of entities (volume, extent, delineation, number of occurrences) in the human body. Normal anatomy that is subject to the quantification varies enormously. This is even moreso the case for pathological deviations. Hence, a major part of the analysis is to acquire, represent, and integrate this knowledge in the image interpretation method.

It is not always necessary to develop an analysis method from scratch. Existing commercial and free software packages provide methods that can be adapted to the purpose of carrying out some specific analysis. They range from parametrisable analysis methods offered through a graphical user interface to class libraries that can be used or extended to serve a developer's purpose for a new method. The question of how to employ which domain knowledge to solve a specific analysis task still resides with the developer when deciding on the use and adaptation of such a method.

1.5   Exercises

• What analysis task would be typical for analyzing a photograph that would be untypical for a medical image?

- What is an example for the kind of information that is measured for a medical image?
- Name at least two analysis tasks that could arise when using images for diagnosis support.
- What is the main problem when validating an analysis method?
- Name a difference between analysis tasks for a clinical study compared to image analysis in computer-assisted surgery.
- Where in a hospital does image analysis take place? Who are the persons involved?
- Name a rapid-prototyping language that could be used for developing an analysis method.
- How can workstation software be used for developing an analysis solution if the workstation software itself does not provide the solution?
- Why is it so important to provide detailed documentation for all information and assumptions used for developing an analysis algorithm?

References

Al-Zubi S, Toennies KD, Bodammer N, Hinrichs H (2002) Fusing Markov random fields with anatomical knowledge and shape based analysis to segment multiple sclerosis white matter lesions in magnetic resonance images of the brain. Proc SPIE 4684:206–215 (Medical imaging 2002)

Admasu F, Al-Zubi S, Toennies KD, Bodammer N, Hinrichs H (2003) Segmentation of multiple sclerosis lesions from MR brain images using the principles of fuzzy-connectedness and artificial neuron networks. In: Proc intl conf image processing (ICIP 2003), pp 1081–1084

Bankman IN (2008) Handbook of medical image processing and analysis, 2nd edn. Academic Press, San Diego

Dhawan AP, Huang HK, Kim DS (2008) Principles and advanced methods in medical imaging and image analysis. World Scientific, Singapore .

Dhawan AP (2011) Medical image analysis. IEEE Press Series on Biomedical Engineering, 2nd edn. Wiley, New York

Ritter F, Boskamp T, Homeyer A, Laue H, Schwier M, Link F, Peitgen HO (2011) Medical image analysis: a visual approach. IEEE Pulse 2(6):60–70

Suri JS, Wilson D, Laxminarayan S (2005) Handbook of biomedical image analysis. Vols I–III. Springer, Berlin

Udupa JK, Samarasekera S (1996) Fuzzy connectedness and object definition: theory, algorithms, and applications in image segmentation. Graph Models Image Process 58(3):246–261

Digital Image Acquisition

2

Abstract

Medical images are pictures of distributions of physical attributes captured by an image acquisition system. Most of today's images are digital. They may be postprocessed for analysis by a computer-assisted method.

Medical images come in one of two varieties: Projection images project a physical parameter in the human body on a 2D image, while slice images produce a one-to-one mapping of the measured value. Medical images may show anatomy including the pathological variation of anatomy if the measured value is related to it or physiology when the distribution of substances is traced.

X-ray imaging, CT, MRI, nuclear imaging, ultrasound imaging, photography, and microscopic images will be discussed in this chapter. The discussion focuses on the relationship between the imaged physical entity and the information shown in the image, as well as on reconstruction methods and the resulting artefacts.

Concepts, notions and definitions introduced in this chapter

›   *Imaging techniques*: x ray, fluoroscopy and angiography, DSA, x-ray CT, CT angiography, MR imaging, MR angiography, functional MRI, perfusion MRI, diffusion MRI, scintigraphy, SPECT, PET
›   *Reconstruction techniques*: filtered backprojection, algebraic reconstruction, EM algorithms
›   *Image artefacts*: noise, motion artefacts, partial volume effect, MR-specific artefacts, ultrasound-specific artefacts

A major difference between most digital medical images and pictures acquired from photography is that the depicted physical parameters in medical images are usually inaccessible for inspection (see Fig. 2.1). Features or quantities determined by computer-assisted analysis cannot easily be compared with true features or quantities. It would be, e.g., infeasible to open the human body to verify whether a tumor

K.D. Toennies, *Guide to Medical Image Analysis*,
Advances in Computer Vision and Pattern Recognition,
DOI 10.1007/978-1-4471-2751-2_2, © Springer-Verlag London Limited 2012

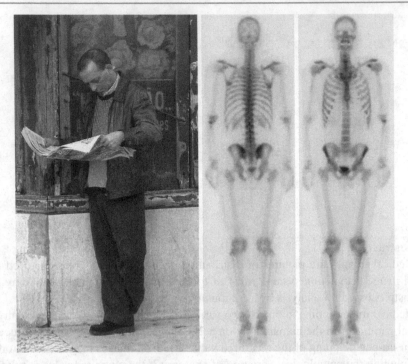

Fig. 2.1 Information from a photography is quite different from that of a medical image (in this case a bone scintigraphy, published under Creative Commons license). While the human depicted in the photo looks familiar, interpretation of the *image on the right* requires expertise with respect to the meaning of the intensities. On the other hand, specific domain knowledge exists as to how to interpret image intensity in the scintigraphy and the image is acquired in a way that makes analysis as easy as possible, all of which cannot be said about the *picture on the left*. Obviously, the kind of task for computer-based image analysis is different for these two pictures

volume measured in a sequence of CT images in some posttreatment confirmation scan corresponds to the true volume.

Fortunately, the physical property depicted, its diagnostic value, and possible artefacts are usually well known. Furthermore, the imaging technique has been chosen on purpose because it is known to produce images that depict diagnostically relevant information. The development of efficient analysis techniques often uses this knowledge as part of the domain knowledge to make up for the inaccessibility of the measured property.

A physical property measured by an imaging device and presented as a picture must meet three conditions to be useful. It has to penetrate the human body, it must not unduly interfere with it, and it must be meaningful for answering some medically relevant question.

With respect to digital imaging, four major[1] and several minor imaging techniques meet these requirements. The major techniques are as follows.

- *X-ray imaging* measures the absorption of short wave electromagnetic waves, which is known to vary between different tissues.
- *Magnetic resonance imaging* measures the density and molecular binding of selected atoms (most notably hydrogen which is abundant in the human body), which varies with tissue type, molecular composition, and functional status.
- *Ultrasound imaging* captures reflections at the boundaries between and within tissues with different acoustic impedance.
- *Nuclear imaging* measures the distribution of radioactive tracer material administered to the subject through the blood flow. It measures function in the human body.

Other imaging techniques include *EEG* and *MEG imaging*, *microscopy*, and *photography*. All the techniques have in common that an approximate mapping is known between the diagnostic question, which was the reason for making the image and the measurement value that is depicted. This can be very helpful when selecting an analysis technique. If, for instance, bones need to be detected in an x-ray CT slice, a good first guess would be to select a thresholding technique with a high threshold because it is known that x-ray attenuation in bone is higher than in soft tissues and fluids.

Many of the imaging techniques come in two varieties: *Projection images* show a projection of the 3D human body onto a 2D plane and *slice images* show a distribution of the measurement value in a 2D slice through the human body. Slice images may be stacked to form a volume. Digitized images consist of a finite number of image elements. Elements of a 2D picture are called *pixels* (picture elements) and elements of stacked 2D slices are called *voxels* (volume elements). We will call pixels or voxels *scene elements* if the dimension of the scene is not known or not important.

2D and 3D images may have an additional time dimension if the variation along the time axis provides additional diagnostic information (e.g., if normally and abnormally beating hearts are compared). Slice images are usually reconstructed from some kind of projection. Reconstruction may cause additional artefacts.

The chapter provides an overview on image acquisition systems for digital images in medicine. Emphasis is put on the semantics of the image and on system-specific artefacts. A more detailed look at the imaging techniques and the reconstruction of medical images is provided by specialized literature such as Prince and Links (2005) or the text of Bushberg et al. (2002) (the latter is more directed toward radiology residents). Imaging techniques in this chapter are listed by the kind of entity that is measured.

---

[1]Imaging techniques are ordered by importance with respect to digital imaging and digital image analysis. Orders of importance with respect to relevance to diagnosis or with respect to frequency of examination are different, of course.

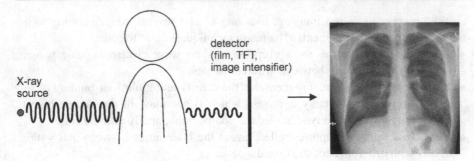

Fig. 2.2 X-rays penetrate the human body and produce an image that shows the integral of tissue-specific absorption along a path from the X-ray source to a detector

2.1   X-Ray Imaging

X rays were discovered in 1895 by Wilhelm Röntgen.[2] He noticed an unknown kind of ray emitted by a cathode ray tube (CRT) that easily penetrated paper, aluminum, and many other materials, but not a lead plate. He also found that this kind of ray is not reflected, refracted, diffracted, or deflected by electrical fields. He discovered that the rays blackened film so that photographic images could be produced. Röntgen called this unknown type of radiation *x rays*.

A material-specific amount of the energy of an x ray is attenuated when penetrating a material. For the first time in history, a technique allowed noninvasive insight into the human body (see Fig. 2.2).

The harmful aspects of x rays were not known in the early years. It was employed for all kinds of purposes without balancing the potential information gain through imaging against the harmfulness of exposure to radiation. For instance, until the 1960s, some shoe stores offered a service by which customer's feet wearing shoes to be fitted were x rayed. Few, if any, precautions were taken to secure operators of x-ray machines from harmful exposure.

2.1.1   Generation, Attenuation, and Detection of X Rays

X rays are electromagnetic waves with a wavelength above the visible spectrum. Electromagnetic radiation has the characteristics of waves, but is actually traveling as clusters of energy called *photons* with a given wavelength. Electromagnetic waves do not need a carrier such as sound waves and travel at the speed of light c. Their wavelength λ and frequency f are related by

$$c = \lambda f. \tag{2.1}$$

---

[2]Carl Wilhelm Röntgen was Professor for physics at the Julius-Maximilian-Universität Würzburg, when he discovered x rays in his experiments with the cathode ray tube in 1895. He received the Nobel price in Physics for his discovery.

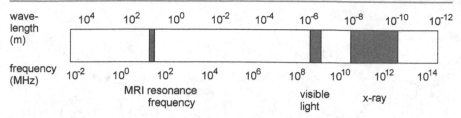

Fig. 2.3 The spectrum of diagnostic X-ray is above the spectrum of visible light in the range of 0.01 to 15 nm (10^{-11} to 1.5×10^{-8} m)

The energy of a photon measured in electron volts (eV) is the energy that a single electron acquires when moving through a potential of 1 V. The energy of a photon is characterized by its wavelength. It is given by

$$e = 1.24/\lambda \tag{2.2}$$

if the unit of measurement is a kilo electron volt (keV) and the wavelength is measured in nanometers (nm).

The wavelength of an electromagnetic wave corresponds to its energy. Examples for electromagnetic waves, in the order of increasing energy, are radio waves (being used for magnetic resonance imaging), visible light, and x rays or gamma rays (see Fig. 2.3). The difference between x rays and gamma rays is not their wavelength, but the fact that gamma rays are created in the nucleus of an atom while x rays are not. The energy of x-ray photons is sufficient to release electrons from an atom, a process which is called *ionizing radiation*.

X rays are characterized by their *exposure*, i.e., the amount of charge per volume of air, which is measured in röntgen (R). Exposure measures the energy of the radiation source, but it does not describe how much of the radiation is absorbed by a body under radiation. Absorption per unit mass is called *dose* and it is measured in radiation absorbed dose (rad) or gray (Gy) with 1 Gy = 100 rad. The ratio between exposure and dose varies with the x-ray energy and is often called the f-factor. The f-factor at low exposure for hard tissues such as bone is much higher than for soft tissues and water. Hence, bone at low doses absorbs a significantly higher amount of radiation than soft tissues.

2.1.1.1 X-Ray Generation

Understanding the different types of x rays requires some understanding about their generation. Electrons in an atom are organized in shells around the nucleus. Since the negatively charged electrons are attracted to the protons in the nucleus, the innermost shell contains electrons with the lowest energy. Energy is needed for moving an electron from an inner shell to an outer shell, which is equivalent to the difference between energy levels of the two shells. If an electron is released from a shell, the required energy amounts to the difference between its current energy level and the level of the outermost shell plus the energy to remove an electron from the outermost shell. Electrons on the outermost shell are thus the easiest to remove and are called *valence electrons*.

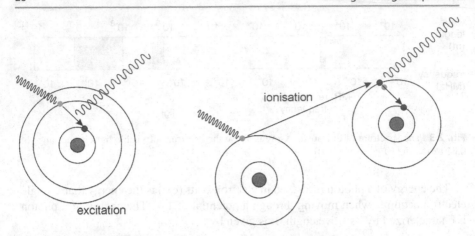

Fig. 2.4 X-ray generation by excitation and ionization. In excitation, external energy pushes an electron from an outer shell to an inner shell. Excess energy is released as x rays. The ionization process is similar, except for the fact that excitation happens indirectly by an electron that is released from an outer shell of a different atom

X rays are generated as excess energy from electrons in the material of a *cathode ray tube* (CRT)[3] when heating the cathode. Energy from heating causes electrons to be released from the cathode and accelerated toward the anode. In the anode, electrons lose their kinetic energy by excitation, ionization, and radiation. *Excitation* and *ionization* cause electrons of the anode material to move from an outer shell to an inner shell (see Fig. 2.4). For excitation, this happens directly, whereas ionization causes the electrons of an outer shell to be released, which then excites the electrons of another atom. The excess energy being released as x rays depends on the energy difference between the outer and the inner shells. Hence, the radiation from this process is monochrome. This kind of x ray is called *characteristic* or *monochrome* x-ray radiation.[4]

Most of the x-ray radiation, however, is *polychrome*. An incident electron is slowed down by passing the nucleus of an atom. Slowing down means that the frequency of the electron changes. The excess energy is emitted as a photon. Its amount depends on how close the incident electron passes to the nucleus. All its energy is released as x rays if it annihilates in the nucleus. If it passes the nucleus, more energy is released for an inner shell passage than for an outer shell passage. This type of radiation is called *bremsstrahlung* and it is inherently polychrome (see Fig. 2.5).

---

[3]The material for anode and cathode is usually Tungsten (also called Wolfram), a chemical element belonging to the metals with the highest melting point of all metals. In CRTs for mammography, another metal, Molybdenum, is used.

[4]The detection of characteristic x ray radiation by Charles G. Barkla in 1905 resulted in another Nobel price in Physics presented to its discoverer in 1917.

Fig. 2.5 Polychrome radiation is a result of a passage of an electron. The frequency of the released radiation depends on the extent to which the electron loses its energy

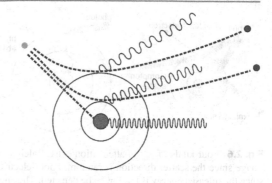

The likelihood of passing an atom at a given distance increases with the distance to the nucleus because the surface of a sphere of a given radius increases with the radius. Thus, the spectrum of the bremsstrahlung of a cathode ray tube should roughly be of a triangular shape. However, the surrounding glass of the tube filters some of the low-energy radiation. Hence, the actual curve is zero at low energy levels, then increases to some maximum at intermediate energy levels and finally decreases to zero at the maximum energy (which is the maximum energy of electrons incident on the anode of the tube). The complete spectrum of a typical x-ray tube is a combination of monochrome and polychrome radiation, where some spikes indicate various characteristic radiation energy levels in the otherwise smooth curve.

X-ray tubes are characterized by the total amount of energy that is emitted as x rays and the quality of the radiation. A high-quality tube has a higher ratio of high-energy radiation and of monochrome radiation. High-quality radiation imposes a lower dose on the patient and generally produces better images.

The quantity and quality of x-ray radiation depend on a number of characteristics of the tube (such as the anode material) and on the parameters to be selected by the operators (such as the potential between cathode and anode, voltage, and exposure time).

The quality of the emitted x rays can be enhanced by a filtering process called *beam hardening*. The glass surrounding the tube already filters some of the low-energy rays of the bremsstrahlung. It reduces the total energy of the emitted x rays, but shifts the spectrum toward the high-quality range. The emitted frequency range can be further improved by the additional filtering of low-frequency components. The amplitude of monochrome radiation is usually higher than that of bremsstrahlung. Beam hardening may thus be used for an overall reduction of x-ray radiation enhancing monochrome radiation in the spectrum as well.

2.1.1.2 X-Ray Attenuation

When x rays enter the human body, four types of attenuation can happen: Raleigh, scatter, Compton scatter, photoelectric absorption, and pair production (see Fig. 2.6). Of these, Compton scatter and photoelectric absorption are the main factors for image generation from medium-range energy x-ray imaging such as that used in diagnostic imaging.

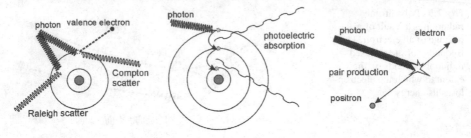

Fig. 2.6 Four kinds of X-ray attenuation exist. Raleigh and Compton scatter causes noise in the image since the scatter direction is random. Photo-electric absorption produces the X-ray image, since the released energy is too low to be detected. The energy levels used in X-ray imaging do not produce pair production

Raleigh scatter mainly happens in low-energy imaging such as mammography. A photon causing Raleigh scatter loses its energy by exciting the whole atom, which immediately releases a photon with almost the same energy, although usually scattered in a different direction.

A photon causing *Compton scatter* will release a valence electron from its shell. It will lose as much energy as was necessary for the release. Scattered photons will change their direction.

Scatter, be it Raleigh scatter or Compton scatter, increases noise and reduces contrast in an image. Noise stems from the randomness of scattering and the random change of direction for scattered photons. Contrast is reduced because scattered photons reaching the receptor do not carry position information of the locus of scattering, thus only increasing the overall brightness in the image.

Photoelectric absorption is the main contributor to imaging even though absorption in diagnostic x rays happens less often than Compton scattering. A photon releases its energy through photoelectric absorption by removing one of the electrons of the inner shells. The photon loses its energy completely. The released electron leaves a vacancy in the shell that is filled by an electron of one of the outer shells. This initiates a cascade of filling in the vacancies from the outer shells. The energy gain from each transition is released as characteristic radiation. The characteristic radiation caused by this process has a much lower energy than that of the incident photon. Hence, it is absorbed by the surrounding atoms and does not contribute to the degradation of the image. Absorption is the cause of a meaningful image, but it also increases the radiation dose absorbed by the tissue.

The probability of absorption increases with atomic number (e.g., the calcium in bone absorbs more than the hydrogen of the cerebrospinal fluid) and decreases with beam energy. Absorption increases dramatically when the photon energy equals the binding energy of an inner electron. This value is called the *absorption edge* and its existence is exploited by *contrast agents*. Contrast agents such as iodine and barium have a high atomic number and an absorption edge in the range of diagnostic x rays (33 and 37 keV). The high atomic number already increases the probability of absorption. Energy in the range of the absorption edge of the radiation spectrum will be further reduced.

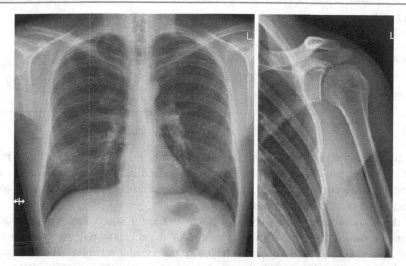

Fig. 2.7 Two radiographs (with kind permission from Siemens Sector Healthcare, Erlangen, Germany). Bone structures in the two images are clearly visible. Differentiating between different soft tissues is more difficult as is the depth order of the projected structures

Pair production, the last of the four effects, happens only if the energy exceeds 1022 keV, which is beyond the usual diagnostic range for x-ray imaging. In pair production, a photon annihilates and produces an electron–positron pair. The positron and electron are sent in opposite directions. Although this is not relevant for x-ray imaging, it should be noted that the opposite process (i.e., the annihilation of a positron when merging with an electron producing two photons with 511 keV) is used for positron emission tomography (PET), an imaging technique that is described later in this chapter.

2.1.2 X-Ray Imaging

X-ray imaging uses the dependency of photoelectric absorption on the atomic number for producing a diagnostically meaningful image (see Fig. 2.7 for examples). Being the oldest technique, a vast number of different imaging methods evolved from the original method presented by C.W. Röntgen. In this section we will only touch on the subject to give an impression of how the images are created and what kind of different x-ray imaging techniques exist. A more detailed treatment can be found in Bushberg et al. (2002) and Prince and Links (2005). Much of this section has been taken from there and from the AAPN/RSNA Physics Tutorial for Residents that appeared in various issues of the Radiographics journal (McCollough 1997; Bushberg 1998; McKetty 1998; Pooley et al. 2001; Wang and Blackburn 2000).

Fig. 2.8 Different sizes of
the focal spot cause different
blurring even if the aperture is
the same

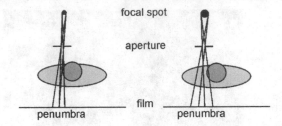

Diagnostic equipment for x-ray imaging consists at least of a cathode ray tube emitting x rays and a receptor with the patient placed between the emitter and receptor. The receptor may be film, an image intensifier, or a flat panel detector with the latter two producing digital images.

If the x-ray tube is assumed to be a point source for x rays and the receptor is planar, the image intensity at every location of the receptor will be proportional to the attenuation along a ray from the x-ray tube to the receptor. The measured intensity for a monochromatic beam at a location (x, y) on the receptor is then

$$I_{out} = I_{in} \cdot \exp\left(-\int_{s_0}^{s_1} \mu(s)\,ds\right), \tag{2.3}$$

where I_{in} is the incident intensity of x rays when entering the body, s is a ray from the x-ray source to (x, y) on the image plane, s_1 is the point where the ray enters the body, and s_2 is the point where it exits the body. The function $\mu(s)$ is the *attenuation*. Attenuation, as pointed out in the previous section, is mainly caused by Compton scatter and photoelectric absorption and to a small extent by Raleigh scatter. The intensity at some location (x, y) is given by x-ray attenuation plus intensity due to scattered photons. If scattered photons are assumed to be distributed evenly over the image, they increase the brightness in the image by a noise component thus reducing contrast.

The imaging process described above is idealized in that it assumes that the x-ray source is a point source. In reality, the *focal spot* of an x-ray source covers a finite area leading to a loss of resolution due to penumbrae. Its extent depends on the distances between the source, object, and receptor, as well as on the diameter of the focal spot (see Fig. 2.8). Regular x-ray CRTs have a focal spot with a diameter of 1 mm, fine focus CRTs have one with a 0.5-mm diameter and microfocus CRT has a 0.2-mm diameter focal spot.

Integrated attenuation along s of polychromatic x rays is different to the monochromatic case described above since low-energy radiation is absorbed earlier than high-energy radiation. Placing the patient between the source and receptor causes additional beam hardening. Continuous beam hardening of an x ray traveling through the body has the effect that attenuation changes depending on the distance traveled in the body. This makes the image content dependent on patient positioning. It also causes some of the low-energy radiation to be absorbed by the patient without having an impact on the images and unnecessarily increases the dose. Prior beam hardening by filtering lessens these unwanted effects.

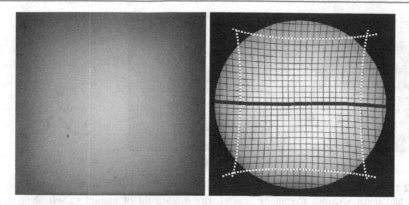

Fig. 2.9 Vignetting causes shading in an image as it can be seen in the picture of homogeneous *material on the left*. The location dependent magnification by a pincushion distortion of an image intensifier is seen on the test pattern of equal-sized *squares on the right* (*dashed lines*). This image also shows the much less prominent deformation due to the earth magnetic field

Of the three types of receptors *analogue film* is the oldest and still the most widespread. Film may be digitized, but receptors such as image intensifiers and flat panel detectors are preferred if computer-assisted postprocessing is desired.

An *image intensifier* produces a visible image from x rays in a similar fashion than a conventional CRT. X rays are turned into visible light on a phosphor screen in a vacuum tube, which is then converted into electrons by a photocathode. The electrons are focused and accelerated—this is the enhancement step—toward the anode and cast onto the output phosphor producing the intensified image. Enhancement through an image intensifier increases the brightness at the output phosphor more than 1000 times with respect to the very weak signal at the input phosphor.

The image intensifier was originally invented for creating a visible signal without the need to use and develop film. It has the additional advantage of enabling the transmittance of the electronic signal and its digitization through an A/D converter.

Images from an image intensifier suffer from a number of artefacts of which the following three are relevant for postprocessing (see Fig. 2.9).

- *Vignetting* is caused by the angle at which rays fall onto the input screen. The angle is perpendicular to the image screen in the center. In this case, the incident x-ray energy is distributed over the smallest possible area. The intensity (i.e., the energy per unit area) is maximal. The angle decreases with the distance to the center, causing the incident x-ray energy to be distributed over a larger area. Hence, the intensity decreases with the distance to the center.
- *Pincushion distortion* is caused by the curvedness of the input screen and results in magnification. Magnification increases with the deviation of the input surface from a tangent plane to the center of the screen.
- The *S-distortion* is caused by external electromagnetic fields that influence the course of the electron beam between the input and output phosphor.

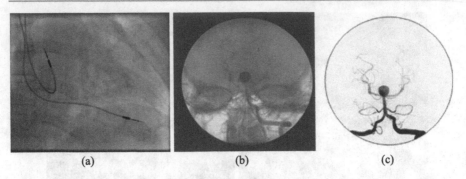

(a)   (b)   (c)

Fig. 2.10 (a) Fluoroscopy guiding pacemaker implanting (from knol.google.com/k/pacemakers, published under Creative Commons license). (b) Angiogram of cranial vessels showing an aneurysm (the eye sockets and parts of the skull are visible as well and hide some of the small vessels), (c) Digital subtraction angiogram of (b)

A completely digital receptor for x rays is the TFT *flat panel detector* that has been developed in recent years. A flat panel detector combines a flat panel scintillator, which turns x rays into visible light with a detector that transforms the light into an analogue electric signal, which then may be digitized. Several studies established the adequateness of using a flat panel detector in diagnostic imaging with the added advantage of lower doses necessary for imaging (e.g., Bacher et al. 2003; Fink et al. 2002; Garmer et al. 2000).

The *blackening curve*, which measures the dependency of incident radiation on the receptor and intensity of the resulting images, has a larger interval of linear increase for flat panel detectors and image intensifiers than for film. This decreases the likelihood of an accidental overexposure or underexposure. The spatial resolution in digital radiography is still lower than that of film. However, recent advances in TFT detector design have pushed the limits of achievable resolution into the range of film (about 4000 × 4000 pixels).

An advantage of digital radiography using either a TFT detector or an image intensifier is that the operator may choose the spatial resolution. If imaging at a lower resolution is sufficient for some diagnostic purpose, this can be achieved by analogue or digital integration over several pixels of the image. Since integration reduces noise, the signal-to-noise ratio increases without having to increase the exposure and, consequently, the dose.

2.1.3 Fluoroscopy and Angiography

Fluoroscopy is a specific kind of x-ray imaging to visualizes moving or changing objects in the human body (see Fig. 2.10a). Examples for using diagnostic fluoroscopy are as follows:
- to follow the heartbeat for detecting abnormal behavior,

- to follow the course of a contrast agent through the colon to detect potential abnormalities such as a tumor,
- to image cardiac or cerebral blood flow by using a contrast agent.

The technique received its name because x rays are turned into visible light using a fluorescent screen. Early fluoroscopy systems placed the screen directly behind the x-ray tube and the patient. The physician was sitting in front of the screen. Fluorescence from the x rays is very weak so that the introduction of the image intensifier made fluoroscopic imaging a much more viable tool.

Most of today's fluoroscopic imaging devices produce digital images and enable the creation of x-ray films as well. Fluoroscopic imaging devices are not necessarily static. When mounted on a C-arm, they can be rotated around the patient for producing projections along arbitrary directions. Fluoroscopic imaging is used for diagnosis and supports surgical interventions. It is an attractive imaging technique for the latter usage because images can be produced during the intervention.

Fluoroscopic imaging of the vascular system using a contrast agent is called *angiography* (see Fig. 2.10b). The contrast agent is applied by a catheter being guided to the location to be imaged (e.g., the brain or the heart wall). Imaging cerebral or cardiovascular flow supports the diagnosis of arteriosclerosis, arterio-venous malformations (AVMs), and so on. Angiographic images show anatomy of the human body with the blood vessels enhanced through the contrast agent. Angiographic images can be acquired in real-time and can be used to guide a surgical intervention (see Fig. 2.11 for a modern angiographic image acquisition system). Such acquisition systems can also be used to reconstruct 3D images from a sequence of projection from different angles similar to the computed tomography (see Sect. 2.1.5).

Anatomic information from all other structures can be removed when an image is subtracted, which was made prior to giving the contrast agent. Although it is possible—and has been done—to do the subtraction mechanically using film, it is now done on digital images. The technique is called *digital subtraction angiography* (DSA, see Fig. 2.10c).

DSA enhances vessels much more when compared to angiography, but the images may suffer from motion artefacts. This is particularly true in cardiac angiography. Cardiac motion is too fast for creating two images without the heartbeat influencing the result. Gated imaging is possible, but it may be still difficult to choose two images with and without the contrast agent that were taken at exactly the same point in the heart cycle. Furthermore, motion due to breathing and patient movement cannot be removed by gating. DSA images from cerebral blood flow are affected to a much smaller extent by motion artefacts from heartbeat and patient motion.

Motion artefacts cannot be corrected easily because of the location dependency between 3D motion and its projection onto a 2D plane. If corrected at all, motion correction consists of selecting an optimal null image (the image without the contrast agent) from several images, which after subtraction minimizes some error measure. Some research work on nonrigid registration between the two images in DSA has been reported, but as far as we know none of this has reached maturity up to a point that the technique is routinely applied (see Meijering et al. 1999 for a review).

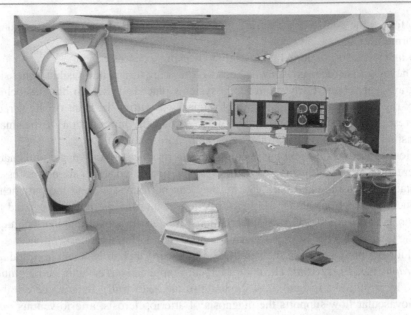

Fig. 2.11 Angiographic imaging device (C-arm) which is used for guiding minimal invasive interventions (Siemens Artis zeego, with kind permission from Siemens Sector Healthcare, Erlangen, Germany)

2.1.4 Mammography

Bremsstrahlung is the major influence in most x-ray tubes with the exception of x-ray tubes for *mammography* (see Fig. 2.12). The purpose of mammography is to detect small, nonpalpable lesions in the female breast. This requires a much higher image quality than normal x-ray imaging with respect to contrast and spatial resolution. Since contrast and resolution are affected by scattering, mammography tubes reduce bremsstrahlung by suitable filtering. Furthermore, mammography tubes use a material (Molybdenum) that produces an almost monochrome x ray with peak energies around 17 to 19 keV. This would be unwanted in regular x-ray imaging as most—if not all—of the radiation would be absorbed and not reach the receptor. For the breast, however, the use of low-energy beams increases the contrast between the subtle differences of different tissues. Using an (almost) monochromatic beam will also reduce scatter, which again increases contrast.

Differences and findings in mammograms are subtle. Hence, *digital mammography* with its potential for postprocessing has received much attention for quite some time (see, e.g., Chan et al. 1987; Dengler et al. 1993; Cheng et al. 1998). Digital mammograms have numerous advantages. They can be easily distributed and accessed in a hospital network. The dynamic range of digital detectors (about 1000:1) is much higher than that of film (40:1). Digital mammograms can be created using currently available TFT flat panel detectors, but owing to the need for a high resolution, the development of techniques reaching an even better resolution is still an active research field.

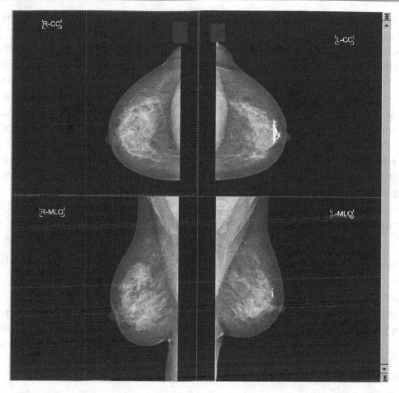

Fig. 2.12 The goal of human or computer-assisted analysis in mammography is to find calcifications which are potential tumor sites (images with kind permission from Siemens Sector Health-care, Erlangen, Germany)

2.1.5   Image Reconstruction for Computed Tomography

The images from x-ray attenuation discussed so far are projection images. The structures are projected on top of each other. High attenuating objects such as bone may hide other objects. In cranial images, for instance, the skull would hide most of the details of the enclosed soft tissue. Furthermore, the cone beam geometry makes the measurement of absolute distances impossible.[5]

Tomography (from the Greek "tomos" = cut, slice) attempts to create an image of one or more slices through the body. A set of slices provides a detailed 3D distribution of x-ray attenuation per volume unit. The name *computed tomography* (CT, also called CAT = computed axial tomography) emphasizes that these images are not acquired directly by some clever imaging device, but are computed from pro-

---

[5]There are exceptions, if, e.g., images are made by two different cone beams of a rotating C-arm where the magnification of objects in the center of both cones can be computed.

jection measurements. X-ray computed tomography was invented in the 1970s by
Godfrey N. Hounsfield based on the work of Alan M. Cormack[6] (Buzug 2008).

Tomography had been known before as an analogue technique. It produced slices
through the body directly on film by moving the film and x-ray source in opposite
directions during exposure (Geluk 1979). Depending on the ratio between the speeds
of the film cassette and x-ray source, a specific single slice parallel to the image
plane was imaged in focus overlaid by blurred layers above and below this slice.

Computed tomography goes a different way. It produces a digitized solution of
the inverse *Radon transform* from projections in a slice without interference from
other slices (see Buzug 2008 for a detailed treatment of reconstruction techniques).
The inversion is computed numerically from projections by the imaging computer.[7]

For a 2D attenuation function $\mu(x, y)$ describing the x-ray attenuation per unit
volume in some slice z in the human body, the Radon transform is given by all line
integrals through this function

$$R(s, \theta)\left[\mu(x, y)\right] = \int_{-\infty}^{\infty} \int_{-\infty}^{\infty} \mu(x, y) \delta(s - x\cos\theta - y\sin\theta)\,dx\,dy, \quad (2.4)$$

where δ is the Dirac-delta function.

In other words, for a given angle θ, the Radon transform produces the projections
onto a line s along rays perpendicular to s with angle θ to the x-axis. The Radon
transform is invertible, which means that $\mu(x, y)$ may be reconstructed from all
projections onto lines s for all angles $0° < \theta < 180°$. This essentially solves the
reconstruction problem. Since

$$I_{\text{out}} = I_{\text{in}} \cdot \exp\left(-\int_{t_0}^{t_1} \mu(t)\,dt\right), \quad (2.5)$$

we have

$$\int_{t_0}^{t_1} \mu(t)\,dt = -\ln\left(\frac{I_{\text{out}}}{I_{\text{in}}}\right) \quad \text{with } t = s - x\cos\theta - y\sin\theta. \quad (2.6)$$

If we assume that no attenuation takes place outside of $[t_1, t_2]$, we can extend the
bounds of the integral to infinity and

$$R(s, \theta)\left[\mu(x, y)\right] = \int_{-\infty}^{\infty} \mu(t)\,dt = \int_{-\infty}^{\infty} \int_{-\infty}^{\infty} \mu(x, y) \delta(s - x\cos\theta - y\sin\theta) \quad (2.7)$$

---

[6]Alan M. Cormack has been a physicist at the University of Cape Town in South Africa when he
developed the theoretical basis for Computer Tomography in the late 1950s. This work was taken
up later by Godfrey N. Hounsfield, an electrical engineer at EMI research lab, who presented the
first whole body CT scanner in 1975. For their invention, both received the Nobel price of Medicine
and Physiology in 1979.

[7]An optical solution for the reconstruction exists as well which has been proposed in the 70s in
order to overcome limitations because of lack of computing power (Geluk 1979).

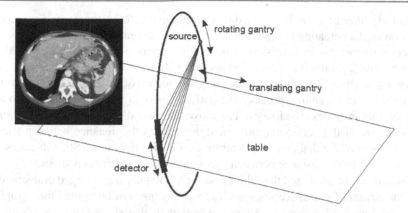

Fig. 2.13 Schematic view of CT image generation. The patient is placed on a moveable table. A CT image is a slice that is reconstructed from multiple projections taken from different angles. A sequence of CTs is created from translating the table and repeating the image acquisition procedure

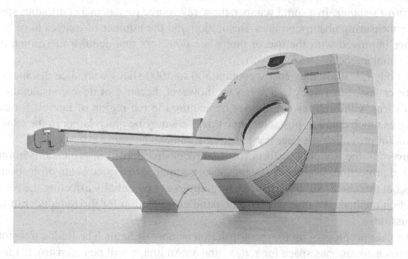

Fig. 2.14 An X-ray CT scanner (Siemens Somatom, image with kind permission by Siemens Sector Healthcare, Erlangen, Germany). Image acquisition takes place in the doughnut-shaped gantry that houses x-ray source and detector rings (which, in this system, can be tilted). The patient is moved through the gantry while slices of CT images are acquired

may be computed from radiographic projections at angles $0° < \theta < 180°$. If we had enough of these projections, the Radon transform could be inverted numerically and a 3D distribution of *attenuation coefficients* is reconstructed.

A CT scanner that acquires projections consists of a single slice or a multiple slice detector ring around which an x-ray source rotates (see Fig. 2.13 for a schematic view and Fig. 2.14 for an image acquisition system). During rotation, detections are constantly made. It can be thought of as a device that creates single or multiple lines of x-ray images from different angles. Measurements are created much faster than creating complete x-ray images from multiple angles.

Reconstruction by the inversion of the Radon transform creates single or multiple slices of voxels containing attenuation per unit volume in the imaged patient.

A stack of slices is produced by scanning a sequence of different slices or groups of slices. For the scanning process, the patient lies on a table that moves into the detector ring in prespecified steps. The movement is called (translational) *gantry*. The step size of the horizontal movement determines the distance between slices. The thickness of the detector ring determines the slice thickness. Slice thickness is often lower than the distance between slices causing a gap between slices.

The number of slices and their thickness for a CT study has changed dramatically with the advent of multislice scanners. In the early times of computed tomography, a slice thickness of 5 mm with a 5 mm gap or even thicker slices was quite common. A brain image data set from CT may have contained less than 20 slices. A detailed analysis (e.g., of the fine structures in the brain) was difficult to impossible. Newer scanners produced thinner slices, but motion during image acquisition often caused artefacts and image quality deteriorated. An advancement was the development of the *spiral scanner*. In a spiral scanner, the x-ray source rotates in a continuous spiral while measuring absorption data. Resolution and the number of images have been further improved with the use of multislice detectors that acquire more than one slice simultaneously (Buzug 2008).

A body CT study may easily contain 500 to 1000 slices with slice distances of 1 mm or less. Slice thickness may vary, however, because of dose considerations. Thin slices with high resolution may be acquired in the region of interest for capturing as much detail as possible. Slice thickness may be much larger in the context region for providing the necessary anatomic context.

Inverting the Radon transform for slice reconstruction from projections implies parallel projection, whereas x-ray images are acquired in a cone beam projection. It turns out that this is solvable by transformations not essentially affecting the reconstruction method. We thus will assume parallel projection for the remainder of this discussion.

Another problem of image reconstruction is more difficult. The Radon transform assumes a continuous space for s, θ, x, and y. An image will be reconstructed from a limited number of projections and a limited number of measurements per projection. Fortunately, just a finite number of voxels needs to be reconstructed with the attenuation coefficients assumed to be constant within the voxel. Nevertheless, the influence of the digitization on the inversion of the Radon transform needs to be investigated.

Inversion is by means of the Fourier transform, which leads to the *filtered backprojection* (FBP) algorithm. The Fourier transform of the Radon transform delivers what is known as the *Central Slice Theorem*. The theorem states that the Fourier transform $M(u, v)$ of a projection of a function $\mu(x, y)$ in a direction with angle θ to the x-axis equals the coefficients on a line with this angle θ in the frequency space of the Fourier transform of μ (see Fig. 2.15). This can easily be shown for a line with $\theta = 0$, where

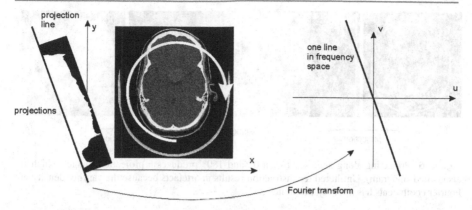

Fig. 2.15 The central slice theorem states that the Fourier transform of a projection onto a line with some angle a equals a line in frequency space of the Fourier transform with equal angle of the image

$$
FFT\big[R(s,0)\big(\mu(x,y)\big)\big] = FFT\left[\int_{-\infty}^{\infty} \mu(x,0)\,dx\right]
$$

$$
= \int_{-\infty}^{\infty}\left[\int_{-\infty}^{\infty} \mu(x,0)\,dx\right]\exp(-ivy)\,dy
$$

$$
= \int_{-\infty}^{\infty}\int_{-\infty}^{\infty} \mu(x,0)x\exp\big(-i(0u+vy)\big)\,dx\,dy
$$

$$
= M(x,0). \tag{2.8}
$$

The theorem is true for all other angles θ as well because of the rotation property of the Fourier transform. Hence, projections of $R(s,\theta)[\mu(x,y)]$ for all angles θ are transformed into one-dimensional (1D) frequency space. The coefficients for a projection $R(s,\theta)$ are mapped out on the corresponding line with angle θ in the 2D frequency space. The inverse Fourier transform is then applied for computing the reconstructed image.

There are two problems with this. First, the Fourier transform from projections is defined in a polar coordinate system, whereas coefficients for carrying out the inverse transform are required in Cartesian coordinates. We need to account for the difference in the size of a unit area in polar and Cartesian coordinates. Otherwise, low frequency components in the image would be overly emphasized (see Fig. 2.16). The correction is done by multiplying the Fourier coefficients with $1/r$, where r is the radial distance of a given location (u, v) to the origin. Hence, it is an application of a radial *ramp filter* (see Fig. 2.17 for a filtered reconstruction).

Second, the distribution of Fourier coefficients from polar coordinates becomes sparser in the high frequency range of the Cartesian coordinate system. It may cause artefacts because noise often predominates in the high frequency range. Hence, projections are usually low-pass filtered, by filters such as the *Hamming window* or *Hamming filter* (see Sect. 4.3 on image enhancement).

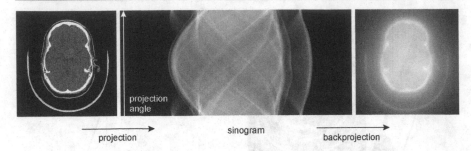

Fig. 2.16 Projecting along angles between 0° and 180° produces a projection image (which is also called sinogram). Unfiltered reconstruction results in artefacts because the varying density of Fourier coefficients has not been accounted for

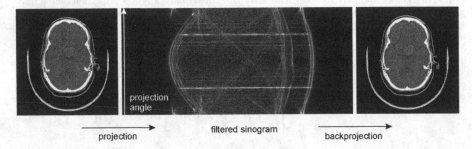

Fig. 2.17 Filtering the projection with a ramp filter that attenuates amplitudes with decreasing frequency removes artefacts from simple reconstruction

The inversion of the Radon transform using the Central Slice Theorem does not really require transforming the projection data into frequency space. The Fourier transform is a linear operator. Adding terms for the Fourier transform or its inverse may be carried out in any order. One particular order would be to transform a line s of the projection data, filter the result and invert the transformation, and then carry on with the next line. If we look at the process more closely, we see that this can be replaced by convolving the projection data of this line with a convolution function that is the spatial domain equivalent of the filter function, and then project the result perpendicular to s onto the image. This is to be done for every projection and gives the method its name *filtered backprojection* or *convolution backprojection reconstruction*.

The reconstruction result is a digital image of attenuation coefficients for each voxel with the thickness of the slice and a size along x and y according to the chosen in-plane spatial resolution. Common image sizes for CT images are 512×512 or 256×256. The size of the voxel along the x- and y-axes depends on the field of view (FOV), which depends on the opening angle of the cone beam scanning the patient. For brain images with an FOV of about 30×30 cm^2, in-plane voxel sizes for a 512×512 image are 0.5×0.5 mm^2.

Table 2.1 Hounsfield units of different tissues. Air, water and bone are well-differentiated, while contrast between different soft tissues is low

Air	Fat	Water	Blood	Muscle	White matter	Grey matter	CSF	Bone
−1000	−100	0	30–45	40	20–30	37–45	15	>150

Attenuation coefficients are normalized for making the result independent of imaging parameters such as beam energy. The scale is called the *Hounsfield scale*. Normalization is based on the attenuation μ_{Water} of water and μ_{Air} of air

$$HU(\mu) = 1000 \cdot \frac{\mu - \mu_{Water}}{\mu_{Water} - \mu_{Air}}. \tag{2.9}$$

Thus, air has −1000 HU (Hounsfield units) and water has 0 HU. Hounsfield units for different tissue types are given in Table 2.1. Hounsfield units are mapped to integers and usually represented in a range from −1000 to 3000. Hence, attenuation coefficients can be represented by two byte integers.

The display software of a scanner system lets the user choose an appropriate HU range to be mapped onto the displayable range of 256 gray values by specifying the *window* (the width of the range to be mapped) and the *level* (the value to be mapped onto the gray value 128). Different window and level settings are used to emphasize different tissues. A bone window, for instance, will have a high level and a large window because attenuation for bone is high and extends over a wide range. A lung window, on the other hand, will have a much lower level since most of the lung is filled with air.

Air, fat, water, and bone have significantly different attenuation, whereas the differences between the various soft tissues are small (see Table 2.1). In fact, the results from the first experiments of CTs of the head were not overwhelming and medical equipment companies were reluctant to build a CT scanner.[8] Scanners have much improved since then in terms of spatial resolution as well as in terms of suppressing noise and artefacts. CT is probably still the most often used digital image device in diagnosis and surgical intervention. Typical application areas for diagnostic imaging are bone CT, CT of the brain, and CT of the parenchyma.

A number of artefacts may occur when creating the image by FBP, which have to be accounted for in a later image analysis.

- *Noise* (Fig. 2.18) is caused from scatter in the patient and at the detector. Since the likelihood of a photon reaching the detector unscattered can be modeled as a Poisson process, the noise is often modeled by a Gaussian function (which is a good approximation of a Poisson distribution for large numbers of events).
- The *partial volume effect* (PVE, Fig. 2.18) occurs because attenuation within a voxel may not be uniform. The PVE within a slice is usually easy to recognize. It is most prominent between adjacent voxels with very different attenuation coefficients such as at the bone-CSF boundary. The reconstructed attenuation coefficient will be a value between that of the two tissues. The PVE occurs between

---

[8]The first CT scanner was built by a record company (EMI).

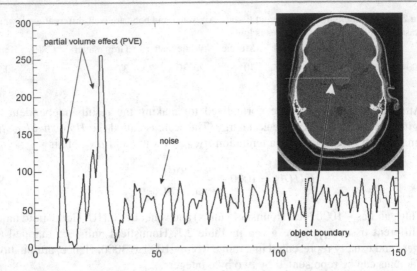

Fig. 2.18 Noise and the partial volume effect (PVE) in CT imaging. The PVE causes blur at skin, fat, bone and CSF boundaries. Noise amplitude in this image is in the range of the signal increase at the object boundary

slices as well and may be less obvious because the object causing the PVE may be in the slice above or below the currently displayed slice.

- *Metal artefacts* are caused by the very high difference between the attenuation of metal and tissue. This makes the reconstruction less robust against other influences such as noise and PVE.[9] It results in severe *streak artefacts*. Such artefacts can be observed at all high contrast boundaries, but are particularly severe in the case of metal artefacts.

- *Motion artefacts* are the result of voluntary or involuntary patient movement (movement due to breathing, heartbeat, etc.) during the acquisition of a single slice. Motion violates the assumption that attenuation at some location (x, y) is the same for every projection and causes blur in the image. Since the influence from motion may be different for different slices, it may cause the so-called *step-ladder-artefact* between slices (visible in reoriented views, see, e.g., Ghersin et al. 2006).

Tomographic imaging using x rays can also be carried out using x-ray equipment for projection images. Early attempts included the use of image intensifiers for rapid imaging of the heart (Mayo Clinic; Robb et al. 1982). Newer developments employed angiographic acquisition systems for reconstruction (Ning et al. 2000; Akpek et al. 2005). Since angiography uses a moveable and rotatable C-arm, projections can be reconstructed from programmed C-arm rotation. The receptor device is a TFT flat panel detector with up to 1000×1000 elements. Each projection si-

---

[9]The problem of image reconstruction can be stated as an algebraic problem of finding unknowns—the attenuation—from linear equations—the projections—and it can be shown that the problem becomes more ill-conditioned when some very high attenuation regions exist.

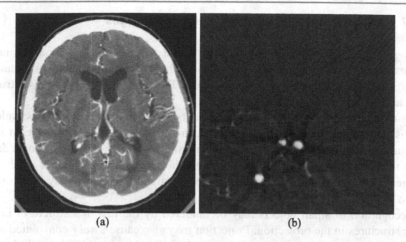

(a)   (b)

Fig. 2.19 CT angiography (**a**) shows contrast-enhanced vessels. While showing also tissue in the context, vessels are more difficult to detect than in reconstructed DSA images (**b**)

multaneously acquires data from 1000 slices with 1000 projections per line. Reconstructed images thus have a higher spatial resolution than ordinary CT images and produce all slices at the same time. It comes at a cost, however. Current systems are not fast enough to generate projections from as many angles as a conventional CT system. In consequence, artefacts due to an insufficient number of measurements increase. The images are noisier and the streak artefacts are more pronounced.

2.1.6 Contrast Enhancement in X-Ray Computed Tomography

The contrast agent used in fluoroscopic imaging or angiography is used in x-ray CT as well. Instead of showing a time-varying function such as in fluoroscopy, the use of a contrast agent in x-ray CT enhances structures that are otherwise difficult to differentiate. A major application is the depiction of vessels (*CT angiography* or CTA; Dillon et al. 1993).

CTA works similarly to ordinary x-ray angiography with the difference being that the images are not projections (see Fig. 2.19a for an example). The 3D nature of CTA images allows quantitative analysis by direct measurement on the image. With the spatial resolution of today's scanners, diagnosis of the extent of a stenosis becomes possible through CTA even for smaller vessels. It needs to be kept in mind, however, that CTA requires a higher exposure to x rays than x-ray angiography. Compared to subtraction angiography (a reconstruction from DSA is depicted in Fig. 2.19b), CTA provides information about soft tissues not visible in DSA. On the other hand, the intensity of vessels filled with the contrast agent is similar to that of bone, making it difficult to separate the vessel structures close to the skull from bone structures.

2.1.7   Image Analysis on X-Ray Generated Images

Radiographs have a high spatial resolution which supports the detection of small lesions such as microcalcifications in mammography, potentially cancerous nodules in lung scans, or small stenoses in angiography. The signal is bright for dense structures and dark for low attenuation objects.

As the image is a projection, no assignments between absolute brightness value and tissue type can be made. Distance measurements are not possible, except for measurements of distance ratios between structures of which the approximate distance to the radiation source is known to the radiologist. Overexposure or underexposure (for digitized film) may reduce the contrast and the images may be blurred due to motion or the size of the focal spot.

Recognition of small objects may be hindered by the fact that structures hide other structures in the projection. Projection may also cause a very convoluted appearance of larger objects (such as complex bone fractures), which bears little resemblance to the actual shape of this object. Deducing the true geometry of such an object from its projection may be easy to the experienced radiologist, but difficult to implement in an algorithm. It requires extensive context knowledge about the projection direction, the orientation of the organs being imaged, and their relative position with respect to the projection direction.

Creating tomographic images reduces or removes some of the problems above, which is one of the reasons for the sudden increase of computer-assisted analysis methods in medicine with the appearance of CT imaging in the 1970s. CT images have a lower spatial resolution than radiographs, which is why radiographs may still be preferred if the diagnosis requires high resolution images.

If noise, partial volume effects, and other artefacts are disregarded, a mapping between the tissue type and attenuation coefficient exists in a voxel of a CT. The normalized attenuation coefficients of the Hounsfield scale make mappings from different images created by different machines comparable. The value of this is not to be underestimated. Even though the mapping is only approximate and distorted by artefacts and even though it is certainly not invertible (i.e., a certain HU value is not uniquely associated with a certain type of tissue), it comes close to the primary goal of imaging (i.e., directly measuring and displaying the tissue and tissue characteristics).

2.2   Magnetic Resonance Imaging

Protons and neutrons of the nucleus of an atom possess an angular momentum that is called *spin*. These spins cancel if the number of subatomic particles in a nucleus is even. Nuclei with an odd number exhibit a resultant spin that can be observed outside of the atom. This is the basis of *magnetic resonance imaging* (MRI) (Liang and Lauterbur 2000). In MRI, spins of nuclei are aligned in an external magnetic field. A high frequency electromagnetic field then causes *spin precession* that depends on the density of magnetized material and on its molecular binding. The resonance of the signal continues for some time after this radio signal is switched off. The effect is measured and exploited to create an image of the distribution of the material.

The resonance effect has been used in MR spectroscopy for quite some time. A detailed description of MR spectroscopy and its clinical applications can be found in Salibi and Brown (1998). However, imaging (i.e., the computation of the spatial distribution of effects from magnetic resonance) did not exist before the 1970s. Image generation with magnetic resonance is due to Paul C. Lauterbur and Peter Mansfield.[10]

Magnetic resonance imaging almost exclusively uses the response of the hydrogen nucleus which is abundant in the human body. Variation of hydrogen density and specifically its molecular binding in different tissues produces a much better soft tissue contrast than CT. MRI has some further advantages if compared with x-ray CT.

- MRI does not use ionizing radiation.
- Images can be generated with arbitrary slice orientation including coronal and sagittal views.
- Several different functional attributes can be imaged with MRI.

In summary, MRI is a remarkably versatile imaging technique justifying an extended look at the technique.

2.2.1 Magnetic Resonance

As mentioned above, nuclei with an odd number of protons or neutrons possess a spin. To produce a resonance image, spins of all nuclei of the body are aligned in a static magnetic field B_0. The strength of the magnetic field is measured in Tesla (T) or gauss (10,000 Gauss = 1 T). Today's MR imaging devices for human full body imaging operate with field strengths between 1 and 3 T.

The static field causes spins to be aligned either parallel or antiparallel to the magnetic field. The strength of the measurable signal depends on the difference between these two types of alignment. This, in turn, depends on the type of atom, on the magnetic field strength and on the temperature at which the measurement takes place. The atom-specific sensitivity is highest for hydrogen.

A precession of spins around an axis parallel to the B_0-field can be induced by a radio signal. The effects of parallel and antiparallel precessing spins cancel. For hydrogen at normal room temperature and a magnetic field of 1.5 T, the ratio between the parallel and antiparallel spins is approximately 500.000:500.001. Hence, the observed net signal from all spins will come from just one in a million protons (see Fig. 2.20).

---

[10]Peter Mansfield is a British physicist who provided the basis for interpreting the signal from resonance. Paul C. Lauterbur is a chemist who first provided the methodology for turning the signal into an image. For their achievement, both received the Nobel price for Physiology and Medicine in 2003.

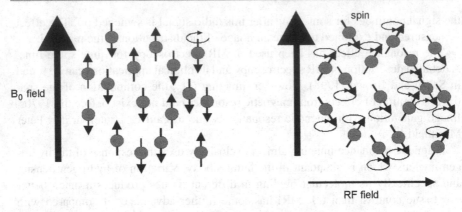

Fig. 2.20 Spins are aligned parallel or anti-parallel to the B_0-field. They produce a signal induced by an RF field. Just a small excess amount of protons aligned parallel produce the signal, since signals from parallel and anti-parallel aligned protons cancel

Given that the hydrogen atom possesses the highest sensitivity of all atoms and that the temperature cannot be increased arbitrarily, the only way to increase the signal is to increase the magnetic field. This is the reason for the exceptionally high magnetic fields that are applied in MRI (for comparison, the strength of the Earth's magnetic field is 0.00003–0.00006 T).

If spins are aligned in the external B_0-field, their angular momentum (i.e., their spin frequency ω) depends on the strength of B_0 and an atom-specific *gyromagnetic constant* γ

$$\omega = \gamma B_0. \tag{2.10}$$

The frequency ω is called the *Larmor frequency*. The gyromagnetic constant for water is 42.58 MHz/T, which translates into a spin frequency of 63.87 MHz for an MRI scanner with a static field with 1.5 T.

To produce resonance, additional energy is supplied causing the spins to precess around the direction of the B_0-field.[11] It is applied by an electromagnetic field that is perpendicular to B_0. The field effects proton spins only if it changes with the same frequency than the rotation frequency of the spins. Hence, if the strength of the B_0-field would be 1.5 T, the required frequency of the resonance triggering field would be 63.87 MHz. This high frequency field (HF) radio wave is supplied by a radio antenna.

The radio signal tilts the spins by an angle $0° < \alpha < 180°$ from their rest direction. The magnitude of the angle depends on the energy of the HF field signal (see Fig. 2.21). After the signal is switched off, the spins slowly return into their rest direction parallel or antiparallel to the B_0-field while still carrying out the precession.

---

[11]The following discussion relates to effects observed in voxels containing a large enough number of photons so that quantum effects can be neglected.

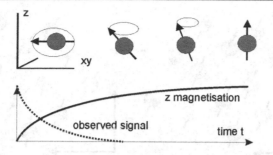

Fig. 2.21 Free induction decay experiment: spins of excited hydrogen atoms are projected into the xy-plane orthogonal to the B_0 magnetic field. After switching of the RF signal, the original z-magnetization is restored with time constant T_1. The observed signal decreases much faster since spins start to dephase

This can be measured by an antenna (which could be the sender of the HF field acting as receiver). The observed decreasing signal is called *free induction decay* (*FID*). Its amplitude depends on several factors.

- The amplitude is proportional to the number of spins. Hence, amplitude per unit volume is proportional to the *proton density*.
- Spins returning to their rest direction will deliver a signal of decreasing magnitude, which will cause the FID signal decay with time. The restoration of the original spin direction is called *longitudinal relaxation*. Magnetization $M_z(t)$ in the z-direction (the direction of the B_0-field) at time t is

$$M_z(t) = M_0\big(1 - c \cdot \exp(-t/T_1)\big), \qquad (2.11)$$

with M_0 being the magnetization in M_0 before excitation. The time constant of the exponential relaxation is called T_1-*time*, *spin-lattice-relaxation time*, or *longitudinal relaxation time*.

- Spinning protons act as magnets and influence the behavior of adjacent protons. The precession of spins will dephase with time and the observable FID signal will vanish long before the original magnetization in the z-direction is restored since the antenna measures a vector sum of all spins (see Fig. 2.22). The signal decay is exponential as well, and is described by a constant that is called T_2-*time*, *spin-spin-relaxation time*, or *transverse relaxation time*. If $M_T(t)$ is the transverse magnetization perpendicular to z at time t, then

$$M_1(t) = M_T(0) \cdot \exp(-t/T_2). \qquad (2.12)$$

T_1 and T_2 constants for the same proton differ depending on the proton's molecular binding. Protons in water have a larger T_1 than in soft tissue, while T_2 is smaller in soft tissue. T_1 and T_2 in water are in the range of seconds.

Additionally to the tissue-specific attributes, an unwanted effect causes a much faster signal decay than T_2 relaxation. Signal generation is made under the assumption that the static B_0 field is constant everywhere in the imaged region. Even small

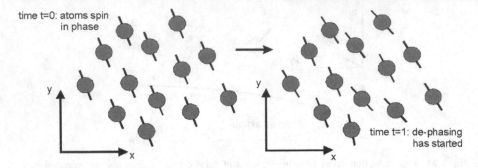

Fig. 2.22 Immediately after the RF signal is switched off, all spins are in phase giving the maximum signal. Locally different magnetization from neighboring atoms causes dephasing as does inhomogeneity of the B_0 field. The observed net magnetization decreases, since its magnitude is the magnitude of the vector sum of all protons in a voxel

field variations cause a much quicker dephasing of spins than dephasing by spin–spin relaxation. Signal decay due to an inhomogeneous magnetic field is exponential with a constant T_2^*. The T_2^* effect is unwanted, as it interrogates the homogeneity of the magnetic field, but not the chemical composition of the probe to be imaged.

The resonance signal allows analyzing the chemical composition of a probe in MR spectroscopy. Instead of exciting just hydrogen, the occurrence and density of other atoms with an odd number of protons or neutrons may be measured by applying a frequency band encompassing all the frequencies necessary to excite the respective atoms. Frequency analysis and the measurement of decay times enables the separation of the signal in constituents caused by the different materials. For imaging, however, additional measures need to be taken to localize the MR signal.

2.2.2 MR Imaging

Extending the MR technique for creating an image is due to the work of Mansfield and Lauterbur. The dependency of the excitability of a proton on the frequency of the HF field is used for the necessary localization. It requires additional *gradient magnetic fields* (called x-, y-, or z-gradient according to the direction of increasing field strength).

If, before applying the HF field, a linear gradient field in the z-direction is overlaid to the B_0-field, the magnetic field strength will linearly increase in the direction of z. Protons will spin with a frequency that depends on their location in z. If an HF field is applied whose frequency range corresponds to the spin frequencies of protons in a slice with $z_1 < z < z_2$, only those protons will be excited and produce a resonance signal (see Fig. 2.23). The process is called *slice selection*. After excitation, the z-gradient is switched off and protons in the selected slice spin with a frequency as determined by the B_0-field.

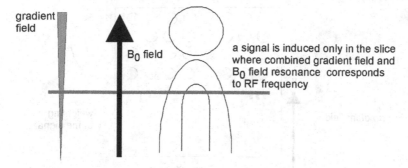

Fig. 2.23 Slice selection is done by selecting an RF band that corresponds to a specific resonance frequency band given by the B_0 field and the slice selection gradient

Fig. 2.24 Frequency encoding of the signal is done by a gradient field in the xy-plane. It causes spins to rotate with different frequencies at readout time, so that atoms can be associated to lines orthogonal to the gradient field

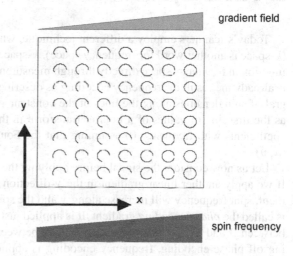

To localize protons within a slice, a similar technique is applied while reading the signal. If a linear gradient field in the x-direction is applied during the observation of the resonance signal, the recorded signal will contain a range of frequencies (see Fig. 2.24). The process is called *frequency encoding*. The gradient is called *readout gradient*. Frequencies w_0 to w_{max} correspond to x-values x_0 to x_{max}. The resonance signal is then transformed into frequency space. The amplitude value at frequency $w_0 + (w_{max} - w_0) \cdot (x_k - x_0)/(x_{max} - x_0)$ corresponds to the response of all protons on the line $x = x_k$.

The technique produces a projection of spin densities along y onto the x-axis. A complete set of projections can be obtained by adding projections at measurements with gradient fields along different directions. Having obtained the data, an image could be reconstructed by filtered backprojection. This was the first technique for reconstructing MR images.

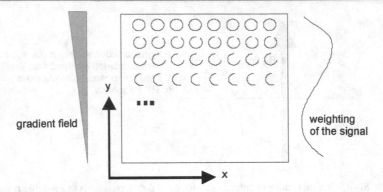

Fig. 2.25 The gradient field for each phase encoding causes a controlled dephasing which acts as a weighting of the observed signal with a cosine function. Phase encoding is done before readout and the phase encoding gradient is switched off before readout

Today's scanners employ a different technique, which is called k-space imaging (k-space is another word for frequency space). k-space imaging generates the image function in frequency space directly through measurements. The first line in k-space is already the result of frequency encoding as described above. It produces the integral of spin densities along the lines of the constant y-value and can be interpreted as the first line of values of a Fourier transform in the u-direction (containing the coefficients with frequency 0) assuming that the Fourier transform maps (x, y) to (u, v).

Let us now consider the signal before applying the frequency encoding gradient. If we apply another linear gradient in the y-direction prior to making the measurement, spin frequency will increase along y and the spins will dephase. The gradient is called the *phase encoding* gradient. It is applied just long enough to dephase spins between 0 and 2π for the range of y-values between y_0 and y_{max}. After switching off phase encoding, frequency encoding is applied and the obtained signal is transformed into frequency space. The results are integrated spin densities along x weighted with a cosine wave of frequency 1 for each line of constant y. In other words, we have produced the real-valued part of the next line in k-space of the Fourier transform in the u-direction (see Fig. 2.25). The imaginary part is computed by weighting the signal with the corresponding sine wave.

The measurement is repeated with phase encoding for the remaining lines in k-space. Once the k-space is filled, the image is generated by transforming it back into the spatial domain.

The image equipment looks similar to CT (see Fig. 2.26). However, the gantry in which the B_0-field is produced is usually smaller than a CT gantry. Image planes need not to be perpendicular to the direction of the B_0-field since the gradients may be generated in arbitrary directions. It is a major difference compared to CT imaging. Also, a variety of different images may be produced of the same patient showing different aspects of the resonance signal. Three different parameters—spin density ρ, spin-lattice relaxation T_1, and spin–spin relaxation T_2—determine the

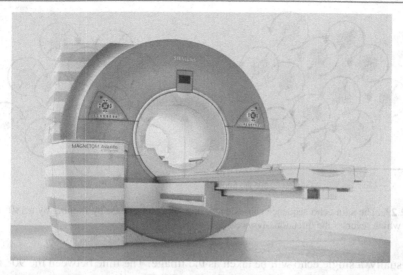

Fig. 2.26 Gantry of an MR imaging device (Magnetom Avanto, with kind permission from Siemens Sector Healthcare, Erlangen, Germany). Images can be produced at arbitrary angles with respect to the gantry by producing appropriate slice selection gradients

resonance signal. Hence, different sequences can be developed for enhancing either of the parameters (some of the major sequences used in MR imaging will be discussed in the next section; a more detailed treatment can be found in Liang and Lauterbur 2000). It changes the appearance of different tissues in images (e.g., water and fat is bright in T_2 images and tissue is darker while the opposite is true for a T_1 image). A normalized scale such as the Hounsfield units of CT does not exist.

2.2.3 Some MR Sequences

T_1 and T_2 time constants cannot be measured directly because signal strength is always influenced by proton density and because field inhomogeneities (the T_2^* decay) hide the T_2 effect. T_2-enhanced images can be generated by the *spin echo* sequence. The sequence uses a clever mechanism to cancel out T_2^* effects. It consists of a 90° impulse that tilts spins into the xy-plane followed by a sequence of 180° impulses producing spin echoes.

After application of the 90° impulse spins start to dephase due to the combined influence of spin–spin relaxation and field inhomogeneities. Spin–spin relaxation continues after application of the 180° impulse since relative spin orientation although turned by 180° remains the same. T_2^* influence is inverted, however, because higher frequency spins, which had a positive phase difference, now have a negative phase difference with respect to spins with lower frequency. Spins will rephase with respect to field inhomogeneities and produce the first echo of T_2-relaxation (see Fig. 2.27). They dephase again until the next 180° impulse causes the next echo. The envelope containing the echoes decreases exponentially with T_2.

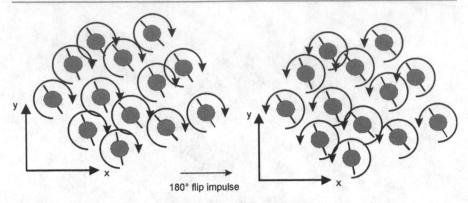

y

x

180° flip impulse

y

x

Fig. 2.27 The spin-echo sequence causes dephasing spins to rephase by flipping by a 180° impulse which reverses the direction of precession

Usually, a single echo will be taken as the image. The time between the 90° impulse and the echo impulse is called *echo time TE*. The time between two measurements is called *repetition time TR*. Short *TE* (20 msec) and long *TR* (2000 msec) will produce a proton-density-weighted image. Using a shorter repetition time (*TR* = 300–600 msec) will produce a T_1-weighted image because T_1 relaxation is generally longer than 200–600 msec. A long *TE* (> 60 msec) and a long *TR* (2000 msec) produces a T_2-weighted image.

The *inversion recovery* sequence is another sequence used in MRI. It produces an image that is strongly influenced by the T_1 time constant. In inversion recovery a 180° impulse is followed by a 90° impulse. The time between the two impulses is called *TI* or *inversion time*. The 180° impulse leads to saturation (i.e., a new impulse would not produce a signal). However, after time *TI* protons have recovered their longitudinal magnetization to an extent that depends on their individual T_1 time. Hence, they are able to produce a resonance signal from the 90° impulse. An echo at echo time *TE* rephases spins that are then read out. Long inversion times (*TI* > 2000 msec) and short echo times (*TE* = 10 msec) produce a proton-density-weighted image. Shorter inversion times (400–800 msec) with the same echo time produce a T_1-weighted image, while choosing a long echo time (*TE* > 60 msec) will produce an image that is T_2-weighted.

MR images of the head created by imagining sequences like the ones above usually have a slice thickness of 1 to 3 mm and 256 × 256 voxels in a slice. Body MR images usually have 512 × 512 voxels per slice. Data acquisition times using either of the sequences are longer compared to CT imaging. For reconstructing an image of size 256 × 256 pixels, 256 lines in *k*-space need to be measured. This requires 256 different measurements. A new measurement is only possible after the effects from the previous measurement have decayed. With T_1-time constants in the range of a second, it results in repetition times in the range of several seconds. It leads to data acquisition times for the image in the range of 10–15 minutes. If the image size doubles, the acquisition time doubles as well. If measurements are repeated to increase the signal-to-noise ratio or if more than one measurement is desired, ac-

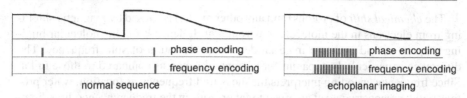

Fig. 2.28 The main difference between normal encoding and a fast imaging sequence is that in fast imaging several to all encodings are done during a single excitation of the resonance signal

quisition times for a full study may easily reach 30–60 minutes. The acquisition of a sequence of slices, however, does not necessarily take much longer. Since slice selection only influences protons of a given slice, signals from several slices may be acquired in an interleaved mode.

In the early 1980s, acquisition times have been a serious drawback. Since the 1990s, a wealth of fast imaging sequences have been developed. *Gradient echo imaging* was one of the first techniques to speed up imaging time. In gradient echo imaging an excitation pulse of α (with $\alpha \leq 90°$) is given. However, instead of using the 180° impulse to produce a rephased spin echo, an inverse gradient is applied to cause the echo. Echo times between applying the second gradient and readout are much faster than echo times of the spin echo sequence. Pulses with α close to 90° produce a T_1-weighted image. Low angle pulses result in a T_2^*-weighted image. The image is not T_2-weighted because, as opposed to spin echo imaging, the gradient echo reverses dephasing from inhomogeneities and spin-spin relaxation in the same way.

Turbo spin echo sequences make several measurements at a time. This is done by applying a sequence of several phase shift gradients during a single echo and reading the signal after each phase shift (see Fig. 2.28). Several lines of k-space are filled at the same time and image acquisition time decreases by a factor of the number of lines acquired per repetition. In its extreme, all lines are acquired from a single excitation (RARE—Rapid Enhancement with Relaxation Enhancement) so that an image can be acquired within time *TE*. RARE is a variant of an older sequence known as Echoplanar Imaging (EPI), a term which simply refers to acquiring the complete k-space in a single resonance experiment.

2.2.4 Artefacts in MR Imaging

Ultrafast sequences such as EPI produce images in less than 100 msec. There are problems, however. While making the measurements from a single echo, T_2^* dephasing continues to occur. Different lines in k-space are measured with a different contrast with respect to T_2^* decay. Moreover, the number of lines to be measured in k-space is usually restricted to 128 or less so that the spatial resolution of a single shot image does not exceed 128 × 128 pixels. Furthermore, artefacts from chemical shift, ghosting, and shading may be particularly pronounced for fast imaging sequences.

The *chemical shift* of protons (and any other nuclei) is caused by magnetic shielding from electrons in the molecular environment. It depends on the molecular binding of protons and causes a material-dependent deviation of spin frequency. The difference is particularly apparent for protons in water, as compared to those in fat. Since frequency encoding interprets the measured frequency as location, water protons will be reconstructed at an offset to fat protons in the frequency encoding direction. Chemical shift is present in all nonshift-corrected images, but is pronounced in EPI (RARE) images where the offset may amount to 8–10 pixels. At 3-mm voxel size this is an offset of about 2.5 cm.

Ghosting appears because of the inaccuracies in the phase encoding. If one or more lines in k-space are phase shifted, the corresponding waves in the spatial domain are shifted as well. Ghost images appear in this direction. Ghosting may also happen in regular imaging if the patient has moved in the phase encoding direction between acquisitions. Motion in the direction of frequency encoding causes the much less prominent blurring artefact similar to this kind of artefact in CT.

Shading is due to the variation of attenuation of the RF signal and an inhomogeneous magnetic field. It causes differences in the resonance signal according to location. It is then turned into different intensities to be reconstructed for the same material at different locations.

Artefacts from noise and PVE are similar to CT imaging. Metal artefacts from paramagnetic materials cause signal deletion. The presence of ferromagnetic materials such as implants is a contraindication for MR imaging as is the presence of implanted electronic devices such as a pacemaker.

2.2.5 MR Angiography

MR angiography (MRA) exists with and without using contrast agents. Contrast-enhanced angiography uses *gadolinium*, an agent that causes a strong decrease of the T_1 relaxation time. Gadolinium-enhanced vessels can be imaged with a T_1-weighted sequence that saturates all other tissues while highlighting the vessels. The resulting contrast is so high that the images look similar to DSA images, but without the necessity of subtracting a null image (see Fig. 2.29a). Vessels may be depicted even if they are smaller than a voxel because of the partial volume effect.

MRA images come as a true 3D volume, but they are often displayed as *maximum intensity projection* images (MIP). This visualization technique projects the brightest voxel along the projection line on a pixel on the output screen. MIP is simple, fast, and produces images similar to digital subtraction angiograms.

MR angiography without the use of a contrast agent exploits two different effects, which are called *flow void* and *phase contrast angiography* (Dumoulin 1995). A flow void occurs when a proton that has been excited by an HF impulse has moved out of the slice before the readout impulse is applied.

Phase contrast angiography uses the motion artefact of moving blood for imaging. If a proton moves in the direction of the phase encoding gradient, it carries its phase with it (see Fig. 2.30). Two different phase encoding gradients are applied at

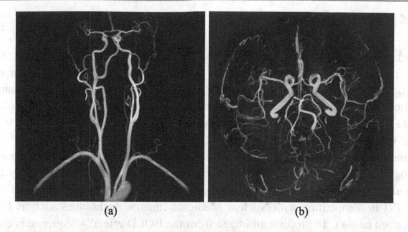

(a)   (b)

Fig. 2.29 Maximum intensity projections of gadolinium-enhanced MRA (*left*) and phase-contrast MRA (*right*). While using gadolinium contrast agent produces images with better resolution, phase contrast imaging is non-invasive and has the potential for computing vessel velocities (images from Siemens Sector Healthcare with permission)

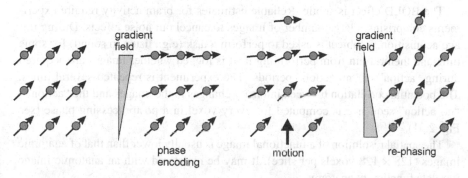

gradient
field

gradient
field

phase
encoding

motion

re-phasing

Fig. 2.30 Principle of phase-contrast imaging: protons are phase-encoded by applying a gradient field. Motion in phase encoding direction leads to dephasing. If a rephasing gradient is applied, dislocated protons cause a signal loss since they are not completely rephased. The amount of signal loss depends on the motion in phase encoding direction

times t_1 and t_2. The second gradient is exactly opposite to the first gradient. The effects of the gradients on protons that have not moved between t_1 and t_2 will cancel. Protons that moved along the gradient direction will acquire a phase shift relative to static protons, which is proportional to the distance traveled between t_1 and t_2 (i.e., proportional to their speed). A 3D velocity vector for moving protons can be created by applying phase encoding in the x-, y-, and z-directions. Velocity indicates the existence of a vessel (see Fig. 2.29b). Suggestions have been made that phase contrast angiography may even enable the analysis of velocity differences in blood vessels (e.g., at a stenosis or in an aneurysm).

2.2.6 BOLD Imaging

Blood supplying the brain carries oxygen via hemoglobin. Oxygenated hemoglobin is diamagnetic such as all the other tissues but deoxygenated hemoglobin is paramagnetic causing a small, local distortion of the magnetic field. The distortions change the measurable signal that can be made visible. The technique is called *Blood Oxygen Level Dependency* (*BOLD*) imaging (see Huettel et al. 2004 for a detailed look and Forster et al. 1998 for a short tutorial).

Since brain activity is associated with the energy supply through oxygenated hemoglobin, BOLD imaging may be used to image brain activity. The ability for measuring functional activity truly differentiates MRI from CT imaging and has put MRI in competition with Nuclear Medicine Imaging techniques such as PET (described below). To produce an image from the BOLD effect, a sequence is chosen that is sensitive to local field inhomogeneities caused by the presence of deoxygenated hemoglobin. The gradient echo imaging with low angles presented in Sect. 2.2.3 is particularly sensitive to inhomogeneities and is often used in *functional MRI* (*fMRI*). It can be carried out using an EPI sequence by which an image is acquired with a single shot. Spin echo EPI can be used as well.

The BOLD effect is subtle. Reliable estimates for brain activity require experiments comprising a large number of images to cancel out noise effects. During image acquisition, a subject is asked to perform a task (e.g., listen to sound) for some time and then refrain from performing it. It is logged whether images are acquired during "action" or "no action" periods. The experiment is repeated several times. The potential correlation between intensity changes in the images and the "action"–"no action" sequence is computed for every voxel in a postprocessing phase (see Fig. 2.31).

The spatial resolution of a functional image is usually lower than that of anatomic images (128×128 voxels per slice). It may be registered with an anatomic image to relate function to anatomy.

Creating an fMRI image study is not easy. Severe distortions due to recording T_2^* images for fMRI need to be corrected properly. Motion artefacts during the study may bias the correlation of the task. Noise further reduces contrast and the resolution of the fMRI images.

Several software packages exist to register anatomic and functional images, to carry out signal analysis, and to enable intersubject studies. The most popular software, SPM, carries out statistic parametric mapping (as presented by Friston et al. (1995), webpage http://www.fil.ion.ucl.ac.uk/spm/). Other commercial as well as noncommercial alternatives exist [e.g., BrainVoyager (Goebel et al. 1998), www.brainvoyager.com, FreeSurfer (Fischl et al. 1999), surfer.nmr.mgh.harvard.edu/]. Despite the complexity of processing the functional data, fMRI is popular and currently the only technique to measure cortical activity at a spatial resolution under 3 mm. Newer scanners such as a 7T scanner, now commercially available, carry the promise of pushing the achievable resolution even further.

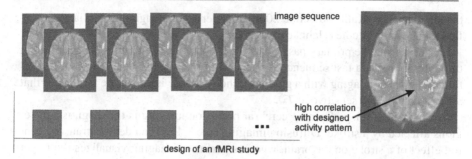

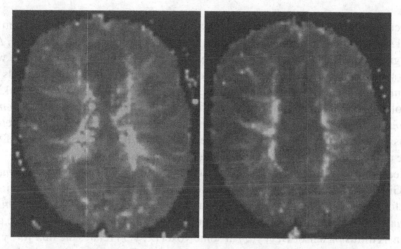

Fig. 2.31 A simple fMRI sequence consists of a sequence of images taking during a time in which a task is either on or off. Locations of which intensity changes correlate with the task design are then emphasized

Fig. 2.32 Perfusion images are not interpreted as raw images. Diagnostically relevant measures such as the regional blood volume, regional blood flow and mean transit time are computed and visualized. The two images here show the mean transit time of two slices of the brain of a normal volunteer

2.2.7   Perfusion Imaging

Gadolinium may be used to measure *perfusion* in MRI. Gadolinium not only reduces the T_1 time, but also shortens the T_2 time (and with this the T_2^* time). The change in T_2^* is related to the amount of gadolinium. Since this is related to the amount of blood passing through the volume of tissue, gadolinium-caused T_2^* contrast predicts blood perfusion.

The main application of perfusion imaging is the depiction of parameters such as the *relative cerebral blood volume* (rCBV), relative cerebral blood flow (rCBF), and the mean transit time (MTT) in the brain (Gillard et al. 2004) (an example for the display of MTT is depicted in Fig. 2.32), perfusion imaging for tumor analysis in the female breast (Kuhl and Schild 2000), and perfusion imaging in cardiac imaging for rest and stress studies (Jahnke et al. 2007).

For observing the primary passage of the blood bolus containing the gadolinium through the tissue, a fast sequence is needed to produce sufficient temporal resolution. Echoplanar imaging with a gradient echo sequence is one of the sequences that are fast enough and sensitive to T_2^*.

An indication for performing cerebral perfusion imaging is the diagnosis of regions affected by a stroke. Diffusion imaging (see below) can demonstrate the central effect of a stroke on the brain, whereas perfusion imaging visualizes the larger "second ring" delineating blood flow and blood volume.

2.2.8   Diffusion Imaging

Molecules in a medium are in constant motion and will stray further away from an initial start location with time. The motion is neither directed nor deterministic. After a given time it can only be said that—with certain likelihood—a molecule will be in some sphere around its initial position. The radius of the sphere depends on the time passed and on a diffusion coefficient. The latter is characteristic of the kind of molecule and the medium in which diffusion takes place. This is called *homogeneous, isotropic diffusion* and requires molecules to be able to move unhindered. Diffusion will be lower if blocked by a cell boundary. It will be anisotropic if the shape of the cell restricts diffusion in some directions more than in others.

Measuring the diffusion coefficient of isotropic diffusion is called *diffusion imaging* (Gillard et al. 2004). A change of the value of the diffusion coefficient may indicate, for instance, the breakdown of cells in the brain after a stroke. *Diffusion tensor imaging* (DTI) relates to the measurement of a tensor that describes anisotropic diffusion. A diffusion tensor $\mathbf{D}(x, y, z)$ at some voxel (x, y, z) relates the flux $\mathbf{j}(x, y, z)$ to the gradient $\mathbf{D}$ of concentration $u(x, y)$ of some diffusing quantity u in the following way:

$$\mathbf{j}(x, y, z) = -\mathbf{D}(x, y, z) \times \nabla u(x, y, z). \tag{2.13}$$

The interesting part is the tensor itself. An eigenvector decomposition of $\mathbf{D}$ will produce an orthogonal system of diffusion directions together with the variance of diffusion (the eigenvalues) in each of the directions. Elongated cells such as a nerve fiber (an axiom) should produce maximal diffusion in one of these directions. This is the direction of the fibers. Diffusion in the other two directions should be much lower (see Fig. 2.33). The knowledge of the local fiber direction is used for *fiber tracking* in the brain (Mori and van Zijl 2002), which—together with fMRI—may be used to infer the configuration of the regions of brain function (see Fig. 2.34). If two adjacent voxels belong to the same fiber bundle, they should exhibit linear diffusion and their main diffusion directions should be similar.

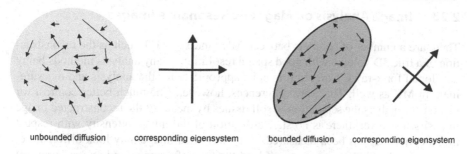

unbounded diffusion   corresponding eigensystem   bounded diffusion   corresponding eigensystem

Fig. 2.33 The diffusion tensor of unbounded diffusion will have equal eigenvalues. If diffusion is bounded, eigenvalues will be lower and if the bounds are anisotropic, at least one eigenvalue will be lower than the others. Furthermore, the first eigenvector will point in the direction in which the bounded volume has its maximal extent

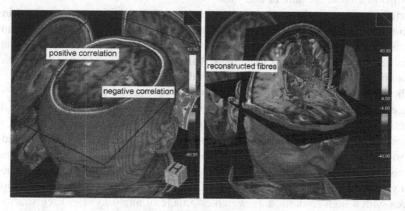

Fig. 2.34 Reconstructed fibers from diffusion MRI depicted on the right can be used with fMRI (depicted *on the left*) to infer configurations of functional regions in the brain (images from Magnetom Verio, with kind permission of Siemens Sector Healthcare, Erlangen, Germany)

Diffusion imaging by magnetic resonance employs a variant of a spin echo sequence. The purpose of the spin echo sequence is to cancel out the effects of magnetic field inhomogeneities given that the protons being imaged are static. Diffusion causes a slight loss of signal that cannot be recovered by the echo because diffusing protons move (as in phase contrast imaging). A diffusion sequence measuring isotropic diffusion emphasizes this signal loss. The amount of diffusion enhancement depends on the strength and duration of the gradient impulses and on the time between the two impulses. The diffusion coefficient can be computed if these are known.

In the case of anisotropic diffusion, the response on the gradient impulse depends on the directions of the gradient field. Elements of the diffusion tensor are computed separately by applying a sequence of different gradient excitations.

2.2.9   Image Analysis on Magnetic Resonance Images

There are a number of parallels between MRI and x-ray CT such as the reconstruction of a true 3D volume with good spatial resolution. Many analysis methods being developed for x-ray CT are, in principle, appropriate for the analysis and measurement in MR as well. There are differences, however. The much better contrast for soft tissue enables the separation of soft tissues by means of the reconstructed image intensity. However, there is no standardization of the image intensity with respect to the entity that has been measured. A T_2-weighted image may look different depending on the kind of sequence used, on the type of scanner, and on measurement parameters such as repetition time or echo time; and it certainly differs from the appearance of a T_1-weighted image. Computer-assisted analysis tools must take this into account either by incorporating scanning parameters into the method (which is seldom done), or by training the appearance from sample images, or by requesting user information at the time of analysis.

Artefacts from shading in a study with known acquisition parameters hinder defining a mapping between tissue type and image brightness within this study. The automatic separation of gray matter and white matter in the brain, for instance, which have excellent contrast in some MR images, may need to deal with the different absolute brightness of the two materials at different locations.

The wealth of different properties that can be imaged through magnetic resonance also increased interest in registration algorithms (discussed in Chap. 10). Sometimes, images showing different properties are already registered (e.g., if two echoes of a spin echo sequence are reconstructed). The first echo is dominated by proton density and the second is T_2-weighted. Clustering and classification in multidimensional feature space may, in such a case, provide further information about the entities being imaged. If registration is required (e.g., when combining functional images with a high resolution T_1-weighted image of anatomy) rigid registration is usually insufficient. Registration has to account for deformation due to the different effects of T_2^* susceptibility in different imaging sequences.

Noise in MR imaging can be a problem if an analysis tool requires the mapping of a tissue type to a small range of brightness values such as in direct volume rendering visualization or in threshold segmentation. Noise removal through the usual set of filters (to be discussed later in Chap. 4) helps, of course. It should be kept in mind, however, that most noise removal techniques operate under the hypothesis that the true image value is locally constant. Local homogeneity is not given if the size of image details reaches the limits of spatial resolution. The accidental removal of such details by noise reduction is critical in MRI since the detection of small objects is often an objective of applying MRI because of its good soft tissue contrast.

2.3   Ultrasound

Sound waves will be reflected at the boundaries between materials of different acoustic impedance. An ultrasound wave sent into the human body will be reflected at organ boundaries. The locus of reflection can be reconstructed if the speed of

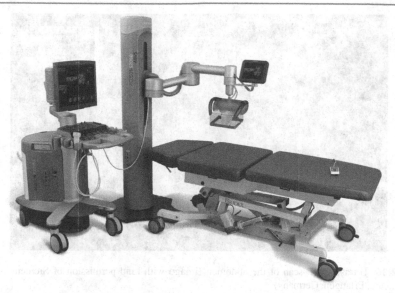

Fig. 2.35 Ultrasound equipment (Siemens Acuson, with kind permission of Siemens Sector Healthcare, Erlangen, Germany)

sound in the material through which the wave travels is known (Szabo 2004). For most soft tissues this speed is around 1500 m/sec.

An ultrasound reflection signal is created using a transducer which acts as the sender and receiver of ultrasound waves (Fig. 2.35 shows typical ultrasound equipment). Frequencies for diagnostic ultrasound range between 1 and 20 MHz. High frequency waves attenuate faster than low frequency waves and do not penetrate the body as good as low frequency waves. High frequency waves resolve smaller structures, however, since the size of a reflecting object has to be larger than the wavelength.

2.3.1 Ultrasound Imaging

An ultrasound *A-scan* sends a single wave with known direction into the body and records the amplitude of reflections as a function of travel time between sending and receiving the signal. It is a one-dimensional probe into the body showing tissue boundaries and other boundaries between regions with different acoustic impedance. *Ultrasound (US) images* (the so-called *B-scans*, see Fig. 2.36) are created from a planar fan beam of differently rotated A-scans. Amplitudes are mapped to gray values for creating the image. They may also be acquired as 3D images with this fan beam rotating around a second axis perpendicular to the first axis of rotation.

Ultrasound imaging (also called *sonography*) happens in real time and is able to show the motion of the organs being imaged. Ultrasound imaging of internal organs is only possible if they are not hidden by bone since bone causes the total reflection

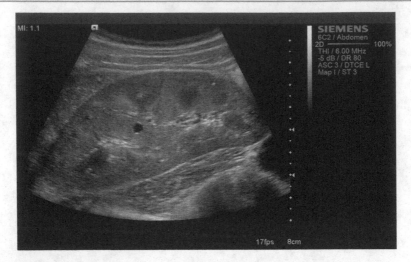

Fig. 2.36 Ultrasound B-scan of the abdomen (image with kind permission of Siemens Sector Healthcare, Erlangen, Germany)

of the incident sound waves. The organs to be imaged include the liver, gallbladder, pancreas, kidneys, spleen, heart, and uterus. Heart imaging may also be carried out by putting the ultrasound device (a transducer sending and receiving sound waves) into the esophagus.

Doppler imaging is a specific technique using the Doppler effect for estimating the speed and direction of moving objects (such as blood) in the ultrasound image (see Fig. 2.37). It is used for diagnosing the effects of vessel blockages or changes of blood flow due to stenosis.

A number of effects cause artefacts in an ultrasound image (see Fig. 2.38).

- Sound waves are attenuated just as electromagnetic waves in x-ray imaging.
- Absorption turns wave energy into heat.
- The wave may be scattered or refracted.
- Interference and a diverging wave cause further deterioration.

Absorption causes a decrease in amplitude with increasing depth. The decrease is exponential with an unknown absorption coefficient of the tissue. It is usually corrected by assuming constant absorption throughout the tissue.

Interference, scatter, and refraction of and between waves lead to the typical speckle artefacts in ultrasound images. It is a nonlinear, tissue-dependent distortion of the signal.

Tissues and tissue boundaries that reflect or attenuate a high amount of the incoming sound energy produce an acoustic shadow behind the tissue. Materials that attenuate little of the incident energy lead to signal enhancement in tissues behind this material. This is, for instance, the case when imaged organs are behind a fluid-filled organ such as a filled bladder. The smaller absorption in the fluid contradicts the hypothetically assumed constant absorption and causes a higher than necessary absorption correction.

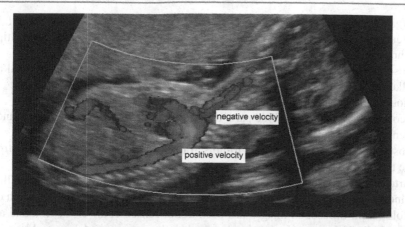

Fig. 2.37 Doppler sonography uses the Doppler effect to depict blood velocity. In its original, velocity is color-coded differentiation between flow direction and velocity (image with kind permission of Siemens Sector Healthcare, Erlangen, Germany)

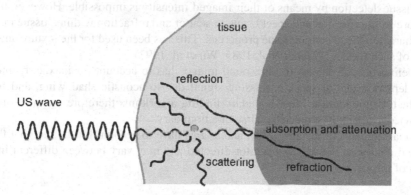

Fig. 2.38 Different effects influence the incident US wave of which only direct reflection is the wanted effect

2.3.2 Image Analysis on Ultrasound Images

Ultrasound is noninvasive and inexpensive. Hence, it is widely used as a diagnostic tool. The artefacts mentioned in the previous section as well as the approximate nature of many of the underlying assumptions for imaging may adversely influence measurements in quantitative analysis.

- Localization in ultrasound imaging assumes that the speed of sound in the material is known. It is usually taken as a constant value of the average speed of sound in soft tissue and causes signal displacement depending on the deviation from this average.
- Refraction that has not been accounted for may lead to a further displacement error.

- Organ boundaries may cause mirror echoes or multiple echoes that appear as false boundaries in the image. Mirror echoes appear behind the true boundary. Multiple echoes appear between the transducer and boundary.
- False, hyperbola-shaped boundaries may be caused by low frequency lateral oscillation of the sound wave.
- Motion artefacts lead to wave-like distortions of boundaries.
- Acoustic shadowing may hide parts of tissues and fluid-induced signal enhancement may lead to a position-dependent signal increase.
- Absorption decreases the signal-to-noise-ratio with respect to the distance from the transducer.

Artefact removal through postprocessing is only partially successful since their nonlinearity and nonstationarity defy common restoration techniques (although deconvolution in ultrasound images has been done; Jensen et al. 1993; Hokland and Kelly 1996). Using standard noise removal techniques to reduce speckle noise would seriously affect the image content since speckle is neither of high frequency nor stationary. Hence, image analysis often proceeds using the unaltered image and analysis methods have to account for this.

Tissue detection by means of their imaged intensity is impossible. However, the texture from reflection and speckle due to scatter and refraction within a tissue may be characteristic to certain tissue properties. This has been used for the texture analysis of such tissues (Wagner et al. 1985; Wu et al. 1992).

Delineation of objects in ultrasound images has to account for inexact boundary depiction due to speckle, missing signal due to acoustic shadowing, and for artefactual boundaries. Most boundary-finding algorithms therefore include some knowledge about the expected course of a boundary.

Measurements of distance, size, and angles have to account for the fact that the slice direction of the scan is operator-directed and may vary between different images of the same patient.

2.4   Nuclear Imaging

Nuclear imaging measures the distribution of a radioactive tracer material and produces images of a function in the human body. The tracer material is injected intravenously prior to the image acquisition and will distribute through blood circulation. Distribution is indicative to the perfusion of organs in the body. Examples for applications are measurements of brain activity, perfusion studies of the heart, diagnosis of inflammations due to arthritis and rheumatism, or the detection of tumor metastases due to increased blood circulation.

Images are created from measuring photons sent by the tracer material through the body. Spatial resolution in nuclear imaging is lower than for the procedures described above since tracer concentration is very low so as to not to interfere with the metabolism. The sensitivity of imaging techniques in nuclear medicine is high since detectors are able to measure a signal from a few photons. Major imaging techniques in nuclear medicine are as follows.

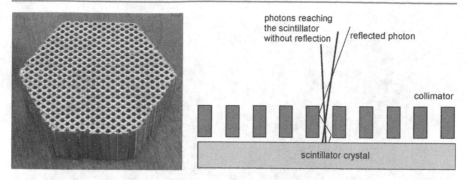

Fig. 2.39 Photons reaching the scintillator are those on (approximately) parallel rays

- *Scintigraphy*, which measures a projection of the tracer distribution with a geometry similar to projection x-ray imaging.
- *SPECT (Single Photon Emission Computed Tomography)*, which is a reconstruction from projections of tracer material producing a 3D material distribution.
- *PET (Positron Emission Tomography)*, which is a tomographic technique as well, but uses a different tracer material that produces positrons. Radiation of positron-electron annihilation is measured and reconstructed.

2.4.1 Scintigraphy

For creating a scintigram, a molecule carrying the radioactive atom 99^{Tc} (Technetium-99) is applied. Photons emitted by tracer radiation are measured by a *gamma camera* (also written as *γ-camera* and sometimes called *Anger camera*; see Mettler and Guiberteau 2005). The camera consists of a collimator that restricts measurements of photons to those who hit the detector approximately at a 90° angle, a *scintillator crystal* that turns incident radiation into visible light, and *photomultipliers* for amplifying the signal.

The camera is usually mounted on a gantry that enables the camera to rotate (around various directions) around the patient. The *collimator* is a thick lead plate with drilled cylindrical holes whose axes are perpendicular to the scintillator crystal. Photons reaching the detector on a path perpendicular to the detector plane will reach the scintillator at a location that is given by the positioning of the detector hole through which it passes. Photons on a path with any other angle are reflected or attenuated by the lead collimator. If they reach the detector crystal through scattering, they have lost too much energy for being detected. Hence, the collimator causes the image to be an approximate parallel projection of photons from tracer material in the body onto the image (see Fig. 2.39).

The scintigram acquired by the gamma camera is a projection of activity weighted by the attenuation that photons experience on their path between emission and detection (see Fig. 2.40 for an example). Photons are attenuated by absorption and scatter. Absorption reduces the signal while scatter reduces contrast and increases noise.

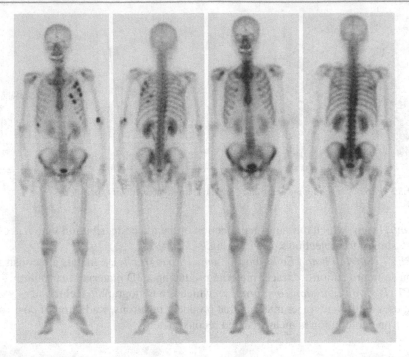

Fig. 2.40 Bone scintigraphy (in this case before and after-treatment bone scintigraphy from Mado et al. 2006, published under Creative Commons license)

Collimator characteristics limit spatial resolution and contrast of the scintigram (see Fig. 2.41). Photons reaching the detector do not exactly follow a path perpendicular to the detector plane. They originate from a cone-shaped volume whose size is determined by the diameter and the length of the cylindrical apertures in the collimator. Reducing the diameter and increasing the length will increase the spatial resolution, but it will also decrease the number of photons that reach the scintillator crystal, hence reducing the signal.

2.4.2 Reconstruction Techniques for Tomography in Nuclear Imaging

Slice computation from multiple views of the gamma camera is done by applying tomographic reconstruction techniques. A sequence of images is acquired while the gamma camera rotates around the patient. If the axis, around which the camera rotates, is taken as the y-axis of a device coordinate system, a slice may be reconstructed from lines with a constant x-value of all projection images made by the camera.

Slice reconstruction of nuclear images from projections for SPECT and PET is similar to reconstruction from x-ray projection but with an important difference, which makes the FBP technique of x-ray CT less suitable for slice reconstruction

Fig. 2.41 The geometry of the collimator limits the spatial resolution of the scinitgram. Resolution decreases with distance to the gamma camera

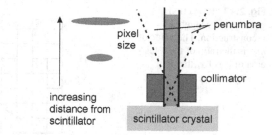

Fig. 2.42 Attenuation that depends on the attenuation coefficients along the path between emission site and detector causes different activity levels to be measured of from the same site if the detection position is different

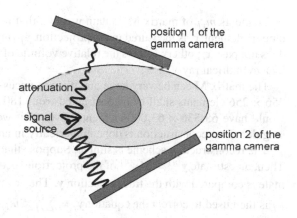

although it is commonly used in commercial software. The aim of reconstruction is to depict the spatial distribution $\mu(x, y)$ of radioactive tracer material. Reconstruction from projection would require projection of this distribution. The measurement, however, consists of projected, *attenuated* activity. Attenuation depends on the material between the emission site and detector. This violates the assumption of the Radon transform since the contribution of $\mu(x, y)$ to a line integral is dependent on the projection direction (see Fig. 2.42).

If attenuation is neglected, filtered backprojection may be used. However, it may lead to signal degradation, which is unwanted in view of the already low signal. If attenuation were known for each voxel (x, y) in any projection direction (θ, s), it could be accounted for, provided a suitable reconstruction algorithm exists.

Such a technique is given by modeling reconstruction as a problem of estimating unknowns (the unknown densities $\mu(x, y)$) from a number of (linear) equations, which are the different projections. The oldest method based on this model, which originally was also used to reconstruct CT images, is the *algebraic reconstruction technique* (ART; Herman et al. 1978). For reconstructing the image, variables are rearranged so that all unknown densities μ are in a 1D vector $\mathbf{x}$. Projections are arranged in another 1D vector $\mathbf{y}$ (see Fig. 2.43). Now, the reconstruction requires finding an $\mathbf{x}$, for which

$$\mathbf{Mx} = \mathbf{y}. \tag{2.14}$$

Fig. 2.43 Projection
geometry for algebraic
reconstruction. The value of
m_{ij} is the ratio of the total
area of pixel x_i that is
covered by ray y_j

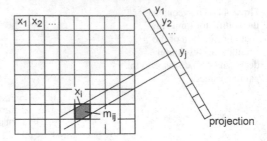

Elements m_{ij} of matrix $\mathbf{M}$ contain weights that represent how much of the volume in element x_i is measured in the projection y_j ($m_{ij} = 0$, if the projection ray y_j does not pass x_i; otherwise it is the relative volume of the voxel x_i, which is covered by a cylindrical ray y_j).

The matrix $\mathbf{M}$ can be very large and it is not necessarily square. If an image with 256×256 elements shall be reconstructed from 180×350 projections, the matrix would have $65{,}536 \times 63{,}000$ elements. Even if it were a square matrix it may be singular. The reconstruction is done numerically in an iterative fashion.

The reconstruction scheme is simple. Suppose that an estimate $\mathbf{x}^{(n)}$ of $\mathbf{x}$ is given. Then, an estimate $\mathbf{y}^{(n)} = \mathbf{M}\mathbf{x}^{(n)}$ of the projection vector can be computed. This estimate is compared with the true projection $\mathbf{y}$. The error $y_j - y_j^{(n)}$ for some projection y_j is then used to correct the equation $y_j = \sum_{j=0}^{N} m_{ij}x_j$ in the following way:

$$x_i^{(n+1)} = x_i^{(n)} + \left(y_j - y_j^{(n)}\right)\frac{m_{ij}}{\sum_{i=0}^{M} m_{ij}}. \tag{2.15}$$

This procedure is repeated for every equation in the system and—since corrections of $\mathbf{x}$ from a later equation will have changed earlier corrections—it will be iterated until the residual error $\|\mathbf{y} - \mathbf{y}^{(n)}\|$ falls below some threshold. The first estimate $\mathbf{x}^{(0)}$ can be simply $\mathbf{x}^{(0)} = \mathbf{0}$ or it may be an estimate from some other reconstruction technique (e.g., FBP).

Algebraic reconstruction takes much longer than FBP and is no longer applied for CT reconstruction. However, it is particularly easy to include effects such as attenuation into the problem. If α_{ij} is the attenuation of photons emitted at x_i and detected at y_j, all that is needed is to weight the m_{ij} (which may be interpreted as the likelihood of an emitted photon at x_i to be detected at y_j) with α_{ij}.

Reconstruction in SPECT and in PET employs this strategy although a different reconstruction strategy is used. Photon detection is treated as a random process with known probability distribution. The method is called *maximum likelihood expectation maximization (MLEM) reconstruction*. For a detailed treatment see Lange and Carson (1984) for an introductory treatment of common reconstruction techniques in nuclear imaging.

To model the problem, we assume that photon emission is a random process and that x_i is the mean number of photons emitted at location i, which is detected at location y_j with probability m_{ij}. It results in the same equation as above, but with a slightly different meaning for **x** and **y**. The number of photons detected at j depends on the probability that it is attenuated on its way, which in turn depends on the density, i.e., the mean number of photons $\bar{y}_j$ along the ray, which is

$$\bar{y}_j = \sum_{i=1}^{M} m_{ij} x_i. \tag{2.16}$$

It can be described by a Poisson process, whereby the probability of detecting y_j photons at j is

$$P(y_j) = \frac{\exp(-\bar{y}_j) \cdot (\bar{y}_j)^{y_j}}{y_j!}. \tag{2.17}$$

The measurements and thus the probabilities are independent. The conditional probability $P(\mathbf{y}|\mathbf{x})$ of observing measurement **y** given the tracer distribution **x** is the product

$$L(\mathbf{x}) = P(\mathbf{y}|\bar{\mathbf{x}}) = \prod_{j=1}^{N} P(y_j) = \prod_{j=1}^{N} \frac{\exp(-\bar{y}_j) \cdot (\bar{y}_j)^{y_j}}{y_j!}. \tag{2.18}$$

The maximum of L is computed by taking the derivative and setting it to zero. To simplify the computation, the derivative is taken on the log-likelihood (maximizing the logarithm l of L also maximizes L)

$$l(\mathbf{x}) = \sum_{j=1}^{N} -\bar{y}_j + y_j \ln(\bar{y}_j) - \ln(y_j!). \tag{2.19}$$

Replacing $\bar{y}_j$ by the right-hand side of (2.16), we get

$$l(\mathbf{x}) = \sum_{j=1}^{N} \left(-\sum_{i=1}^{M} m_{ij} x_i + y_j \ln \left(\sum_{i=1}^{M} m_{ij} x_i \right) - \ln(y_j!) \right). \tag{2.20}$$

Taking the partial derivatives with respect to the x_i (using the chain rule and remembering that the derivative of $\ln x$ is $1/x$), we get

$$\frac{\partial l(\mathbf{x})}{\partial x_i} = -\sum_{i=1}^{M} m_{ij} + \sum_{j=1}^{N} \frac{y_j}{\sum_{i=1}^{M} m_{ij} \bar{x}_i} m_{ij} x_i = 0. \tag{2.21}$$

Multiplying both sides with x_i and resolving for x_i, we receive

$$x_i = -\frac{x_i}{\sum_{i=1}^{M} m_{ij}} \cdot \sum_{j=1}^{N} \frac{y_j}{\sum_{i=1}^{M} m_{ij} \bar{x}_i} m_{ij}, \tag{2.22}$$

which can be turned into the iteration step

$$x_i^{(n+1)} = -\frac{x_i^{(n)}}{\sum_{i=1}^{M} m_{ij}} \cdot \sum_{j=1}^{N} \frac{y_j}{\sum_{i=1}^{M} m_{ij} \bar{x}_i^{(n)}} m_{ij}. \tag{2.23}$$

This is the MLEM algorithm. Again, *attenuation correction* may be added by modifying the likelihoods m_{ij} with the attenuation weight. Other effects such as the loss of resolution with distance to the detector can be included in the weighting as well. Even scatter interaction can be included although this is not possible by simply adopting the weighting since interactions between sites have to be modeled (Shcherbinin et al. 2008).

A variant of the MLEM algorithm is *OSEM* (*ordered subset expectation maximization*), by which the order in which equations are updated is changed (Hudson and Larkin 1994). If projections are taken from 96 angles, projection angles may be ordered in, say, 16 subsets with projections 1, 17, 33, . . . , in the first subset, projections 2, 18, 34, . . . , in the second subset and so on. This reconstruction strategy has been shown to speed up convergence. The factor by which convergence increases is in the order of numbers of subsets.

Image reconstruction with EM increases noise in later iterations because noise characteristics are not accounted for. This means that it can be difficult to decide when to stop the algorithm. *MAP-EM* (*maximum a posteriori expectation maximization*) remedies this by including *a priori* knowledge about desired smoothness in the model. Different versions of MAP-EM exist. They have in common that smoothness is described by making constraints about activity differences in adjacent pixels. An algorithm by Green (1990), which is called the *OSL* (*one-step-late*) algorithm, for computing the MAP-EM estimate is similar to the EM algorithm. The term $\sum_{i=1}^{M} m_{ij}$ in (2.23) is replaced by

$$\sum_{i=1}^{M} m_{ij} + \beta \frac{\partial}{\partial x_i} U\left(\bar{x}_i^{(n)}\right), \tag{2.24}$$

where $\frac{\partial}{\partial x_i} U(\bar{x}_i^{(n)})$ is an energy term enforcing smoothness, e.g.,

$$\frac{\partial}{\partial x_i} U\left(\bar{x}_i^{(n)}\right) = \sum_{k \in Nbs(i)} w_{ik}\left(\bar{x}_i^{(n)} - \bar{x}_k^{(n)}\right), \tag{2.25}$$

and *Nbs*() refers to some neighborhood around a site i. The weighting term w_{ik} balances different types of neighboring pixels (e.g., neighbors at different distances).

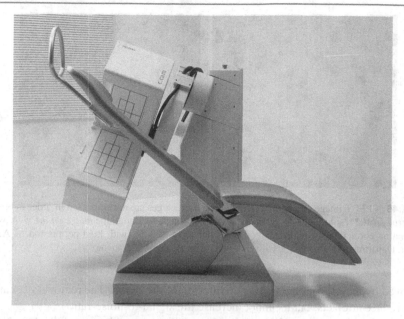

Fig. 2.44 Two-plane SPECT imaging system used in cardiac imaging (with kind permission from Siemens Sector Healthcare, Erlangen, Germany)

2.4.3 Single Photon Emission Computed Tomography (SPECT)

SPECT uses projection images from the gamma camera to create an image of the radioactive tracer distribution (Mettler and Guiberteau 2005) (see Fig. 2.44 for an example of the image acquisition system used in cardiac SPECT). Images without attenuation correction can be reconstructed by FBP yielding a spatial resolution of approximately 3 to 6 mm side length of a pixel. Image sizes vary between 64 × 64 and 128 × 128 voxels per slice with 25 to 35 slices to be reconstructed. Using iterative reconstruction, attenuation correction and smoothness constraints may be included, leading to a better image quality at the expense of longer reconstruction times if compared to FBP (see Fig. 2.45). Attenuation maps can be generated from the reconstruction of a transmission scan taken prior to imaging.

The acquisition of SPECT images can be carried out by a single rotating gamma camera. However, modern systems use *3-head cameras* for capturing three projections at a time. The acquisition time for a single projection is about 15 to 20 seconds, which amounts, for a 3-head system, to total acquisition times between 5 and 10 minutes.

Scatter in SPECT decreases contrast and causes noise in the image. Due to the small number of photons measured, scatter may also cause artefacts since scattering in dense materials with a high uptake of radioactive material may be falsely attributed to nearby regions. Scattered photons due to Compton scattering can be identified due to the energy loss of the scattered photon. Scattered photons may be

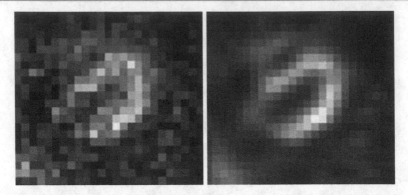

Fig. 2.45 SPECT image of the left ventricle. The two images are not smoothed in order to reveal their true spatial resolution. The *left image* was reconstructed without, the *image on the right* with attenuation correction using the method of Celler et al. (2005) (with kind permission of Anna Celler, Department of Radiology, University of British Columbia, Vancouver)

removed by the appropriate frequency filtering of the signal. The removal of scatter does reduce artefacts, but it cannot increase the signal-to-noise-ratio.

Artefacts due to motion during image acquisition cause blurring of the data. Non-gated cardiac SPECT is not able to show the heart motion because of the long acquisition time, but produces an average image over the complete heart cycle.

Major application fields for SPECT imaging are the imaging of ventricular perfusion and ejection fraction of the heart, scans of lungs, kidneys, liver, and bone for tumor detection, and brain perfusion studies.

2.4.4 Positron Emission Tomography (PET)

PET uses positron emitters for producing the image (Mettler and Guiberteau 2005). Radioactive isotopes of atoms such as oxygen or fluoride emitting positrons are administered to the human body. If distributed in the body, emanating positrons annihilate if they meet an electron and produce two photons that are emitted in the near-opposite direction. Photon energy is 511 keV. Events are measured by a *detector ring* and do not require collimators. An annihilation event is registered if two photons are detected at nearly the same time (within nanoseconds). The event is attributed to a location on a line connecting the two detection sites (see Fig. 2.46). This line is called the *line of response (LOR)*.

PET is an expensive technique if compared to SPECT because positron emitting isotopes have a short half-life and need to be generated in a cyclotron in close neighborhood to the PET scanner. The scanning technique is demanding, requiring a fixed detector ring that is capable of analyzing events according to synchronicity of measurement. The image quality of PET is better than SPECT. The number of attenuated photons decreases without collimation, the higher energy of the photons reduces attenuation loss in the body, and the near-parallelism of the path of the two

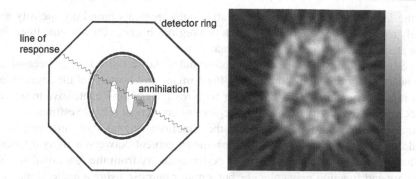

Fig. 2.46 Schematic view of a PET scanner (*left*) and resulting image of measured activity in the brain

protons focuses the ray better than the cylindrical aperture of the collimator in a gamma camera.

The spatial resolution of PET is in the range of 2 to 5 mm side length of a voxel. The signal-to-noise level is low due to the low number of counts. The true spatial resolution (i.e., the closest distance between two discernable objects) is often sacrificed to reduce noise by smoothing the data during or after reconstruction. PET, similarly to SPECT, does not produce anatomic information. Metabolic function as imaged by PET is best evaluated if registered with some anatomic scan (e.g., from CT or MRI). Registration algorithms for the registration of PET with anatomic imagery were developed in the 1980s and 1990s (Pelizzari et al. 1989). The technical problems of registration at the resolution of PET images can be considered to be solved. Some of today's PET machines are combined with a multislice CT scanner for creating anatomic and functional images almost simultaneously and in close registration.

One of the many uses of functional imaging using PET is to observe brain activity using an oxygen isotope as a tracer. Being able to resolve cortex activity at resolutions of 5 to 10 mm stipulated much activity beginning in the late 1980s because PET, for the first time, allowed to observe activity at a resolution that is comparable to the size of major substructures—such as the visual cortex—in the brain (Senda et al. 2002). Presently, functional brain imaging through PET is challenged by fMRI, which is able to measure activity at an even higher spatial resolution than PET although being only an indirect indicator using the BOLD effect.

Further applications for PET imaging are the analysis of tumor metabolism in oncology or the tracing of labeled neuroreceptors in psychiatry.

2.4.5 Image Analysis on Nuclear Images

Images come as projection images as well as slice images sharing the advantages and disadvantages of such kinds of images, as explained in the section on computed tomography. The signal strength in the images depends on the amount of tracer given and the individual metabolism. Quantitative measurements based on intensity are usually a comparison of activity between two regions because the absolute intensity value at some location depends on external factors.

The image quality (i.e., resolution and signal-to-noise ratio) is poor because of the low number of photons contributing to an image and because of the restrictions from image acquisition. This sometimes requires integrating quantitative measurements of relative activity over a larger region for arriving at reliable estimates.

Analysis often requires correlating the functional signal with anatomy. One should never be tempted to take the apparent agreement between activity distribution and expected anatomy as reason to derive anatomy from the functional signal. Anatomy and function may coincide, but a major purpose using a nuclear imaging technique is to identify and analyze regions where this is not the case. If analysis has to be carried out with respect to anatomy (e.g., "which part of the cardiac ventricle in a SPECT image is perfused normally?"), anatomical information has to be supplied by other means such as registering the data with anatomic images or an anatomic model of the organ to be imaged.

2.5   Other Imaging Techniques

The image modalities discussed so far make up the majority of images that are subjected to computer-assisted analysis. We will conclude this chapter with a brief discussion of some other methods that—although in part quite common in clinical practice—are not often subject to image analysis methods. The reasons for this are that, at present, most of them are diagnosed quite satisfactorily by inspection by a human expert.

2.5.1   Photography

An example for diagnosis using photography is the depiction of vascular processes in retina photography (see Fig. 2.47). The retina is the only location in the human body where vessels are visible on the surface (Saine and Tyler 2002). Another application is the diagnosis and staging of skin tumors (Malvehy 2002) or burn scars (van Zuijlen et al. 2002). Photography in this field is sometimes replaced by dermoscopy (Bowling 2011) which produces microscopic images of the skin surface with a magnification factor of 1:10.

In treatment planning, photography may be used for estimating the effects of plastic surgery. Digital photographs are usually high quality and high resolution color images.

A photographic image is a projection of some opaque surface, so that similar rules with respect to measurement and analysis apply than for x-ray projection images. If, for instance, distances on the retina surface shall be measured, the curvedness of the retina and the magnification factor due to the distance between the camera and retina has to be considered. When using intensity or color in digital pho-

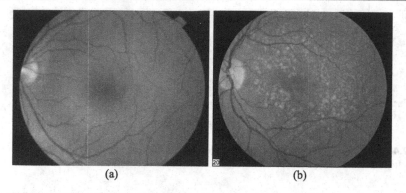

(a)   (b)

Fig. 2.47 Examples of retina photography (note that the original images are in color): (**a**) retina of a normal (**b**) degeneration of the macula (with kind permission of the National Eye Institute http://www.nei.nih.gov)

tographs for analysis, effects from external lighting, shading, or the camera position need to be accounted for.

2.5.2   Light Microscopy

Microscopes in medical imaging are often light-optical microscopes, which are able to analyze living structures of sizes between 0.1 μm and 1 mm. Magnification is generated through a system of lenses. Photosensitivity decreases with increased spatial resolution. Microscopic images are often used for the diagnosis of pathology in a tissue specimen on the cell level (see, e.g., Fig. 2.48). Images are usually color images with good contrast and signal-to-noise ratio. Microscopic images are used for cell counting, shape analysis of cells, and structural analysis of cells and cell distribution (Török and Kao 2008).

Microscopic images are good quality high resolution images, which may suffer from blurring due to defocussing. Since color staining in cells is done on purpose, color-based segmentation and classification are often appropriate strategies for successful analysis. Cell classification and the detection of the structural arrangement of cells may require quite elaborate segmentation techniques and a very good understanding of the often qualitative criteria to categorize cells.

A variant of cell microscopy is fluorescence microscopy. Instead of using reflection and absorption, the signal is generated by the fluorescence response of the living material to incident laser light. Since the response is at a different wavelength than the evoking laser light, influences from light reflection and absorption can be filtered so that the image only shows the fluorescence of the reacting material (Fig. 2.49 shows examples of fluorescence microscopy of the synaptic vesicles from drosophila larvae).

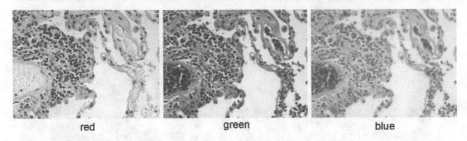

red   green   blue

Fig. 2.48 Red-, green- and blue-channel of a color-stained microscopic image of lung cells (image taken from Rogers 2004 published under Creative Commons license)

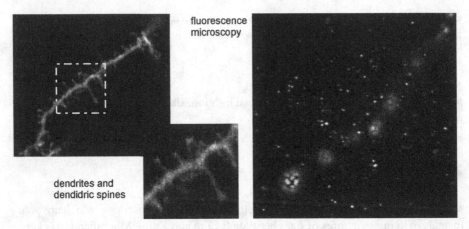

Fig. 2.49 Dendritic spine (*left*) and fluorescence microscopy (*right*) of the synapses of drosophila larvae, see Bachmann et al. (2004). It is characteristic for fluorescence images that only fluorescent particles are visible while influence from the incident illumination is filtered out (the original images are in color showing different types of particles in different color channels). Hence, the dendrite is not visible in the *image on the right*

2.5.3 EEG and MEG

For creating an *electroencephalogram* (*EEG*) a number of electrodes (16 to 25) are placed on the scalp to detect electrical impulses caused by brain activity. The impulses are amplified and represent an array of brain activity curves indicating the function of the human brain. Brain activity happens in gray matter, which—for the most part—is close to the scalp. Hence, EEG provides a brain map of functional activity (Chambers and Sanei 2007).

Spatial resolution is poor, but the temporal resolution of EEG is excellent (see Fig. 2.50 for an example of EEG time curves). Hence, EEG is a potential candidate to supplement methods with good spatial resolution and low temporal resolution of imaging (such as fMRI). An EEG measures neural activity directly whereas other methods such as fMRI, SPECT, or PET deduce brain activity from secondary signals (such as the blood oxygen level). Currently, the main activity in processing EEGs is

Fig. 2.50 An EEG consists of a set of time signals that are acquired from different locations on the head surface. Lines of the original EEG were dilated in this picture for enhanced visibility (EEG entry of www.wikipedia.de from user "Der Lange", published under Creative Commons license)

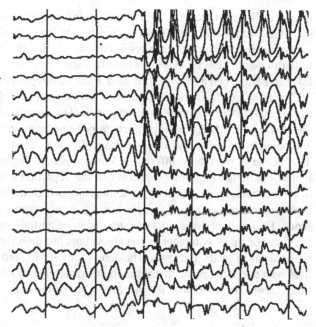

signal analysis and pattern recognition of the temporal image. Image analysis plays a lesser role due to the poor spatial resolution of the signal.

A *magnetoencephalogram* (*MEG*) measures a similar effect as EEG through the magnetic field of neural brain activity (Hämäläinen et al. 1993; Papanicolaou 1995). MEG requires a system for recording very small magnetic fields (10^{-15} T) and requires a special kind of recording magnet that is sensitive to such small fields (it is called *SQUID—superconducting quantum interference device*). Measuring a magnetic field that is more than a billion times smaller than the Earth's magnetic field requires excellent shielding of the examination room. Compared to EEG, requirements for applying MEG are much higher. However, the achievable spatial resolution of about 2 mm is much better than in EEG. The temporal resolution is 1 ms and in the same range as EEG.

MEG is a very new technique and does not produce images yet. Hence, not much can be said about its potential and of the properties of such images. So far, spatially resolved MEG was mainly used for the exact localization of a certain activity. However, acquiring a surface map of the cortex is possible in principle and may provide excellent spatiotemporal resolution.

2.6   Concluding Remarks

Image acquisition methods presented in this chapter can be grouped by acquisition technique into projective and nonprojective methods, by the imaged parameters into physiological and functional imaging techniques, and by the physical effect that is measured. Each of the techniques produces information that is related to physiological and/or functional attributes in a known way. It can be assumed that the selection of an imaging technique is always intentional so that this relation can be exploited for subsequent analysis. Artefacts are often specific to an imaging technique so that this knowledge can and should be used when developing an analysis method.

The term "medical image" comprises a wide variety of different acquisition techniques and different signals to be acquired. Hence, understanding the semantics of the image will require a new effort every time that a new analysis task shall be solved with the help of a semi-automatically or automatically working algorithm. This is one of the major differences between processing medical images and other pictures. Another important aspect is that the depiction is usually not the projection of mostly opaque materials, but either a projection of transparent materials (such as in x-ray imaging or in scintigraphy) or a full reconstruction of a 3D (or even 4D) scene. Recovery of distances or the treatment of partially hidden structures being in the focus of many computer vision algorithms are therefore not a major concern of the analysis of medical images. The main problems in medical image analysis are to deal with the incomplete differentiation of structures of interest, with artefacts from image acquisition and with the inaccessibility of the data to be analyzed.

2.7   Exercises

- Why is it impossible to measure distances in projections images?
- Why is angiography in cardiac imaging more popular than digital subtraction angiography?
- Explain the difference of the imaging technique between standard x-ray imaging and mammography.
- Explain the image acquisition process for digital radiography.
- What is meant by vignetting in radiographic imaging and what are the effects of this artefact?
- What is the partial volume effect and how does it affect the image?
- Why is it necessary to filter the projection data in filtered backprojection?
- Explain the backprojection procedure.
- What is the major difference between CT angiography and 3D reconstructed digital subtraction angiography?
- What is the purpose of filtering with a Hamming window filter when reconstructing CT images?
- What is meant by window and level in displaying CT images? Why is it needed?
- What is the typical spatial resolution of a body CT scan?
- Name three typical artefacts that occur in CT and MR imaging.
- What is the entity in the body that gives rise to the signal in MR imaging?
- Explain the meaning of the three components (ρ, t_1, t_2) that make up the MR signal.
- Explain the steps of slice selection, phase, and frequency encoding in MR imaging.

- What is the difference between t_2-relaxation and t_2^*-relaxation in MR imaging?
- How does the spin-echo sequence in MR imaging avoid adverse effects from t_2^*-relaxation?
- Why is most MR image acquisition much slower than CT image acquisition?
- What is the principle of fast MR imaging techniques such as EPI imaging?
- Name and explain the differences between the different kinds of angiogtaphic imaging in MRI. Which of the techniques can be used to recover velocity information?
- What is meant by ghosting in MR imaging and when does it occur?
- What imaging technique uses Hounsfield units for normalization and what are the two reference values for normalization?
- What is the purpose of MR perfusion imaging? How is the perfusion information generated?
- What is the BOLD effect and how is it used in functional MRI?
- Why is it necessary to acquire a time sequence of images in functional MRI?
- What is measured in diffusion imaging? Why and how can this information be used for fiber tracking?
- What are A- and B-scans in ultrasound imaging?
- How is spatial information about the depth of a reflection generated in ultrasound imaging?
- Name some typical artefacts in ultrasound images.
- What imaging techniques are subsumed under the term "nuclear imaging"? Which of the techniques produces projection images?
- Explain the design of a gamma camera. What is the purpose of the collimator in this design?
- What are the adverse influences for reconstructing SPECT images?
- What are the reasons for SPECT having a low spatial resolution compared to, e.g., CT imaging?
- What are potential diagnostic questions that require a scintigraphy?
- What are the advantages and disadvantage of MRI opposed to x-ray CT?
- Why is filtered backprojection not always appropriate to reconstruct SPECT images?
- Why is the spatial resolution of PET generally higher than the one of SPECT?
- What generates the signal in PET imaging? How does PET compare with functional MRI?
- What are the applications for using photography in diagnosis?
- What are the potential applications of using light microscopy?
- What is measured by an EEG? What is the spatial resolution of the signal?
- Name a potential application for acquiring an EEG?
- What other imaging techniques produce similar information as that generated by EEG?

References

Akpek S, Brunner T, Benndorf G, Strother C (2005) Three-dimensional imaging and cone beam volume CT in C-arm angiography with flat panel detector. Diagn Intervent Radiol 11:10–13

Bacher K, Smeets P, Bonnarens K, De Hauwere A, Verstraete K, Thierens H (2003) Dose reduction in patients undergoing chest imaging: digital amorphous silicon flat-panel detector radiography versus conventional film-screen radiography and phosphor-based computed radiography. Am J Radiol 181:923–929

Bachmann A, Timmer M, Sierralta J, Pietrini G, Gundelfinger ED, Knust E, Thomas U (2004) Cell type-specific recruitment of Drosophila Lin-7 to distinct MAGUK-based protein complexes defines novel roles for Sdt and Dlg-S97. J Cell Sci 117(10):1899–1909

Bowling J (2011) Diagnostic dermoscopy: the illustrated guide. Wiley, New York

Bushberg JT (1998) X-ray interaction. Radiographics 18(2):457–468

Bushberg JT, Seibert JA, Leidholdt EM (2002) The essential physics of medical imaging, 2nd edn. Lippincott Williams and Wilkins, Philadelphia

Buzug TM (2008) Computed tomography—from photon statistics to modern cone-beam CT. Springer, Berlin

Celler A, Dixon KL, Chang Z, Blinder S, Powe J, Harrop R (2005) Problems created in attenuation-corrected SPECT images by artefacts in attenuation maps: a simulation study. J Nucl Med 46(2):335–343

Chambers JA, Sanei S (2007) EEG signal processing. Wiley, New York

Chan HP, Doi K, Galhotra S, Vyborny CJ, MacMahon H, Jokich PM (1987) Image feature analysis and computer-aided diagnosis in digital radiography. I. Automated detection of microcalcifications in mammography. Med Phys 14(4):538–548

Cheng HD, Lui YM, Freimanis RI (1998) A novel approach to microcalcification detection using fuzzy logic technique. IEEE Trans Med Imaging 17(3):442–450

Dengler J, Behrens S, Desaga JF (1993) Segmentation of microcalcifications in mammograms. IEEE Trans Med Imaging 12(4):634–642

Dillon EH, van Leeuwen MS, Fernandez MA, Mali WP (1993) Spiral CT angiography. Am J Roentgenol 160(6):1273–1278

Dumoulin CL (1995) Phase contrast MR angiography techniques. Magn Reson Imaging Clin N Am 3(3):399–411

Fink C, Hallscheidt PJ, Noeldge G, Kampschulte A, Radeleff B, Hosch WP, Kauffmann GW, Hansmann J (2002) Clinical comparative study with a large-area amorphous silicon flat-panel detector—image quality and visibility of anatomic structures on chest radiography. Am J Radiol 178:481–486

Fischl B, Sereno MI, Dale AM (1999) Cortical surface-based analysis. II. Inflation, flattening, and a surface-based coordinate system. Neuroimage 9:195–207

Forster BB, MacKay AL, Whittall KP, Kiehl KA, Smith AM, Hare RD, Liddle PF (1998) Functional magnetic resonance imaging: the basics of blood-oxygen-level dependent (BOLD) imaging. Can Assoc Radiol J 49(5):320–329

Friston KJ, Holmes AP, Worsley KJ, Poline JP, Frith CD, Frackowiak RSJ (1995) Statistical parametric maps in functional imaging: a general linear approach. Hum Brain Mapp 2(4):189–210

Garmer M, Hennigs SP, Jäger HJ, Schrick F, van de Loo T, Jacobs A, Hanusch A, Christmann A, Mathias K (2000) Digital radiography versus conventional radiography in chest imaging— diagnostic performance of a large-area silicon flat-panel detector in a clinical CT-controlled study. Am J Radiol 174:75–80

Geluk RJ (1979) Transverse analogue tomography (TAT): a new method for cross-sectional imaging using X-rays. J Mod Opt 26(11):1367–1376

Ghersin E, Litmanovich D, Dragu R et al (2006) 16-MDCT coronary angiography versus invasive coronary angiography in acute chest pain syndrome: a blinded prospective study. Am J Roentgenol 186(1):177–184

Gillard JH, Waldman AD, Barker PB (2004) Clinical MR neuroimaging: diffusion, perfusion and spectroscopy. Cambridge University Press, Cambridge

Goebel R, Sefat DK, Muckli L, Hacker H, Singer W (1998) The constructive nature of vision: direct evidence from functional magnetic resonance imaging studies of apparent motion and motion imagery. Eur J Neurosci 10(5):1563–1573

Green PJ (1990) Bayesian reconstructions from emission tomography data using a modified EM algorithm. IEEE Trans Med Imaging 9(1):84–93

Hämäläinen M, Hari R, Ilmoniemi RJ, Knuutila J, Lounasmaa OV (1993) Magnetoencephalography—theory, instrumentation, and applications to noninvasive studies of the working human brain. Rev Mod Phys 65(2):413–497

Herman GT, Lent A, Lutz PH (1978) Relaxation methods for image reconstruction. Commun ACM 21(2):152–158

Hokland JH, Kelly PA (1996) Markov models of specular and diffuse scattering in restoration of medical ultrasound images. IEEE Trans Ultrason Ferroelectr Freq Control 43(4):660–669

Hudson HM, Larkin RS (1994) Accelerated image reconstruction using ordered subsets of projection data. IEEE Trans Med Imaging 13(4):601–609

Huettel SA, Song AW, McCarthy G (2004) Functional magnetic resonance imaging. Palgrave Macmillan, Basingstoke

Jahnke C, Nagel E, Gebker R, Kokocinski T, Kelle S, Manka R, Fleck E, Paetsch I (2007) Prognostic value of cardiac magnetic resonance stress tests: adenosine stress perfusion and dobutamine stress wall motion imaging. Circulation 115:1769–1776

Jensen JA, Mathorne J, Gravesen T, Stage B (1993) Deconvolution of in-vivo ultrasound B-mode images. Ultrason Imag 15(2):122–133

Kuhl CK, Schild HH (2000) Dynamic image interpretation of MRI of the breast. J Magn Reson Imaging 12(6):965–974

Lange K, Carson R (1984) EM reconstruction algorithms for emission and transmission tomography. J Comput Assist Tomogr 8:306–316

Liang ZP, Lauterbur PC (2000) Principles of magnetic resonance imaging: a signal processing perspective. IEEE press series on biomedical engineering. Wiley, New York

Mado K, Ishii Y, Mazaki T, Ushio M, Masuda H, Takayama T (2006) A case of bone metastasis of colon cancer that markedly responded to S-1/CPT-11 combination chemotherapy and became curable by resection. World J Surg Oncol 4:3

Malvehy J (2002) Follow-up of melanocytic skin lesions with digital total-body photography and digital dermoscopy: a two-step method. Clin Dermatol 20(3):297–304

McCollough CH (1997) X-ray production. Radiographics 17(4):967–984

McKetty MH (1998) X-ray attenuation. Radiographics 18(1):151–163

Mettler M, Guiberteau MJ (2005) Essentials of nuclear medicine imaging. Saunders, Maryland Heights

Mori S, van Zijl PCM (2002) Fiber tracking: principles and strategies—a technical review. NMR Biomed 5(7–8):468–480

Meijering EHW, Niessen WJ, Viergever MA (1999) Retrospective motion correction in digital subtraction angiography: a review. IEEE Trans Med Imaging 18(1):2–21

Ning R, Chen B, Yu R, Conover D, Tang X, Ning Y (2000) Flat panel detector-based cone-beam volume CT angiography imaging: system evaluation. IEEE Trans Med Imaging 19(9):949–963

Papanicolaou AC (1995) An introduction to magnetoencephalography with some applications. Brain Cogn 27(3):331–352

Pelizzari CA, Chen GTY, Spelbring DR, Weichselbaum RR, Chen CT (1989) Accurate three-dimensional registration of CT, PET, and/or MR images of the brain. J Comput Assist Tomogr 13(1):20–26

Pooley RA, McKinney JM, Miller DA (2001) Digital fluoroscopy. Radiographics 21(2):512–534

Prince JL, Links J (2005) Medical imaging signals and systems. Prentice Hall, New York

Robb RA, Sinak LJ, Hoffman EA, Kinsey JH, Harris LD, Ritman EL (1982) Dynamic volume imaging of moving organs. J Med Syst 6(6):539–554

Rogers A (2004) T cells cause lung damage in emphysema. PLoS Med 1(1):e25

Saine PJ, Tyler ME (2002) Ophthalmic photography: retinal photography, angiography, and electronic imaging, 2nd edn. Butterworth-Heinemann, Stoneham

Salibi N, Brown MA (1998) Clinical MR spectroscopy: first principles. Wiley, New York

Senda M, Kimura Y, Herscovitch P (2002) Brain imaging using PET. Academic Press, San Diego

Shcherbinin S, Celler A, Belhocine T, Vanderwerf R, Driedger A (2008) Accuracy of quantitative reconstructions in SPECT/CT imaging. Phys Med Biol 53(17):4595–4604

Szabo T (2004) Diagnostic ultrasound imaging: inside out. Academic press series in biomedical engineering

Török P, Kao FJ (2008) Optical imaging and microscopy. Techniques and advanced systems, Springer series in optical sciences

van Zuijlen PPM, Angeles AP, Kreis RW, Bos KE, Middelkoop E (2002) Scar assessment tools: implications for current research. Plast Reconstr Surg 109(3):1108–1122

Wagner RF, Insana MF, Brown DG (1985) Unified approach to the detection and classification of speckle texture in diagnostic ultrasound. Int Conf Speckle 556:146–152

Wang J, Blackburn TJ (2000) X-ray image intensifiers for fluoroscopy. Radiographics 20(5):1471–1477

Wu CM, Chen YC, Hsieh KS (1992) Texture features for classification of ultrasonic liver images. IEEE Trans Med Imaging 11(2):141–152

Image Storage and Transfer

3

Abstract

Medical images are created, stored, accessed, and processed in the restricted environment of a hospital. The semantic of a medical image is driven by the particular purpose for creating it. This results in specific solutions for the archiving of medical images. Transfer is different for medical images as well as it is driven by the technical specification of the various image acquisition systems and the particular requirements of the users of these images.

The archiving and transfer of images is governed by two standards (HL7 and DICOM) that will be discussed in this chapter. The goal of the presentation is to enable the reader to understand the way images are stored and distributed in a hospital. It should further enable the reader to access images if some analysis method shall be applied to it and to decide how to implement such an analysis method in a clinical environment.

Concepts, notions and definitions Introduced in this chapter

› Information systems: the role of HIS, RIS, and PACS
› Basic concepts of HL7
› Introduction to the DICOM standard: information objects and services, establishing DICOM connectivity, the DICOM file format
› Technical properties of medical images
› Medical workstations

It is likely that the first problem encountered when processing a digital medical image is how to access the image within the framework of information systems in the hospital. It will be difficult to set up a useful software module for postprocessing images without some basic understanding as to how they are archived and transferred. Although experienced users in the hospital may be able to help, an image processing expert is generally assumed to be sufficiently knowledgeable with respect to data bases and information systems.

K.D. Toennies, *Guide to Medical Image Analysis*,
Advances in Computer Vision and Pattern Recognition,
DOI 10.1007/978-1-4471-2751-2_3, © Springer-Verlag London Limited 2012

Medical images differ from other images in several aspects. This has an impact as to how they can be accessed. The most obvious of these aspects is that medical images receive their semantics only within the context in which they were created. Context information includes, for instance, demographic information about the person who was imaged, technical details about the image acquisition system, or the reason for the examination. Context information about medical images is much more extensive than for other images, where information about the size and quantization may suffice. For reasons of data integrity and data security, context needs to be firmly associated to the image.

A second important difference is that medical images are mappings of measurements of very different origins into a pictorial representation. Although photographs are used in diagnosis and treatment planning as well, medical imaging goes far beyond this, hence adding to the requirements for image meta-information. An unknown number of details about different image acquisition techniques have to be stored with the image. Storing meta-information describing the different parameters related to some image acquisition system efficiently leads to image formats that are different from conventional formats such as JPEG or PNG.

A third aspect that differentiates medical images from other pictures is that the use of medical images is highly constrained and regulated. Medical images contain sensitive personal information of which misuse must be prevented. Images have often been acquired for justifying quite invasive actions (a decision in diagnosis or therapy with its consequences) that have to be executed with care and responsibility. A system where such images are created, stored, and accessed must be designed in a way that actively supports these goals. In consequence, images must not be accessed out of a framework that guarantees that the purpose of image access serves the intention for creating and keeping the image.

If a user intends to apply computer-based analysis techniques on a medical image he or she should be aware of the points raised above. Hence, we will give an overview about storing and accessing medical images in a hospital. The chapter is not meant to be a comprehensive description about information systems in a hospital in general. We will mainly focus on topics that are directly related to images in the information system.

3.1   Information Systems in a Hospital

Images may be generated from patients who are either admitted to the hospital or who are sent in for outpatient examination. In either case, information is acquired that is necessary for the management of the actions performed while the patient is in the hospital. Hence, this information has to be accessible at various places (see Fig. 3.1). This includes information

- which is necessary for administrating the patient's stay such as patient demographics, billing information, and so on;
- which is necessary for performing the examination to which the images belong such as patient demographics, anamnesis, reports, and so on;

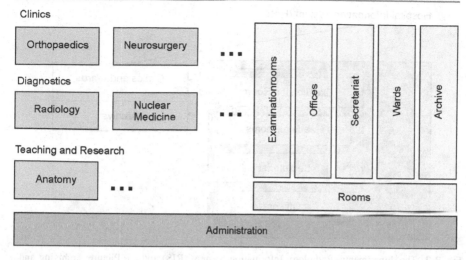

Fig. 3.1 Schematic view at functions and location in a hospital that deal with images or information related to images

- which is necessary for interpreting the images such as patient demographics, reports, imaging device information, the images themselves, and so on.

The information is kept in different information systems in the departments of the hospital. Patient administration data are kept in the *hospital information system* (HIS). The HIS maps the internal structure of a hospital (its departments, clinics, its access points for getting administrative information) into a data base representation and governs access to this information. Ideally, a HIS would replace all paper files documenting a patient's stay. Any authorized person at any location in a hospital would have immediate access to this information. It requires that a modern hospital is equipped with the necessary network infrastructure, storage devices, and access points (such as PCs on the network). Such an environment exists in many modern hospitals. Communication is often realized as a type of intranet solution to prevent unauthorized access. With increasing decentralization (outpatient care, outsourcing of administrative and technical support, teleradiology, etc.), the secure and authorized access to this and other information systems from the outside world has become necessary and possible.

Data about radiological examinations are kept in a different system, which is called a *radiology information system* (RIS, see Fig. 3.2). The reason for this and other independent subsystems within the hospital is the complexity of the information structure and information flow. Modularization keeps the information where it is needed with well-defined interfaces governing the information exchange between systems. It also helps to prevent unauthorized access. Department policy may prohibit, for instance, that an image created in a Radiology Department may be accessed without having a report from the Radiology Department associated to it.

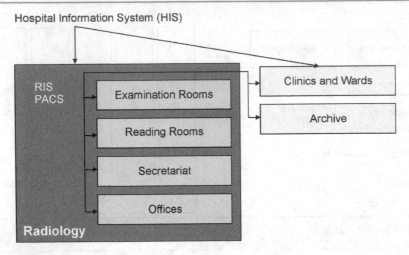

Fig. 3.2 The departmental Radiology Information System (RIS) and the Picture Archiving and Communication System (PACS) are responsible for organizing, transferring and archiving image data and image meta data

Hospital information systems evolved from the need to create a paperless administration of inpatients and outpatients in a hospital. Development was initiated from the hospital administration and in many cases evolved from data base systems for patient data administration. In early times, these systems were in-house adaptations of data base systems or completely locally developed solutions. With information stored in such a system being increasingly used for administrating and scheduling services performed in patient stay, they have evolved into fully grown hospital information systems accessible by all departments of a hospital.

Radiology Information Systems are built to manage information about services that are connected with a radiological examination. This includes information about

- examinations ordered,
- patient scheduling information,
- images created as part of an examination,
- reporting.

RIS and HIS are similar in that they mainly cover the administrative aspects of the patient's stay. If a patient is transferred to a radiology department, his or her demographic data are entered into the RIS together with all the information about the services requested from the department. The RIS is then responsible to guide the patient's stay in the department. Examinations requested are scheduled, reports on examinations performed are kept and transferred to authorized requesters, services rendered are reported to the hospital information system, and so on.

The images themselves are not included in an RIS because of historical as well as practical reasons. Administrative data on the patient were digitized well before the majority of images became digital. Images were linked to the RIS by means of an identification code referring to the pictures kept on film in some archive. The management of these pictures—e.g., ensuring that they actually were in the archive

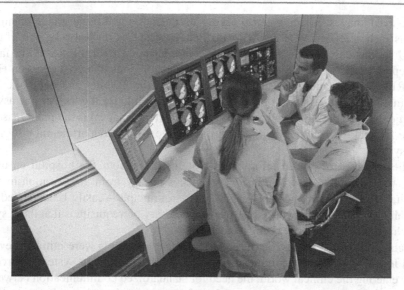

Fig. 3.3 In a PACS, the user has access to images from acquisition systems, workstations and the archive. It usually requires a specific monitor configuration to render images, meta-information, and the interface to administer data access in a suitable way (with kind permission of Siemens Sector Healthcare, Erlangen, Germany)

or, if not, that it was known where they could be found—was a nondigital and only partially computer-supported task.

The situation changed dramatically in the last three decades. In the 1970s, the majority of images created in a radiology department were still analogue x-ray images. Thus, the preferred mode of access and display used analogue means. With the advent of x-ray computed tomography in the 1970s and that of magnetic resonance imaging in the 1980s, images were generated whose primary representation was digital. Even x-ray images, still making up the bulk of the images generated in a hospital, are more and more created digitally. In the foreseeable future, most if not all of the images created in the departments of a hospital will be digital.

It gave rise to the introduction of another image information system, which is called a *picture archiving and communication system* (PACS, see Fig. 3.3). First PACSs were introduced in the early 1980s. A PACS should archive and distribute pictures together with the related information within radiology and to the departments who ordered the images. Besides the images, this information includes patient demographics, information about reports, as well as technical information about the images such as the imaging device and its technical parameters.

RIS and PACS are the two information systems that a computer scientist is most likely to encounter when images in a hospital need to be accessed. The RIS contains information about the specific examination and associated previous examinations. This may also concern nonpicture-based examinations. The brief description above already indicated that RIS and PACS share a lot of information (such as patient demographics). Hence, the RIS sometimes serves as the primary access mechanism to archived images. It then governs access authorization and basic image manipulations such as retrieving or anonymizing images. The task may also be part of the PACS. In this case, access requires only communication with the PACS. In fact, the separation between RIS and PACS is much less obvious than that between HIS and RIS. For the latter, a clear hierarchy between the hospital and departmental information systems is reason for different systems, while for the former one asynchronicity of the development and type of data (text vs. images) is the main reason. In the future, PACS and RIS will probably fuse into a single departmental information system.

The existence of digital information systems throughout the hospital ensures that—in principle—authorized access to images is easy from any location in the hospital. Using the internet, this can—again, in principle—easily be extended to virtually any place in the world. However, a necessary prerequisite is that these systems have export interfaces fitting to each other.

This is not self-evident. The different information systems were initially developed locally with local requirements in mind. With information systems increasingly entering the clinical world, the need for standardized communication between information systems arose. It became clear that much of the information is needed multiple times (such as the patient demographics). Entering such information again every time a patient is admitted to a different department with its own departmental information system is tedious and error-prone.

Two different communication standards evolved: the HL7 messaging standard and DICOM. HL7 was developed for standardizing communication between clinical information systems, whereas DICOM is specifically targeted at standardizing the communication of images. The former plays a role when connecting HIS, RIS, and PACS systems and it will be briefly reviewed here. The latter mainly standardizes image communications between the components of a PACS system. As such, it will be a likely interface encountered by somebody wishing to access images stored in some picture archiving system. It will be reviewed in more detail in the next section.

HL7 is a standard developing organization that is accredited by the American National Standards Institute (ANSI). It is devoted to developing standards for communication in the health care business. The name HL7 stands for Health Level 7 and it refers to the application layer (the seventh layer) of the OSI (open systems interconnect, see Fig. 3.4) model.

The OSI model is a framework for layered protocols in network communication. The application layer provides application-specific protocols for communication including information about the authentification of communication partners, quality of service of the communication, and syntax of the messages exchanged. HL7 is not a complete specification of such a protocol (such as DICOM, see below), but describes the syntax and semantics of messages on this layer. For establishing communication a layer-7-protocol is still to be agreed upon by which these messages are exchanged (such as, e.g., FTP).

An HL7-conform system typically means that HL7-conform messages are created by an interface by which a system (archive, workstation, etc.) communicates

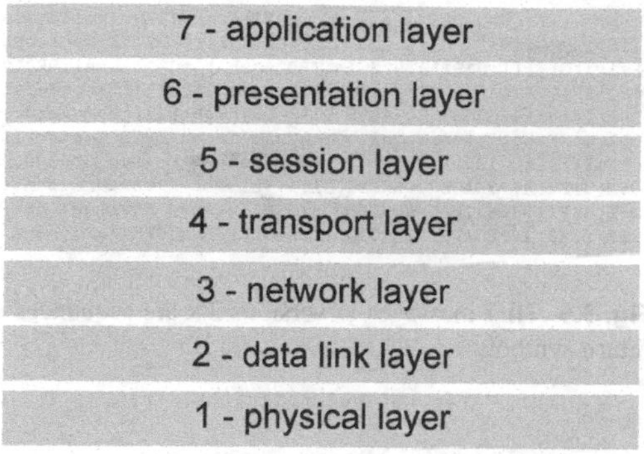

Fig. 3.4 The layers of the OSI model

7 - application layer
6 - presentation layer
5 - session layer
4 - transport layer
3 - network layer
2 - data link layer
1 - physical layer

with other systems. It generally does not mean that a system internally uses the HL7 standard to exchange information. This has consequences for accessing information in an HL7-conform system. Even if the module that uses the information is part of the system, it will need to be defined as an external partner communicating through the HL7 interface. If this is infeasible for reasons of performance, access through internal, often vendor-specific interfaces is needed.

HL7 messages are based on the HL7 *reference information model* (RIM), which is the main contribution of the HL7 organization. In a heroic undertaking they succeeded in mapping most of the clinical information entities onto one big, generic, relational model. Within the RIM, six different stereotypes are specified, four of which refer to the nodes and two of which refer to the relations between nodes of the RIM as follows:

- entity,
- act,
- role,
- participation,
- role-relationship,
- act-relationship.

A specific HL7 message is an instance of a representation of this model. In HL7 versions 2.x, it is a sequence of ASCII characters which consists of segments that in turn consist of composites (see Fig. 3.5). The segments are delimited by "carriage return" (\r) symbols, the components are delimited by other delimiter symbols. The segments or components are either mandatory or optional accommodating a wide range of different messages while still conforming to the HL7 model. The segments may be repeated.

Choosing ASCII was intentional to make the messages readable by humans (although this may require some practice). The new HL7 Version 3 standard replaced the somewhat outdated way of structuring the data. XML-tags are used to tag information units, but the basic structure of the syntax remains the same (see Fig. 3.6).

The semantic of an HL7 message is determined by the first and mandatory identifying component. The current standard defines more than 100 different segments

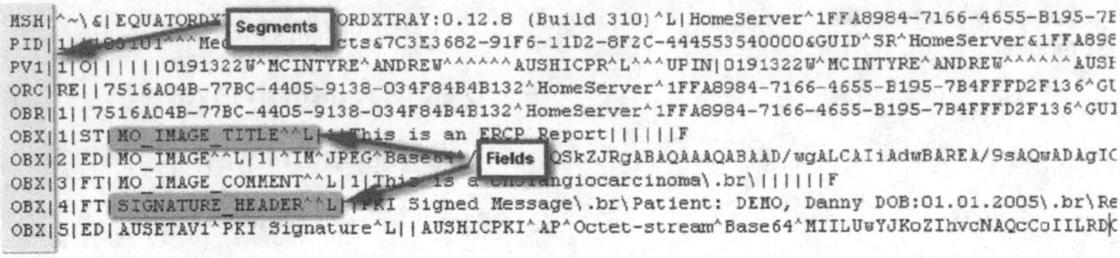

```
MSH|^~\&|EQUATORDX        ORDXTRAY:0.12.8 (Build 310)^L|HomeServer^1FFA8984-7166-4655-B195-7E
                  Segments
PID|1|                  Me      cts&7C3E3682-91F6-11D2-8F2C-444553540000&GUID^SR^HomeServer&1FFA898
PV1|1|O||||||0191322W^MCINTYRE^ANDREW^^^^^^AUSHICPR^L^^^UPIN|0191322W^MCINTYRE^ANDREW^^^^^^AUSF
ORC|RE||7516A04B-77BC-4405-9138-034F84B4B132^HomeServer^1FFA8984-7166-4655-B195-7B4FFFD2F136^GU
OBR|1||7516A04B-77BC-4405-9138-034F84B4B132^HomeServer^1FFA8984-7166-4655-B195-7B4FFFD2F136^GUI
OBX|1|ST|MO_IMAGE_TITLE^^L|     This is an ERCP Report||||||F
OBX|2|ED|MO_IMAGE^^L|1|^IM^JPEG^Base64        QSkZJRgABAQAAAQABAAD/wgALCAIiAdwBAREA/9sAQwADAgIC
                                       Fields
OBX|3|FT|MO_IMAGE_COMMENT^^L|1|This is a  cholangiocarcinoma\.br\|||||||F
OBX|4|FT|SIGNATURE_HEADER^^L|PKI Signed Message\.br\Patient: DEMO, Danny DOB:01.01.2005\.br\Re
OBX|5|ED|AUSETAV1^PKI Signature^L||AUSHICPKI^AP^Octet-stream^Base64^MIILUwYJKoZIhvcNAQcCoIILRDK
```

Fig. 3.5 HL7 messages in versions 2.x are sequences of ASCII characters delimited by carriage return symbols

```
<?xml version="1.0" encoding="ISO-8859-1"?>
  <message>
    <segment name="msh" >
    <field name="field_separator" len="1" >|</field>
    <field name="encoding_characters" len="4" >^~\&amp;</field>
    <field name="sending_application" len="180" >SENDAPP</field>
    <field name="sending_facility" len="180" >SENDFAC</field>
    <field name="receiving_application" len="180" >007</field>
    <field name="receiving_facility" len="180" >007</field>
    <field name="date_time_of_message" len="26" >200601212140</field>
    <field name="security" len="40" ></field>
    <field name="message_type" len="7" >ORU^R02</field>
    <field name="message_control_id" len="20" >HL7777</field>
    <field name="processing_id" len="3" >P</field>
    <field name="version_id" len="8" >2.3</field>
    <field name="sequence_number" len="15" >3434</field>
    <field name="continuation_pointer" len="180" ></field>
    <field name="accept_acknowledgement_type" len="2" ></field>
    <field name="application_acknowledgement_type" len="2" ></field>
    <field name="country_code" len="2" ></field>
    <field name="character_set" len="6" ></field>
    <field name="principal_language_of_message" len="60" ></field>
  <segment name="pid" ><field name="set_id" len="4" >1</field>
```

Fig. 3.6 In version 3 of the HL7 standard XML tags are used to structure the message

that may then follow. A specific implementation may still require a message part, which is not yet standardized. To let a message adhere to the standard nonetheless, the standardization committee allowed user-defined "Z" messages (named after the identification key). It is a potential source of incompatibility between two HL7-conform systems, as it—for instance—allows a vendor to hide nonmandatory information in a "Z" message. Other reasons for incompatibility are the use of different versions of the standard and various violations against the standard that are difficult to detect, such as missing fields (in versions 2.x fields are identified by their position in the segments which means that the missing, nonmandatory fields must be made identifiable by the delimiter symbol) or wrong data formats.

3.2   The DICOM Standard

When digital image acquisition systems such as x-ray computed tomography appeared in the clinics, the medium for data exchange and archival was film. Even though the data were created digitally, they were printed on film when sent away for reporting, for transferring them to the referring physician, or for archiving. Digital images were stored digitally as well, but mainly for internal reasons related to the local infrastructure around the image acquisition system. There, digital images could be displayed on a local workstation, simple image analysis tools could be applied, or images could be selected that should be printed on film.

Initially, digital communication with other systems was not considered. Consequently, most vendors developed their own formats to store information deemed necessary for the purposes mentioned above. The decision about what information to store was dictated by the need to preserve the semantically relevant information produced. This includes the following.

- Patient information: Name and demographic information, identification in other information systems in the hospital, and so on.
- Examination information: Referring clinic and/or physician, examination type, and so on.
- Technical information: Many image acquisition systems require careful parameter selection controlling the acquisition process. A description of an x-ray CT, for instance, would include the wavelength and amplitude of radiation, number and spacing of slices, spatial resolution within slices, reconstruction method and reconstruction kernel, and so on.
- (Auxiliary) reporting information: Measurements and annotations being created during reporting, and so on.
- The image or image sequence.

If sequences of images are generated, this information is often tagged to every single image of the sequence. The kind of information to be stored depends on the type, make, and version of the acquisition system.

With the number and variety of digital imaging systems increasing there was a growing need to manage images digitally. Preventing the digital communication of the images inhibited the inclusion of them into the information system infrastructure of the hospital. This motivated the development of the DICOM 3.0 standard (and its predecessors ACR-NEMA 1.0 and 2.0). DICOM stands for *digital image communication in medicine* and is a full-fledged specification of the application layer of the OSI model. For the communication of medical images it replaces other file communication protocols such as, e.g., FTP.

The DICOM standard and its two predecessors evolved from a joint effort of the American College of Radiology (ACR, http://www.acr.org) and the National Electrical Manufacturer's Association (NEMA, http://www.nema.org). Resources may be found on the home page for DICOM on the NEMA website (http://medical.nema.org).

Initially, DICOM was adopted only reluctantly by the industry. An open system standard supports multivendor environments in a hospital, which automatically increases competition. It was also feared that a multipurpose standard would be inferior to the highly specialized single purpose interfaces of image acquisition systems. On the other hand, DICOM-conform machinery greatly simplifies the connectivity between the imaging components and the hospital information system. Today, it will be difficult to sell a major imaging device that does not conform to the standard.

DICOM is an interface standard similar to HL7. Internal communication is still vendor-specific. DICOM is designed to standardize communication between components such as imaging systems, printers, archives, and workstations. Formerly, these were often stand-alone system clusters communicating through specialized interfaces. This meant, for instance, that a CT image acquisition device of manufacturer X and an MRI device of manufacturer Y both required their own printer, archive, and workstation. Not only does this inhibit combined access to images from both devices, it also results in an inefficient use of hardware resources.

At present, it seems that the potential disadvantages from communication overhead generated by a multipurpose standard are outweighed by the advantages of the open system architecture. It simplifies component sharing in a multivendor environment and ensures system compatibility when adding new components.

DICOM specifies a protocol for communicating objects between devices. Two different types of objects, *composite* and *normalized*, may be exchanged. An image is a typical composite object since it consists of several different entities such as various text entities (e.g., the patient name), numerical entities (e.g., the number of pixels), and the image itself. Normalized objects, on the other hand, consist only of a single entity such as a report. For each of the two types the standard defines the number of services associated with it.

Services were first defined for composite objects, as DICOM was developed to support image communication. Four services, C-STORE, C-FIND, C-GET, and C-MOVE are designed to exchange images. A service for updating an image is not provided to prevent the intentional or unintentional alteration of an acquired image. In practice, this means that every change of an image (e.g., by some image enhancement procedure) will add a new image to a study.

Normalized services apply to single real-world entities. Four general services, N-CREATE, N-DELETE, N-SET, and N-GET, as well as the two specialized services N-ACTION and N-EVENT-NOTIFY were defined. The latter need to be specified within their specific context (e.g., printing a sheet of film followed by notifications of events that are caused by this request).

Service classes describe services that may be rendered to representations of information entities. Such an information entity could be, for instance, an MRI image with all its associated information (patient demographics, technical information about the acquisition, etc.). Classes of information entities in the DICOM world are templates that are called *information object description* (IOD, see Fig. 3.7).

An instance of an IOD is an *information object*. Information objects are uniquely identified. DICOM has adopted the ISO concept of the *unique identifier* (UID) which is a text string of numbers and periods with a unique root for each organization that is registered with ISO and various organizations that in turn register others in a hierarchical fashion.

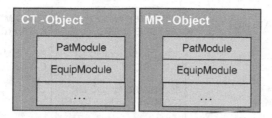

Fig. 3.7 An Information Object Description (IOD) is defined for each information object. Different object classes may have different variants of the same modules. In the example above, for instance, the equipment module will contain different descriptions for CT and MR objects

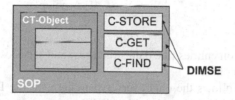

Fig. 3.8 A service-object pair combines an IOD (such as the CT object in this example) with services that are offered for this object. The services are called DICOM Message Service Elements (DIMSE)

For a given information object, the left-hand part of a UID is prespecified by the vendor. It may be decomposed into its hierarchical components. The right-hand part is generated when an information object is created. It is usually a combination of hospital, device, and patient identification together with a time stamp of the examination. This part is not intended to be parsed to regain the components. Its sole purpose is uniqueness. All relevant semantic information may be found in the information object itself.

Information objects are composed of sets of *modules*. Each module contains a specific set of data elements that is present or absent according to specific rules defined by the standard. Modularization supports the reuse of information specifications that are shared among different IODs. For example, a CT Image Information Object contains among others, a Patient module, a General Equipment module, a CT Image module, and an Image Pixel module. An MR Image Information module would contain all of these except the CT Image module, which would be replaced by an MR Image module.

For a given IOD, several composite or normalized services may be useful. A service is defined as a *DICOM message service element* (DIMSE) that invokes an operation or notification across the network. A DIMSE service group is a collection of DIMSEs applicable to an IOD (see Fig. 3.8). An information object description and the set of services operating on it are called a *service object pair* (SOP) class (see Fig. 3.8). An SOP class using composite services is called a *composite SOP class* and an SOP class using normalized services is called a *normalized SOP class*. An instance of such a class is called a composite or normalized object (or, more correctly, a composite or normalized SOP instance). DICOM classes are static, which

Fig. 3.9 Different
application entities (AE) offer
different services

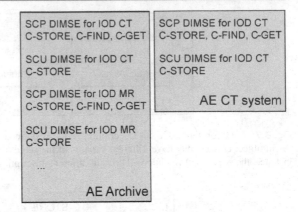

means that information entities (the data structures) and services (i.e., the methods) are provided as a template.

Communication follows the client-server paradigm. In the DICOM world, the server is called the *service class provider* (SCP) and a client is called the *service class user* (SCU). Communication between two components supporting the DICOM standard may be established in different ways between a server and a client. They have in common that messages are created as part of the external interface. A communication session between two components, which are called *application entities* (AE), is initiated by establishing a DICOM association (see Fig. 3.9). Basic understanding is established as to what information objects are to be exchanged and what services are to be invoked.

If communication is established such that full interoperability is ensured, components may exchange messages via DIMSEs. DICOM service classes support five different general application areas for communication:

- network image management,
- network image interpretation management,
- network print management,
- imaging procedure management,
- offline storage media management.

Of these five the first application area is most relevant for accessing images in a hospital environment and thus will be explained in more detail. Network image management involves sending images between two devices. This could be, e.g., a scanner generating images and an external workstation or a digital image archive somewhere in the hospital network.

Two different kinds of communication are supported (see Fig. 3.10). In *push mode*, images are sent from one device to another device. This basic service would be appropriate, e.g., for sending images from a scanner to an archive. DICOM does not specify the timing behavior of the sending device, which means that the scanner could send images whenever the system is ready to do so. The receiver acts as a listener that has to accept information at any time during which a DICOM association is established.

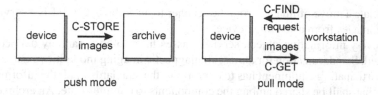

Fig. 3.10 In push mode images are transferred without request, while pull mode only transfers requested images

Pushing images may also be appropriate for communication to a workstation. This could be the case if the workstation serves as a reporting station where all images should be present. It could also be intended for sending images to a departmental workstation of a referring clinic.

Often, however, the push service is not adequate. If a subset of images from an archive or from a scanner shall be processed on some workstation, it makes little sense to send all images over the network and to decide then which of those are actually to be used. Alternatively, the *pull mode* may be used for information exchange. It allows querying the sender first about its images. Selected images may then be pulled by the receiver.

The pull mode consists of two phases. First, the requesting component sends a query to the sending component. The prospective sender matches the keys of the query with images in its data base and returns the number of information objects that match the keys together with their UIDs. The receiver then selects images from this list that he or she wishes to receive and requests them from the archive. Finally, these images are sent to the workstation.

The transfer of information is similar to that using other file transfer protocols such as FTP, however, with one important difference. The establishment of communication includes a common understanding between the sender and receiver about the basic properties of the kind of information exchanged such as keys to request in a pull service. Hence, the sender and receiver know how to interpret such relevant information before a data transfer takes place. This enables the organization and presentation of data according to such criteria. Instead of listing data by file names, which, in the case of the DICOM images, are their UIDs and difficult to interpret anyway, images can be presented in a more meaningful fashion. The result of a query may be structured by listing image data by patient name, patient ID, and study ID. Such organization by clinically relevant categories substantially enhances the use of transferred information.

DICOM network management services are specified in the service, query/retrieve, and storage commitment service classes. They are defined for composite objects only. The storage service class specifies the C-STORE service for pushing data to a client. The query/retrieve service class specifies C-MOVE, C-FIND, and C-GET services. With C-FIND, the sender is queried using the number of keys sent to him. With C-MOVE, a third party may invoke transferring images between two locations. A workstation, e.g., may query a scanner using the C-FIND service and then initiate a move of images from the scanner to an archive. C-GET is a service to retrieve images from a sending device.

For every information object, service classes have to be separately defined and supported. Standardization for almost all diagnostic imaging modalities exist, but all of the participating equipment has to conform to the standards of all the information objects that shall be shared among the components to communicate. An archive, for instance, that supports the storage service class for MRI images will not be able to receive images from a CT scanner if it does not conform to the standard for CT images as well.

The storage commitment service class specifies the quality of storage provided by a device. Medical images are sensitive information and it is to be assured that images are stored reliably for a given amount of time. Reliability means that images must not get lost in the time span to which a storage device has committed itself. Such commitment was part of an analogue archiving system as well. However, digital image archiving required such commitment to be formalized so that it can be converted into a technical solution. Long-term storage devices such as long-term image archives commit to store an image permanently while short-term storage devices such as a departmental image archive commit to a specified amount of time.

3.3   Establishing DICOM Connectivity

This book is not intended to serve as a reference to image networking in a hospital. However, a computer scientist working in medical image analysis in a hospital may encounter a situation where he or she has to participate actively in establishing communication for accessing images in the hospital network. Hence, we will give a short overview on aspects of transferring such images.

With DICOM as accepted standard it would seem that the only question to ask is whether communication of a piece of equipment conforms to DICOM. Unfortunately this is not true. DICOM needs to be highly modularized to accommodate the large variety of information objects to be exchanged in a hospital and the wide range of services requested. DICOM conformity without further specification just means that the piece of equipment conforms to communication according to at least one of the many parts of the standard. Somebody who has to access images from a DICOM-conform image acquisition device, a DICOM archive, or a DICOM workstation needs to know just to which part of the standard this device conforms. For this purpose, every piece of equipment that is said to conform to the DICOM standard has to provide a *DICOM conformance statement*.

A DICOM conformance statement consists of four parts: problem statement, application entity specifications, communication profiles, and specialization. In the *problem statement*, the vendor states the purpose of communication for his piece of equipment (e.g., a DICOM conform CT scanner would state that its communication purpose is to transfer images to a storage device).

The major part of the conformance statement is the *application entity specification*. An application entity is a software module of the equipment implementing a specific application on the equipment. Several application entities may be imple-

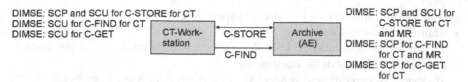

DIMSE: SCP and SCU for C-STORE for CT
DIMSE: SCU for C-FIND for CT
DIMSE: SCU for C-GET

CT-Work-station → C-STORE → Archive (AE)
← C-FIND

DIMSE: SCP and SCU for C-STORE for CT and MR
DIMSE: SCP for C-FIND for CT and MR
DIMSE: SCP for C-GET for CT

Fig. 3.11 It should be possible to decide whether two application entities are able to exchange information by comparing the desired service for the exchange with services offered by the AEs

mented. An entity that is intended to communicate using the DICOM standard will offer one or more services for one or more information objects. Information objects and the services to be provided are described here.

The *communication profile* then describes how services are communicated. Remember that DICOM specifies just the seventh layer of the ISO/OSI layered model. For successful communication, the lower layers have to be specified as well. The conformance statement will list and specify the necessary details such as supported media access protocols (FDDI, Ethernet, etc.) or supported physical media (fiber, coaxial cable, etc.).

The *specialization* part of the conformance statement relates to extensions and vendor-specific specializations. DICOM is designed to be extensible to support new types of equipment or new uses of equipment without invalidating the standard. This policy is implemented by allowing a certain degree of freedom in designing and filling templates of information objects. The subject will be discussed further when we explain the format of DICOM files, but it is of utmost importance that any of such extensions are described in detail in the specialization part of the conformance statement.

It should be possible to decide whether two pieces of DICOM-conform equipment can communicate based on the information in the conformance statements (see Fig. 3.11). If a CT system is SCP for C-STORE of CT information objects and some workstation is an SCU for the same service and information object and if the two components communicate using the TCP/IP protocol and are connected by an Ethernet connection, then the scanner should be able to send images to the workstation.

However, while it is true that the conformance statement greatly simplifies the installation of DICOM communication, it does not guarantee it. By comparing conformance statements, it may tell the engineer whether communication is possible at all. If, for instance, a new CT scanner should send images to an already installed archive, this will be only possible if common intermediate layers 1 to 6 of the OSI model exist and if the conformance statements of the two devices both implement at least the Storage Service class for CT images. Communication may still be impossible or limited for several reasons, including the following.

- Conformance has not been thoroughly tested and fails to establish in the specific environment.
- Information that is optional in the information object may be expected, but is not present.

- Optional information may be present in specialized fields.
- Claimed conformance is erroneous.

Hence, the compatibility of DICOM conformance statements does not ensure plug-and-play behavior of the equipment.

If devices of two different vendors shall be connected, it is sometimes difficult to establish who is violating the confirmations in the respective conformance statements. The search for necessary adjustments may be simpler if new equipment can be tested against some reference DICOM installation. Reference installations are open source software that do not only provide a standardized communication interface, but also allow insight in the communication process itself. It may help an experienced user to determine and fix possible problems for DICOM-based communication.

Client and server software for various DICOM services may be found at the DICOM website of OFFIS (DICOM Test Kit DCMTK, http://dicom.offis.de) or at the Mallinckrodt Institute of Radiology (DICOM Test Node DTN, http://milan.wustl.edu/DICOM/). These two testing modules have been used for several years as vendor-free installations for various demonstration projects and are the base for many of the open-source implementations of DICOM viewers.

3.4   The DICOM File Format

User-implemented image analysis methods usually are not directly integrated into software on a medical workstation communicating via DICOM with an archive or the image acquisition system. In most cases, the images to be analyzed are accessed as files stored on some offline medium. Chapter 10 of the DICOM standard describes a file format standard for communication using offline media. A description is found on NEMA's DICOM pages (http://medical.nema.org).

Since the file format has to support the storage of many different types of information objects, it has to be highly variable. On the other hand, the necessary effort for reading a file should be minimal. The two goals have been achieved by choosing a tagged format. Each tag relates to some data element (e.g., the patient name) of an information object. Its description can be found in a *data dictionary*.

The name of the DICOM file is its UID. Its content consists of a header of a fixed length followed by a sequence of tagged data elements. The header contains the following.

- A 128-byte preamble, which is meant to support specific DICOM implementations. It does not have to follow the tagged structure of the DICOM file. If it is not used, it should be filled with zeroes.
- A four byte identification by the ASCII codes of the letters "D," "I," "C," and "M." Again, this information is not tagged.
- A mandatory set of data elements containing meta-information about the file. Each of the data elements has to follow the tagged file format described below.

A data element consists of three parts: the *tag*, the *length* of the data element specified by the tag, and the *information* itself. The tag consists of a 4-byte *group*

Fig. 3.12 The tagged file
format makes interpretation
simple. Even if some data
elements are unknown, others
can be read, since unknown
elements are simply skipped

```
while not eof do begin
    int t_group = read_tag_group (file)
    int t_element = read_tag_element (file)
    int length = read_length (file)
    Interpret_Data (t_group, t_element, length, file)
endwhile

Interpret_Data()
        if t_group is even and exist(t_group, t_element) then
            interpret according to data dictionary
        else
            skip length bytes
```

number and a 4-byte *element number*. The length of the tag is a 4-byte element following the tag and indicates the number of bytes reserved for the following information.

An information object must contain all mandatory data elements as specified in the standard for this type of object. The standard may also list a number of optional data elements. The information object may be encapsulated according to the meta-information to provide possibilities for encrypting and/or compressing the data. If it is neither encrypted nor compressed, it consists of a sequence of tagged data elements similar to the ones in the meta-information.

Tags are listed by their group and element number in the data dictionary. The data dictionary is part of the DICOM standard and can be found on NEMA's website. It also describes how data are represented (bytes may be interpreted as ASCII code or as various types of integers).

Odd group numbers are reserved for allowing vendor-specific adaptations or specializations. Hence, tags with odd group numbers will not appear in the data dictionary. These groups are also called *shadow groups*. Sometimes, shadow groups are used to represent nonmandatory data elements, which is an efficient way to hide this information. It is possible that the same tag of a shadow group may describe different information for files stemming from different systems because group and element numbers of shadow groups need not be unique.

The semantic of tags from shadow groups must be explained in the conformance statement. Only then will it be possible to interpret all the information contained in transmitted or stored data. Even then the interpretation of the data may be difficult because files may be exchanged without sharing the conformance statement.

Data elements of which the tag definition is missing may be skipped by a DICOM reader since the length of information of a data element is part of the representation. This helps in dealing with unknown shadow groups and it enables reading data without a data dictionary (see Fig. 3.12 for a simple DICOM reader). For the latter, tag interpretation of only the most vital information for reading the data is hard-coded into the reader program. This is a solution of some software products that read the DICOM file format. The advantage is its simplicity although it is clearly insufficient for a DICOM reader within a PACS.

3.5 Technical Properties of Medical Images

Medical images differ from ordinary images taken by a camera in several aspects because they are visualized measurement values (as explained in Chap. 2). This has consequences on the technical properties of these images. With technical properties we mean attributes that result from the image acquisition technique and that are independent of the image's semantics.

Medical images may come with two, three, or four dimensions. 2D images may be slices of the human body such as an ultrasound image or a single CT slice. They may also be projections of a 3D scene such as an x-ray image or a scintigram. 3D images are volumes of the human body such as a 3D sequence from computed tomography, or time sequences of 2D images. 4D images are 3D volumes acquired over time. The DICOM file format in which images are stored often treats 2D images as an information unit even if they are part of a 3D or 4D sequence. A 3D data set is then treated as a sequence and a 4D data set is treated as a study of several sequences.

Images may be differentiated into projection and slice images. In projection images, image attributes are integrated along rays and projected on a single pixel. The type of projection is important, if measurements in such images shall be made. For a cone beam projection such as in x-ray radiography an unambiguous relationship between distance in the image and distance in imaged space cannot be established.

Images may be acquired at several signal bands (e.g., in MRI imaging, see Chap. 2). If done so, these bands are stored separately. Two different bands may even be stored as separate studies. Interpretation is only possible if the image file information about the semantic of each image with respect to the signal can be retrieved.

Image sizes given in the DICOM tags relate to the number of pixels per column or row. The true physical size of a pixel or voxel (in mm or cm) are mandatory data elements that can be found if the tag identification is known (either from the data dictionary or hard-coded in the image reading program).

Pixel values of medical images are quantized. The quantization often differs from digital photos. The range may exceed 256 values when the information acquired by the imaging device justifies a bigger quantization range. Pixel values are stored as integers. The storage reserved for a single pixel is one or two bytes depending on the quantization range. For 2-byte-per-pixel images often only 12 bits are used. Sometimes negative values are stored (e.g., to represent Hounsfield units which begin at -1000).

The user should be aware that there is no guarantee that different vendors represent values in the same fashion. This is especially true if the file format for data exchange is nonstandard. Hounsfield units, e.g., may be represented on a scale from -1000 to 3000 or—shifted—as unsigned integers on a scale from 0 to 4000.

Transferring digital image files between systems may involve changing between big-endian and little-endian notation of the two bytes. This refers to whether the first or the last byte is the most significant byte in a 2-byte-word. It should be no problem if communication is standardized, but needs to be considered otherwise. It is easily recognized when looking at the images (see Fig. 3.13). Endianity may also be different for the bit-order in a byte.

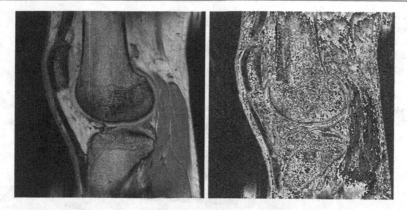

Fig. 3.13 MR image with correct endianity (scaled from its original range 0...4000 to 0...255) and the same image with endianity reversed

Sometimes, pixels or voxels of images presented for postprocessing are reduced to single bytes. This is the case when images are transferred via formats that do not support a wider range. The mapping from 2 to 1 byte may have been created expertly and intentionally to highlight specific details in an image. It may support human capabilities of recognizing important aspects in an image, but computer-based methods operate on very different assumptions than human vision. The reduction, while being supportive for human perception, may be counterproductive to computer-based image interpretation.

3.6   Displays and Workstations

Traditionally, many medical images—x-ray images, computer tomograms, MR images— are viewed as hard copies. Hard copies are readily transportable and readily readable. No specific equipment is needed to perceive a hard copy radiograph although a light box system is required for professional reading.

For reading an image by a radiologist, the film is placed in front of a light box (see Fig. 3.14). Reporting or other evaluation tasks are carried out there. Film has a number of advantages. Backlit light boxes allow for a good control of perceived contrast. This is further supported by the fact that most light boxes are large and are at a fixed position where lighting conditions can be controlled. A modern light box system can easily carry several hundreds of films. On such a system, films are mounted beforehand. Several of the films may be presented simultaneously. They can be selected at the push of a button from the set of films mounted.

Replacing analogue data transfer and display by a PACS has advantages. Most notably, digital data can be easily copied and transferred to any location reachable on the network. Transfer may also be extended to long distances in a short time (teleradiology). Replacing the analogue archive by a digital archive also makes localizing images easier. It has been reported that accessibility increased from 70%

Fig. 3.14 Light box in a traditional reading room: The system can be loaded with several hundreds of films. Films to be read are loaded immediately using a handheld or a foot control (with kind permission of Planilux, Warstein, Germany)

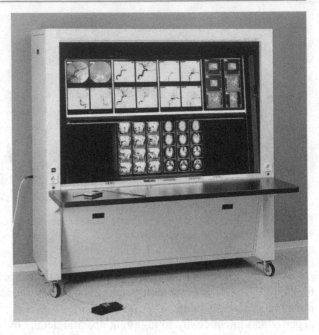

to 98% after switching from analogue to digital archives. Another advantage is that image enhancement techniques such as magnification or contrast enhancement may support image interpretation.

Replacing film viewing by displaying images on a screen should preserve most of the advantages of a film-based reporting. The first problem to be solved relates to image transfer. The capacity of the "muscle net" (i.e., carrying films around) can be surprisingly high and may compare favorably to digital transfer capacities if the network infrastructure is poor.

Although this is becoming a problem of the past with improvement of the network infrastructure, perceived transfer capacity may still be unsatisfactory. Conventionally transported radiographs are "invisibly" transferred to places, i.e., the user does not perceive transport time as waiting time (although he or she may get upset about pictures not or not yet delivered). Once pictures are present, all of them are immediately at his or her disposal.

In a digital environment, the user initiates the image transfer. The time span between the request and completion of an image transfer is perceived as waiting time. Although an 80% decrease in preparation time has been reported after switching to digital reporting, this includes time spent by technicians and archive support staff. The radiologist may still feel that the waiting time increased with the introduction of a digital system. With increased data sizes—a CT study from a modern multislice CT scanner may contain more than 1000 slices—the situation may worsen, as even a fast network may need several minutes to transfer the data. Faster networks and intelligent solutions similar to those preparing a conventional reading session can help to reduce this problem.

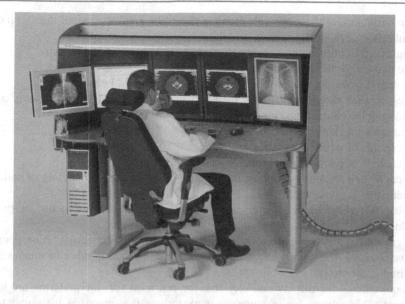

Fig. 3.15 A reading room as part of a PACS displays images on monitors instead of light boxes. Active and passive components of the depicted system control the lighting situation (with kind permission of Planilux, Warstein, Germany)

Another problem is the limited spatial and contrast resolution of a monitor. The contrast range of today's TFT monitors is quite satisfactory, but monitor placement and the influence from external lighting can reduce perceived image contrast. A professional reading system will allow to control such influence (see Fig. 3.15 for an example).

The spatial resolution of a conventional monitor is about 2 megapixels, whereas a digital radiograph may contain up to 4096×4096 pixels ($=16$ megapixels). There are few monitors that are able to display such a resolution. Hence, a professional reading station is much more expensive than a conventional TFT monitor.

Furthermore, a reading room usually contains several light boxes that are able to display several images at the same time. Using several monitors instead is only a partial replacement since there will never be enough monitor space to display as many images as can be displayed on a big light box (see Fig. 3.15 for an example and compare it to Fig. 3.14). A suitable user interface for switching between views has to make up for this deficiency.

There are no legal standards for the display of digital radiography, but the American College of Radiology (ACR) has developed some recommendations. The ACR distinguishes between the images used for diagnosis (interpretation) and those used for other purposes (clinical review, teaching, etc.). According to ACR, the image quality should be sufficient to satisfy the needs of the clinical circumstances if images are meant for display use only. Their recommendations for display and display software are as follows.

- The luminance of the gray-scale monitor should be greater or equal than 50 foot-lamberts.
- Controlled lighting should enable eliminating reflections in the monitor.
- The ambient light level should be as low as feasible.
- A capability for the selection of image sequences should be provided.
- The software should be capable of associating the patient with the study and demographic characterizations with the images.
  The rendering software for images should
- be capable of window and level adjustment,
- be capable of pan and zoom (magnification) functions,
- be capable of rotating or flipping the images, provided correct labeling of patient orientation is preserved,
- be capable of calculating and displaying accurate linear measurements and pixel values,
- be capable of displaying prior image compression ratio, processing, or cropping,
- have available the matrix size, the bit depth, and the total number of images acquired in the study.

Requirements for display consoles that are not used for interpretation are less stringent. This relates, for instance, to workstations that are used for computer-assisted procedures. There are two places where such work can take place:
- workstations as part of the image acquisition system,
- independent workstations in the hospital network.

Most vendors sell workstations and workstation software for postprocessing image data. These workstations are a part of the imaging system and as such may communicate with image acquisition devices in some nonstandard fashion. Standardized communication is not really necessary unless such a workstation is meant to be connected to the network. Methods for image processing are predefined by the vendor of the imaging device (a typical user interface for such a workstation software is depicted in Fig. 3.16). They are generally not open (i.e., they are neither adaptable nor extendable). Software being delivered with such a workstation falls in six different groups.
- Image display: Retrieval and display of images, setting window and level of the mapping between image values and rendered intensities, printing of images.
- Image enhancement: Magnification, contrast enhancement, noise filtering.
- Image annotation.
- Image analysis: Measurements of distances and angles, volume estimation or volume measurements, simple segmentation techniques.
- 3D imaging: Slice view in cine mode, maximum intensity projection, surface and volume rendering.
- Specialized interpretation or support to a specific planning task (e.g., surgical, radiotherapeutical).

Workstations at imaging devices support the radiologist in interpreting the images. If the results of such postprocessing of images are exported, it is carried out by using the DICOM standard or by creating hard copies. Analysis results may not be mandatory data elements of the DICOM standard. Tags for their description may belong to the shadow groups.

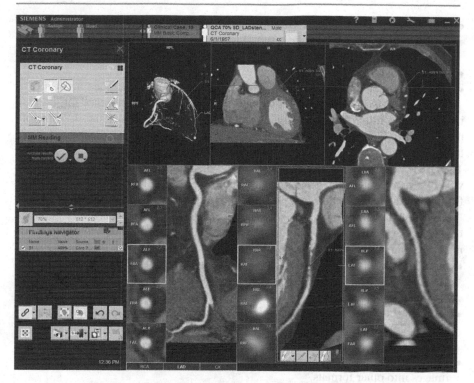

Fig. 3.16 Example of a user interface of a DICOM viewer software. The software is able to interpret the information in the DICOM header and organizes images accordingly. Viewing software includes display and simple tools such as setting window and level or annotating the image (with kind permission of Siemens Sector Healthcare, Erlangen, Germany)

Workstations elsewhere in the network and independent of the image acquisition system may be used for postprocessing image data as well. Such workstations were first offered by vendors selling archiving equipment. An image archive is intentionally meant to make images accessible and it was an obvious strategy to provide processing methods as well.

Images in the archive are associated with records in the RIS. Access to them may be realized through the RIS or PACS interface. Communication with such a workstation is carried out using the DICOM standard and/or the RIS interface. Such a workstation allows radiologists or clinicians anywhere in the hospital direct access to images, provided that they have been granted access to the RIS/PACS.

Images may also be accessed from other workstations connected to the network. DICOM client software such as contained in the DICOM Test Kit (see Sect. 3.3) is needed that pulls images from the archive, the imaging device, or some other workstation. A more comfortable solution is a DICOM viewer, which is able to query other modalities and display the results in some organized fashion. The functionality of a DICOM viewer should consist of the following.

- An implementation of a query to the data base of a DICOM sender (C-FIND).

- An implementation of the C-GET to retrieve images.
- An interface for displaying the result of a query and for selecting queried images to be fetched.
- A rendering module to display retrieved images.
- A storage module that stores retrieved images on the local machine.

Free DICOM viewers can be found on the internet. A good reference for searching a viewer is http://www.idoimaging.com already mentioned in Chap. 1. Some of the viewers only support accessing DICOM files on a local storage device and need to be combined with suitable client software to transfer images to local storage. The DICOM viewer may be used for selecting images for further processing (which would have to be developed and implemented by the user). The viewer may contain further routines that support interpretation or computer-based analysis.

Selecting an appropriate viewer can be difficult. Some viewers are very good in reading and exporting images while others have many useful modules to display and manipulate images. Our current favorites are the following.

- microDicom (http://www.microdicom.com/) is sufficient to display images and view tags. Since it has been implemented as a 64-bit version it is able to handle large data sets (large 3D studies, 4D data sets).
- ezdicom (http://sourceforge.net/projects/ezdicom) is fast and appropriate for displaying images. Tags are not always interpreted correctly. DICOM studies cannot be read.
- dicomWorks (http://dicom.online.fr) reads DICOM studies and is able to export images into other formats.
- MeVislab (http://www.mevislab.de) is—as detailed in Chap. 1—much more than a DICOM viewer, but also displays images, interprets DICOM tags, and exports images.
- OsiriX (http://www.osirix-viewer.com) is software for MAC OS.

The suggestions have to be taken with a grain of salt, however. The selection reflects the current interest of our group when dealing with DICOM images. Furthermore, open-source software may improve rapidly. Some research and experimentation with the software listed on the website mentioned above will always be necessary to find the current best software for a specific purpose.

3.7   Compression of Medical Images

DICOM supports data compression. Images may be compressed lossless or lossy. Lossless compression such as entropy encoding or run-length encoding typically result in compression rates of 1:2 to 1:3. Lossy compression achieves much higher compression rates in the range 1:10 to 1:30. Anybody who ever created a JPEG image knows that most images contain much psychovisual redundancy since data reduction does not automatically reduce the perceived image quality.

Regarding medical images, lossy compression is a difficult issue. Laws in most countries require that medical images are to be saved for a given time. The intention of these laws is that decisions that have been based on these images can be reviewed based on the original data. If data have been compressed for saving storage space, their original content must be retrievable, which prohibits lossy compression.

However, there are other reasons for image compression. If images are transferred in a teleradiology network, their purpose is to provide the person at the receiving end with additional information. This person may be a senior radiologist at home who has to decide whether attendance in the hospital is required. It may also be a transferring radiologist at a small clinic who receives images from one of his patients taken and interpreted in a medical center. In such cases, image compression may be lossy if the partners in the data exchange have agreed that this loss does not constitute a loss of information for the kind of purpose.

There are no general rules as to the quality of such images since image interpretation is to be carried out or confirmed by reading the original images. A recommendation of the American College of Radiology states, however, that, clinically, diagnostic image quality must not be reduced. While this does not rule out lossy compression it is not clear whether it can be established statistically by means of readability studies or whether it requires expert decisions for every individual image.

Compression is part of the DICOM standard. Among others, the JPEG and JPEG2000 standards have been adopted by the DICOM standardization committee. The DICOM committee does not make a decision about the type of compression, whether lossless or lossy. Not all DICOM viewers, however, can read compressed DICOM images. It may also be an obstacle to a self-written DICOM image interpreter when the data have first to be uncompressed before they can be interpreted.

3.8   Concluding Remarks

There are a plethora of resources regarding the two standards HL7 and DICOM, their development, and their role in the clinical environment. Good sources for getting a grip on this topic are the Journal of the American Medical Informatics Association, the Journal of Digital Imaging, Radiology, and the European Journal of Radiology.

A short description of the HL7 protocol is given by Hammond (1993). The new version 3 of HL7 is described in Beeler (1999). The complete description is available at the HL7 website http://www.hl7.org.

An introductory text about the requirements and current state of Picture Archiving and Communication Systems is Bick and Lenzen (1999). Tutorial publications on the DICOM standard directed towards nonexperts in information systems are the papers of Bidgood et al. (1997) and Horii (1997). Honeyman et al. (1996) and Mulvaney (2002) described the current state of integrating DICOM-based PACS with HL7-based RIS systems. The annual SPIE conference Medical Imaging has a conference devoted to PACS and Medical Informatics, where numerous reports about introducing DICOM-based PACS in hospitals have been published. The same is true for the InfoRAD section of the annual RSNA meetings. While the challenges and problems of introducing a PACS may be more of interest for scientists dealing

with clinical information systems, knowledge about the transfer and representation
of images is vital for developing and using image-processing methods. Manufacturers usually do not publish their format specifications, but David Clunie (2005)
maintains an extensive website about medical image formats. Detailed descriptions
of several proprietary data formats as well as about the DICOM file format can be
found at his site.

3.9   Exercises

- What is the difference between an HIS and an RIS? Why is it useful to have
  several different information systems in a hospital?
- Which information systems communicate via the HL7 standard?
- Which aspect of the seventh level of the ISO/OSI standard is not included in the
  HL7 standard?
- What is the main difference between the versions 2.x and 3 of HL7?
- Name potential reasons for the failure to connect via the HL7 standard.
- What is the purpose of a PACS? What is the difference to a RIS?
- What is an information object in the DICOM standard?
- What are the names for client and server in DICOM terminology?
- Where is information to be found that is necessary to connect a new piece of
  equipment to a system that supports DICOM?
- What are potential reasons for the failure to establish connectivity under DICOM?
- When is it useful to use DICOM test nodes and what kind of information can be
  gained from such use?
- Why is the DICOM file format a tagged format?
- Explain the structure of a DICOM file. What are the general components and how
  is the structure of a tagged information entity in the file?
- What information is contained in the data dictionary and how does this support
  reading DICOM files?
- How can DICOM files be interpreted without the use of a data dictionary? What
  are the disadvantages of this?
- What do shadow groups mean? Why are they necessary and what are the disad-
  vantages of this?
- What is the range of values of a CT image?
- What are the differences when reading film as opposed to reading digital images?
- What are the requirements for displays of a medical workstation?
- List a number of image manipulation methods that can be expected to be offered
  in a medical workstation.
- What are the reasons for avoiding or even prohibiting lossy compression of med-
  ical images? When could it be used nonetheless?

References

Beeler GW (1999) Taking HL7 to the next level. Comput Med Pract 16(3):21–24

Bick U, Lenzen H (1999) PACS: the silent revolution. Eur J Radiol 9(6):1152–1160

Bidgood WD, Horii SC, Prior FW, van Syckle DE (1997) Understanding and using DICOM, the data interchange standard for biomedical imaging. J Am Med Inform Assoc 4(3):199–212

Clunie DA (2005) Medical image format FAQ. http://www.dclunie.com/medical-image-faq/html/

Hammond WE (1993) Health level 7. A protocol for the interchange of healthcare data. Stud Health Technol Inform 6:144–148

Honeyman JC, Frost MM, Moser R, Huda W, Staab EV (1996) RIS requirements to support a PACS infrastructure. Proc SPIE 2711:120–125 (Medical imaging 1996)

Horii SC (1997) Primer on computers and information technology. Part 4: A non-technical introduction to DICOM. Radiographics 17(5):1297–1309

Mulvaney J (2002) The case for RIS/PACS integration. Radiol Manage 24(3):24–29

Image Enhancement

4

Abstract

Two reasons exist for applying an image enhancement technique. Enhancement can increase the perceptibility of objects in an image to the human observer or it may be needed as a preprocessing step for subsequent automatic image analysis. Enhancement methods differ for the two purposes.

An enhancement method requires a criterion by which its success can be judged. This will be a definition of image quality since improving quality is the goal of such a method. Various quality definitions will be presented and discussed.

Different enhancement techniques will be presented covering methods for contrast enhancement, for the enhancement of edges, for noise reduction, and for edge-preserving smoothing.

Concepts, notions and definitions introduced in this chapter

> Measures of image resolution and contrast
> The modulation transfer function
> Signal-to-noise ratio
> Contrast and resolution enhancement
> Noise reduction and edge enhancement by linear filtering
> Edge-preserving smoothing by median filtering, diffusion filtering, and Bayesian image restoration

A seemingly simple operation on digital images is to enhance the image or features in the image. The main purpose of it is to map a given image to another image such that the content to be depicted is now easier to recognize. In medical imaging, image enhancement essentially enhances contrast by reducing any artefacts or noise in the image or by emphasizing the differences between objects.

The reason for enhancement is to make structures more easily detectable by a human observer. It may also serve as some necessary preprocessing step for further automatic analysis. While in the latter case success or failure may be found by ex-

K.D. Toennies, *Guide to Medical Image Analysis*,
Advances in Computer Vision and Pattern Recognition,
DOI 10.1007/978-1-4471-2751-2_4, © Springer-Verlag London Limited 2012

perimenting (e.g., does some image processing task perform better with or without the enhancement step?), deciding on the effectiveness of the former can be difficult because it requires modeling the human observer.

Quantitative measures of image quality will help as they describe the aspects of an image that are relevant to human or computer analysis independent of an observer. The improvement of quality measures is then evidence for the success of an enhancement procedure. Some of the measures can also be used to construct a method that only improves this measure.

It should be noted that image quality for visual inspection by human or computer vision depends on many influences that require knowledge of the specific detection task. These include image content, observation task, visualization quality, and performance of the observer. Measures that can be computed a priori make assumptions about these aspects or exclude them from the definition of quality.

4.1   Measures of Image Quality

4.1.1   Spatial and Contrast Resolution

The spatial and contrast *resolution* already being used in Chap. 2 to characterize images, determine the smallest structure that can be represented in a digital image. These two measures are easily computable and relevant to digital image processing. Structures can only be analyzed (delineated, measured, etc.) if they appear in the image. Spatial resolution describes this directly since the sampling theorem states that no detail with a frequency less than twice the sampling distance can be represented without aliasing. The contrast resolution is an indirect measure of the perceptibility of structures. The number of intensity levels has an influence on the likelihood with which two neighboring structures with similar but not equal appearance will be represented by different intensities.

Subsequent enhancement steps such as noise removal (described below) can reduce intensity differences further, which may have consequences for the recognizability of structures if the original intensity difference was small.

Technical measures of resolution do not, however, relate directly to the ability of humans to recognize a structure. Human visual processing involves a combination of various enhancement techniques such as smoothing, edge enhancement, contrast enhancement at edges, and the like. Hence, perceived resolution, as opposed to technical resolution, cannot easily be reduced to a single cause such as spatial resolution.

Perceived resolution may be measured experimentally by treating the human visual system as a black box system with images as input and recognized objects determining resolution as output. The same kind of measure is also used when loss of resolution by transfer of information through a technical system shall be documented (such as creating a radiograph from a scene). The quantity that is measured is called *line pairs per millimeter* (lpmm), which refers to the thinnest pair of parallel black and white lines that can be differentiated (either by a human observer or by an image analysis algorithm). A sequence of parallel pairs of black and white lines

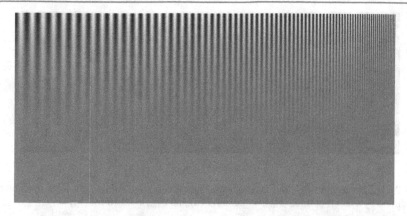

Fig. 4.1 A test pattern for determining perceived resolution in line pairs per millimeter (lpmm). The number of line pairs per millimeter increases *from left to right* while the contrast decreases *from top to bottom*. It can be seen that perceived resolution depends on the contrast in the image and also that this relationship is non-linear

with decreasing line thickness is displayed (see Fig. 4.1). The apparent resolution is $1/x$ lpmm if the thickness of the thinnest line pair is x mm. The measure is proportional to frequency, but it is a more figurative expression and easier to understand.

Perceived resolution by a human is not independent of contrast. An object stands out less against the background if the intensity difference between the object and background is low. Perceived resolution may sometimes be even higher than technical resolution because decreasing contrast may be interpreted as PVE due to the subvoxel size of the object. For instance, vessels are visible in contrast-enhanced MR angiography that are smaller than the voxel size because of the PVE.

4.1.2   Definition of Contrast

Determining contrast requires knowledge about what is an object and what is background. Since this is unknown prior to analysis, a number of measures for calculating image contrast exist that makes implicit assumptions about image content. Examples for object-independent contrast measures are global contrast, global variance, entropy, and contrast from the co-occurrence matrix.

Global contrast $C_{\text{Michelson}}$ according to the Michelson equations (Peli 1990) simply compares the ratio of difference between the highest and the lowest intensity values l_{max} and l_{min} of an image to the average intensity level given by the sum of l_{max} and l_{min}:

$$C_{\text{Michelson}} = \frac{l_{\text{max}} - l_{\text{min}}}{l_{\text{max}} + l_{\text{min}}}. \tag{4.1}$$

The measure assumes a simple image in which the number of foreground pixels approximately equals that of the background pixels. *Michelson contrast* ranges from 0 to 1. It is 1.0 if the full range of intensity values is used and less than 1.0 otherwise.

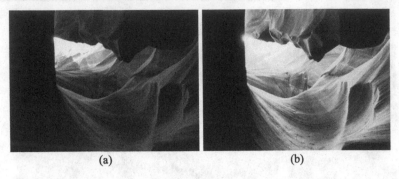

(a)   (b)

Fig. 4.2 The two images have the same global contrast $C_{\text{Michelson}}$, while their local rms contrast C_{rms} differs by a factor of three ($C_{\text{rms}} = 0.006$ for (**a**) and $C_{\text{rms}} = 0.018$ for (**b**))

It is a useful measure to quantify the inefficient usage of the available intensity range. However, it does not account for the distribution of intensities in the image (see Fig. 4.2a). An image could be highly underexposed with most of the pixels having intensities below some low threshold but having just one pixel with value I_{max}, possibly caused by an artefact. The image would be perfect according to global contrast.

A somewhat better approach for measuring global contrast is the *root-mean-square (rms) contrast* (see Fig. 4.2b). Given an image (x, y) with $M \cdot N$ pixels and intensities $l(x, y)$, the expected value of l is

$$\bar{l} = \frac{1}{MN} \sum_{i=0}^{M-1} \sum_{j=0}^{N-1} l(i, j),$$ (4.2)

and the *rms* contrast is

$$C_{\text{rms}}(f) = \sqrt{\frac{1}{MN - 1} \sum_{i=0}^{M-1} \sum_{j=0}^{N-1} \left(l(i, j) - \bar{l} \right)^2}.$$ (4.3)

The measure takes all pixels into account instead of just the pixels with maximum and minimum intensity values.

C_{rms} does not differentiate well between different intensity distributions. Assuming $l_{\text{min}} = 0$, an image containing just two intensity levels $0.75 \cdot l_{\text{max}}$ and $0.25 \cdot l_{\text{max}}$ would have approximately the same variance than another one that contains all intensities between 0 and l_{max} equally distributed. If both are images of the same scene, the latter may show more details than the former.

Entropy as a contrast measure includes histogram characteristics into the measure. It is computed from the normalized histogram of image intensities. A histogram $H(l)$ of an image $l(x, y)$ gives the frequency of occurrence for each intensity. A *normalized histogram* $H_{\text{norm}}(l)$ is computed from $H(l)$ by

$$H_{\text{norm}}(l) = \frac{H(l)}{\sum_{k=I_{\text{min}}}^{I_{\text{max}}} H(k)}. \tag{4.4}$$

It gives the probability of l to appear in an image. If $H_{\text{norm}}(20) = 0.05$, the probability is 0.05 that the gray value of a randomly picked pixel is 20.

Entropy is computed from H_{norm}. It is being used in information theory for determining the average information capacity of a pixel. Entropy is a convenient measure for estimating compression rates for images for a type of lossless compression,[1] but it may also be interpreted as representing the amount of information contained in an image. Increased entropy of an image would indicate enhanced contrast.

Information capacity is defined assuming that information $I(l)$ of a pixel with intensity l is inversely proportional to the probability of its occurrence. Thus,

$$I(l) = \left(H_{\text{norm}}(l)\right)^{-1}. \tag{4.5}$$

If information is stored in a binary number, the number of required digits would be

$$SI(l) = \log_2 \frac{1}{H_{\text{norm}}(l)} = -\log_2 H_{\text{norm}}(l). \tag{4.6}$$

The distribution of intensities of all pixels in the histogram can be used to compute the total number of digits needed to encode the image

$$SI_{\text{total}}(H) = -\sum_{k=I_{\text{min}}}^{I_{\text{max}}} H_{\text{norm}}(k) \log_2 H_{\text{norm}}(k). \tag{4.7}$$

The entropy C_{entropy} is then the average signal length needed (see Fig. 4.3 for an example):

$$C_{\text{entropy}}(H) = -\frac{1}{MN} \sum_{k=I_{\text{min}}}^{I_{\text{max}}} H_{\text{norm}}(k) \log_2 H_{\text{norm}}(k), \tag{4.8}$$

where MN is the number of pixels in f.

Entropy still does not account for the fact that contrast should measure intensity differences between some foreground and background object. This can be computed using a *gray-level co-occurrence matrix (GLCM)*. Co-occurrence calculates the normalized rates of co-occurring intensity values in a given neighborhood. The neighborhood is defined by the distance and direction between the two pixels. Hence, co-occurrence $C_{\alpha,d}$ is a two-dimensional function of intensities l_1 and l_2. $C_{\alpha,d}(l_1, l_2)$

---

[1]Compression rates of a lossless compression method using signal compression are bounded by the entropy. These methods compress pixels independent of their neighborhood. It can be shown that the maximum compression rate is the ratio of bits per pixel in the image to bits per pixel as predicted by entropy. Lossless compression using other kinds of methods such as run-length encoding may achieve higher compression rates.

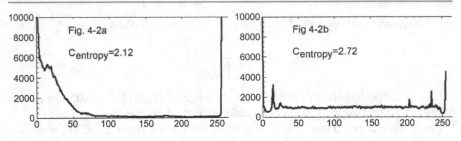

Fig. 4.3 Histograms of the pictures in Fig. 4.2 and entropy-based contrast measure

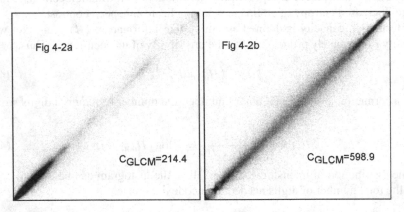

Fig. 4.4 Coocurrence matrices for the two pictures in Fig. 4.2 and entropy-based contrast measure C_{GLCM}

is the probability with which pixels with intensities l_1 and l_2 occur such that pixel l_1 and l_2 are d units apart at an angle of α with the x-axis. Co-occurrence matrices can be computed with different distances and different directions representing intensity changes between structures at different angles and with different sharpness at the edge.

For measuring contrast in a given image, co-occurrence is computed for a fixed distance (e.g., $d = 1$ pixel) and for arbitrary angles. $C_d(l_1, l_2)$ is then the co-occurrence of pixels with gray levels l_1 and l_2 at distance d with an arbitrary angle (Fig. 4.4 shows an example for the two images in Fig. 4.2). For $d = 1$ this would be the four pixels of the 4-neighborhood. Contrast C_{GLCM} is then defined as

$$C_{\mathrm{GLCM}} = \frac{1}{I_{\max}^2} \sum_{i=0}^{I_{\max}} \sum_{j=0}^{I_{\max}} C_d(i, j)\big(1 + (i - j)^2\big) - 1. \qquad (4.9)$$

Contrast thus weights the co-occurrences of two intensities by the difference between the two. Higher differences indicating edges receive higher weights.

4.1.3   The Modulation Transfer Function

To a large extent, the improvement of contrast and resolution are constrained by technical parameters of an imaging modality. Artefacts, noise, and approximations in the reconstruction may reduce contrast in the original measurement due to reconstruction. The degradation that an image suffers through reconstruction, transfer, or any other process that changes contrast, is described by the modulation transfer function (MTF). An MTF is a function of frequency (or of resolution in lpmm), which describes the extent of signal loss (damping) with respect to frequency. It is used, for instance, to describe the loss of contrast, when creating an x-ray image. It can also be used to describe the discrimination performance of human vision with respect to varying contrast. Curiously enough, the human observer MTF does not exhibit a monotone decrease with frequency, but peaks at some low frequency. In other words, contrast at low frequency needs to be higher for recognizing an object than in midrange. This justifies edge sharpening (described below) for enhancing perceived resolution.

4.1.4   Signal-to-Noise Ratio (SNR)

Noise in an image is another factor limiting the perceptibility of objects in an image. So far, all information in an image is assumed to be useful. Noise is an unwanted, image-corrupting influence. Noise $n(i, j)$ in an image is usually described as a random fluctuation of intensities with zero mean. If noise is assumed to be normally distributed, variance $\sigma^2(n)$ or standard deviation $\sigma(n)$ characterizes the noise level. Object detection depends on the ratio of object-background-contrast to noise variance. The former is called the difference signal between the object and background and it is related to noise in the *signal-to-noise ratio (SNR)*:

$$SNR(f) = S(f)/\sigma(n). \tag{4.10}$$

Various specifications exist of what the difference signal should be leading to different definitions for measuring the signal-to-noise ratio in an image. In the simplest case, signal $S(f)$ is defined to be the largest intensity f_{max} (*peak SNR*) or the average intensity $E(f)$. The two measures take the maximum or average image contrast between all objects in the image into account. They can be computed without analysis as to which objects should be recognized in the image.

A common measure, which is measured in dB, is given by the logarithm of the ratio of signal and noise variance

$$SNR_{dB} = 10 \cdot \log_{10}\left[\frac{1}{MN} \frac{\sum_{i=0}^{M-1} \sum_{j=0}^{N-1} (f(i, j) - \bar{f})^2}{\sigma^2}\right]. \tag{4.11}$$

The increase in *SNR* may indicate the enhancement of the image. If *SNR* shall be used as an absolute quantity to determine the perceptibility of objects, the difference signal has to reflect the difference between the object and background intensity.

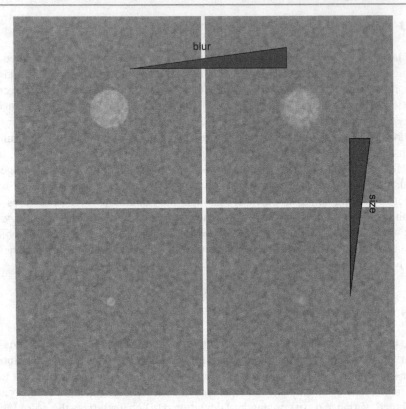

Fig. 4.5 The four images have the same noise level, noise characteristics and contrast. Object-dependent features such as the size of the object or the sharpness of boundaries still cause differences in the perceptibility of depicted objects

None of the quantities listed covers the dependency of recognizing objects based on their size, shape, sharpness of edges, and texture as it would require prior detection of the object in the image. This should be kept in mind. Two images with equal contrast or noise characteristics may still be perceived as being of different quality (see Fig. 4.5).

The dependency of recognizability on object shape exists sometimes for a computer algorithm as well. It is possible, for instance, to recognize an object with $SNR < 1$ (i.e., where the noise exceeds the signal) if the object is large enough. Human vision and also some computer-based enhancement techniques are able to reduce noise in such a case while leaving the signal more or less intact. The potential for such recognition ability cannot be measured or deduced from the image unless the kind of structures to be recognized are known.

4.2   Image Enhancement Techniques

Originally, image enhancement methods were meant to enhance the perceptibility of information. Hence, contrast or edge enhancement improve the image for inspection by a human observer. This should be kept in mind when considering an enhancement procedure. Although most of the methods are also valuable and necessary preprocessing steps for automatic analysis, some of them—such as contrast enhancement—are not since they do not improve the relation between information and artefacts in the image.

4.2.1   Contrast Enhancement

Some of the contrast enhancement techniques can be directly related to contrast measures described in the previous section. The simplest method increases global contrast. If the range of possible intensity values I_{min} to I_{max} exceeds the range of intensities f_{min} to f_{max}, *linear contrast enhancement* is carried out creating new values g from intensities f for every pixel by

$$g(f) = (f - f_{min}) \frac{I_{max}}{f_{max} - f_{min}} + I_{min}. \tag{4.12}$$

The function to map f on g is called the *transfer function*. Contrast enhancement in an arbitrary intensity window w_{min} to w_{max} with $I_{min} < w_{min} < w_{max} < I_{max}$ can be achieved with a similar transfer function. As there may be pixels with values f outside the window, (4.12) is changed to (see Fig. 4.6)

$$g(f) = \begin{cases} I_{min}, & \text{if } f < w_{min}, \\ (f - w_{min}) \frac{I_{max}}{w_{max} - w_{min}} + I_{min}, & \text{if } w_{min} \le f \le w_{max}, \\ I_{max}, & \text{if } f > w_{max}. \end{cases} \tag{4.13}$$

The output intensity of structures with input intensities outside of $[w_{min}, w_{max}]$ is either I_{min} or I_{max} so that they are no longer recognizable. Contrast is improved for all other structures. This kind of enhancement is routinely used for mapping a 16-bit-per-pixel intensity image (such as CT or MRI) onto an 8-bit range. It is called *windowing* with window size $w_{max} - w_{min}$ and level $(w_{max} + w_{min})/2$.

Entropy is enhanced using *histogram equalization*. Assuming that intensities of some image f with normalized histogram $H_{norm}(f)$ are defined on a continuous domain, histogram equalization maximizes entropy by creating a new image g with a constant histogram. The transfer function is

$$g(f) = \int_{I_{min}}^{f} H_{norm}(f) \, df. \tag{4.14}$$

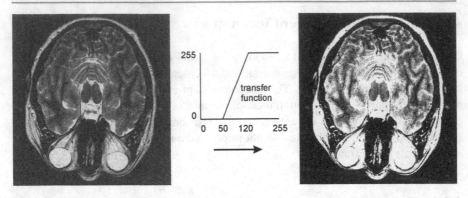

Fig. 4.6 Linear contrast enhancement in a window (50, 120) for enhancing soft tissue differences in an MR image. The enhancement comes at the cost of reducing contrast in regions outside of the window (such as the water in the eye balls)

Intensities are quantized and, hence, histogram equalization is approximated by

$$g(f) = \left| (I_{\max} - I_{\min} + 1) \sum_{i=I_{\min}}^{f} H_{\text{norm}}(i) \right| - 1. \tag{4.15}$$

Histogram equalization does not always achieve the desired effect. Using entropy as a measure for information content implies that information of often occurring intensities should be increased by spreading them over a larger range. It comes at the cost of reduced information for intensities that rarely occur. Entropy does not consider any information about objects in an image and each pixel is equally important. For instance, the large and dark background region of the MR image in Fig. 4.7 is to be enhanced at the cost of reducing contrast in the foreground.

Histogram equalization can be improved by making it locally adaptive. In *adaptive histogram equalization*, local histograms are computed separately for every pixel from the intensity distribution in some neighborhood around this pixel. The resulting mapping is carried out separately for each pixel. This definitely improves local contrast because a large region in some location of the image no longer influences contrast of some small detail at another location. However, it does no longer guarantee that $f(i, j) \leq f(k, l)$ implies $g(i, j) \leq g(k, l)$ for all locations (i, j) and (k, l) in the image, which may confuse the observer and will confuse most computer algorithms as well.

4.2.2 Resolution Enhancement

None of the sections above dealt with enhancing the spatial resolution, although contrast enhancement and noise removal will certainly improve the perceived resolution. Improving the spatial resolution within an image is often avoided because information needs to be added for up-sampling a given image.

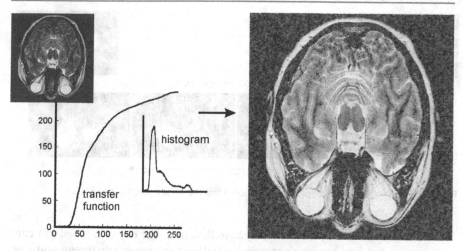

Fig. 4.7 Histogram equalization may produce unwanted effects since it enhances contrast on the assumption that often occurring gray values carry the most information. In the case depicted in this figure it leads to the enhancement of background while reducing foreground contrast

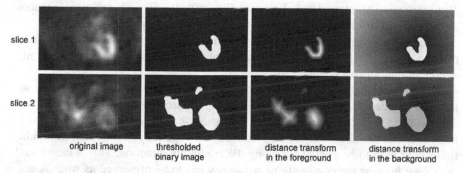

Fig. 4.8 Preparations for shape-based interpolation between two binary images: Computation of the binary image from the original (in this case SPECT *images from the left* ventricle of the heart), computation of a distance transform in the foreground (positive distance values) and in the background (negative distance values)

Slice interpolation is a case where interpolation after reconstruction may be needed. The resolution within an image is sometimes much better than the inter-slice resolution. Most algorithms perform better on isotropic voxels, however.

In its simplest variant, interpolation is carried out as a 1D linear or cubic inter-polation in the direction of the z-axis. Interpolation is improved if structures to be interpolated are already segmented and the data are binary. Then, shape-based in-terpolation on the segment boundary can be carried out (Raya and Udupa 1990). Shape-based interpolation consists of three steps.

1. Creation of a *signed distance map* from every slice (see Fig. 4.8 for an exam-ple): For every voxel, a signed distance map contains a distance to the closest boundary. Voxels inside the object have a positive distance assigned to them.

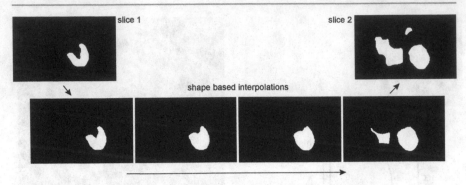

Fig. 4.9 Result of interpolated intermediate slices from the binary images in Fig. 4.8

Voxels outside the object have a negative distance. The distance transform can be carried out, e.g., by using a morphological erosion operator on foreground and background voxels.
2. Linear (or cubic) *interpolation of distance maps*: Interpolation is carried out along the z-axis.
3. *Binarization* of interpolated slices (see Fig. 4.9): Voxels with negative distances are mapped to a background and all other are mapped to foreground voxels.

Shape-based interpolation requires segmented data. It avoids many artefacts from partial volume effects under the assumption that objects in two adjacent slices only overlap if they share a common surface.[2]

For the interpolation of nonsegmented data, a model for continuity based on intensities (instead on boundaries such as in shape-based interpolation) between two slices is needed. A criterion, which has been used, is to assume that structure continuity between two slices may be derived from the continuity of intensity. Interpolation would have to be carried out along the continuity direction. This is easier said than done because the continuity of adjacency has to be preserved as well. A displacement field $\mathbf{d}(i, j) = (u(i, j)v(i, j))$ between two slices with images $f_1(i, j)$ and $f_2(i, j)$ is sought such that

$$\sum_{i=0}^{M-1}\sum_{j=0}^{N-1}\left(f_1\left(i + u(i, j), i + v(i, j)\right) - f_2(i, j)\right)^2 = \min \qquad (4.16)$$

and

$$\sum_{i=0}^{M-1}\sum_{j=0}^{N-1}\left(u(i, j) - u_{\text{avg}}(i, j)\right)^2 + \left(v(i, j) - v_{\text{avg}}(i, j)\right)^2 = \min, \qquad (4.17)$$

[2]The actual definition is a bit more complex. It essentially says that only those objects in two adjacent slices should overlap for whom the shortest distance on the surface between any two points on the two slices should not intersect any other slices.

Fig. 4.10 The gradient is a vector that is always orthogonal to an edge. The length of the gradient depends on the strength of the edge

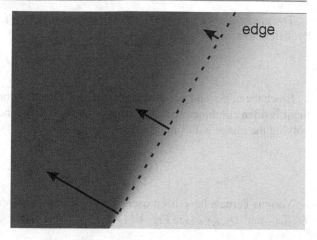

where $u_{\text{avg}}()$ and $v_{\text{avg}}()$ are the average values in some neighborhood around (i, j). The solution can be found using optical flow techniques. Interpolation is then carried out along displacement vectors. Using the quadratic (4.17) for enforcing smoothness of the displacement field will create a smooth interpolation. This behavior is desired if slices are not too thick and a smooth variation of displacement within a slice is the norm. For thick slices, two neighboring pixels in one slice may be displaced to different sites in the next slice (e.g., if a new structure appears in the next slice between them). In such a case, discontinuity-preserving constraints such as the one presented in Sect. 4.3.4 may be more appropriate for achieving the desired results.

4.2.3   Edge Enhancement

Enhancing the edges improves recognizing structures in images. Since automatic or interactive object delineation is a frequent task in image analysis, edge enhancement is often a prerequisite for tracking object boundaries.

Edges are closely associated with the *intensity gradient* because the existence of an edge implies a local change of intensity. For a 2D image with continuous domain (x, y), the gradient is a vector (see Fig. 4.10)

$$\nabla f(x, y) = \left(\frac{\partial f}{\partial x}(x, y) \quad \frac{\partial f}{\partial y}(x, y) \right)^{\text{T}}. \tag{4.18}$$

The *length* (the norm) of the gradient is the change of intensity in the direction of steepest ascent, hence characterizing the strength of the edge at (x, y). The gradient points in the *direction* of steepest ascent, which is perpendicular to the edge orientation at (x, y).

The gradient does not exist in the discrete domain (i, j), but can be approximated by differences

$$\nabla f(i, j) \approx \begin{pmatrix} f(i, j) - f(i - 1, j) \\ f(i, j) - f(i, j - 1) \end{pmatrix}. \tag{4.19}$$

Since the edges and noise both have high frequency components, edge enhancement is often combined with smoothing. The two differences are computed by convolving the image with smoothing difference kernels

$$\nabla f(i, j) \approx \begin{pmatrix} [f * D_x](i, j) \\ [f * D_y](i, j) \end{pmatrix}. \tag{4.20}$$

Various kernels have been used. Examples are the *Sobel operator* with kernels $D_{\text{Sobel},x}$ and $D_{\text{Sobel},y}$ (see Fig. 4.11)

$$D_{\text{Sobel},x} = \begin{pmatrix} -1 & 0 & 1 \\ -2 & 0 & 2 \\ -1 & 0 & 1 \end{pmatrix} \quad \text{and} \quad D_{\text{Sobel},y} = \begin{pmatrix} -1 & -2 & -1 \\ 0 & 0 & 0 \\ 1 & 2 & 1 \end{pmatrix}, \tag{4.21}$$

or the use of a Gaussian kernel. The partial derivatives of the Gaussian with standard deviation σ are

$$D_{\text{Gauss},x} = \frac{\partial f_{\text{Gauss}}}{\partial x}(x, y) = -\frac{x}{\sigma^3 \sqrt{2\pi}} \exp\left(-\frac{x^2 + y^2}{2\sigma^2}\right) \tag{4.22}$$

and

$$D_{\text{Gauss},y} = \frac{\partial f_{\text{Gauss}}}{\partial y}(x, y) = -\frac{y}{\sigma^3 \sqrt{2\pi}} \exp\left(-\frac{x^2 + y^2}{2\sigma^2}\right). \tag{4.23}$$

For computing the two filters $D_{\text{Gauss},x}$ and $D_{\text{Gauss},y}$, the derivatives are digitized and cut off using a suitable window size.

Edge enhancement using first derivatives produces information about the strength and direction of edges, but it does not tell the location of an edge very well. This information is delivered from computing the second derivative. If edges are located at positions where the edge strength has a local maximum, then the edge location is at the zero crossing of the second derivative.

A zero crossing is located between two adjacent pixels if one pixel has a second derivative with value 0 or if the second derivatives of the two pixels have different signs. Zero crossings are computed by the *Laplace operator* (or Laplacian). The Laplacian ∇^2 is the sum of all unmixed second derivatives,[3] i.e.,

$$\nabla^2 f(x, y) = \frac{\partial^2 f}{\partial^2 x} + \frac{\partial^2 f}{\partial^2 y}. \tag{4.24}$$

---

[3]The Laplacian may also be computed as divergence of the gradient, denoted as $\nabla^2 = \nabla \cdot \nabla$, hence the symbol ∇^2.

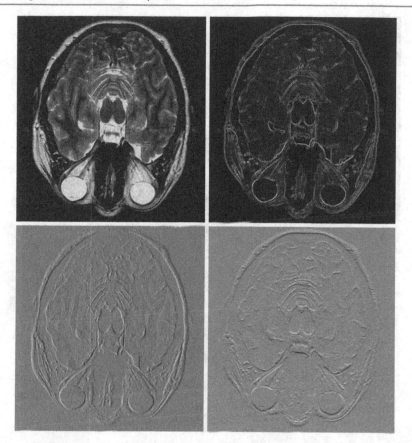

Fig. 4.11 Gradient filters produce approximations of the partial derivatives in x- and y-direction (the *two pictures in the second row* show the result from applying the Sobel operator). The length of the gradient (*upper right*) can be used for computing edge features

For discrete images it is approximated by differences, leading to a convolution with one of the following two kernels

$$D_{\text{Laplace\_4}} = \begin{pmatrix} 0 & -1 & 0 \\ -1 & 4 & -1 \\ 0 & -1 & 0 \end{pmatrix} \quad \text{or} \quad D_{\text{Laplace8}} = \begin{pmatrix} -1 & -1 & -1 \\ -1 & 8 & -1 \\ -1 & -1 & -1 \end{pmatrix}. \quad (4.25)$$

The former approximates (4.24) and the latter adds the two mixed derivatives to (4.24).

The Laplacian is often used in conjunction with a smoothing kernel because it is very sensitive to noise. A well-known kernel is the *Laplacian of Gaussian* (LoG) filter, which computes the Laplacian of a Gaussian function

$$LoG(x, y) = -\frac{1}{\pi \sigma^4}\left(1 - \frac{x^2 + y^2}{2\sigma^2}\right)\exp\left(-\frac{x^2 + y^2}{2\sigma^2}\right), \quad (4.26)$$

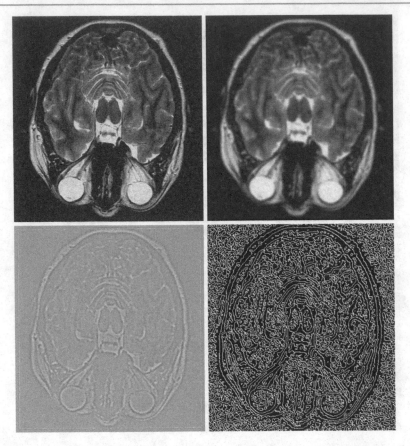

Fig. 4.12 The Laplacian of Gaussian combines a Gaussian smoothing (*upper right*) with a Laplacian to arrive at the result depicted in the *lower left image*. Zero crossings of the Laplacian indicate edge locations in the image (shown in the *lower right image*)

and then uses the result to convolve the image (see Fig. 4.12). The filter is sometimes called the *Mexican hat filter* because of its shape. It is also known as the *Marr-Hildreth filter* after David Marr and Ellen Hildreth, who showed that early edge enhancement in human vision can be modeled by an LoG filter.

The four second derivatives of a 2D image that are summed in D_{Laplace8} are components of the *Hessian* matrix

$$H = \begin{pmatrix} \dfrac{\partial^2 f}{\partial^2 x}(x, y) & \dfrac{\partial^2 f}{\partial x \partial y}(x, y) \\[2mm] \dfrac{\partial^2 f}{\partial y \partial x}(x, y) & \dfrac{\partial^2 f}{\partial^2 y}(x, y) \end{pmatrix}, \tag{4.27}$$

which may be used for enhancing corners. The value of the determinant of the Hessian increases at corner points. The eigenvalues indicate whether a point in the image is a local maximum, minimum, or saddle point. If the two eigenvalues are positive, it is a local maximum, if they are negative, it is a local minimum. Otherwise, it is a saddle point.

Edges may also be enhanced in a directionally sensitive fashion by combining a difference operator with a directionally sensitive smoothing operator. A filter that has been shown to be a model for directionally sensitive cells in the primary visual cortex is the *Gabór filter*. In continuous space (x, y), it is defined as

$$G_{\sigma,\alpha,\gamma,\lambda,\psi}(x, y) = \exp\left(-\frac{s^2 + \gamma t^2}{2\sigma^2}\right) \cos\left(2\pi \frac{s}{\lambda} + \psi\right), \qquad (4.28)$$

with

$$s = x \sin\alpha + y \cos\alpha, \qquad t = x \cos\alpha - y \sin\alpha. \qquad (4.29)$$

The exponential term is a smoothing function that is wider along s (i.e., in a direction α with respect to x) than along t perpendicular to s. The parameter γ determines the elongatedness of the function. The cosine term produces the difference of values along s. Its wavelength is given by λ. It controls the width of the range along which the difference is taken. The parameter ψ is an offset for the difference function.

Filter banks of Gabór filters can be used to enhance and group edges by direction, curvedness, and steepness.

4.3   Noise Reduction

Noise is usually modeled stationary, additive, and with zero mean. A noisy image g is related to the unknown noise-free image f through $g = f + n$, where n is the zero mean noise. Noise removal through linear filtering consists of estimating the expected value $E(g)$. Since $E(n) = 0$, we have

$$E(g) = E(f) + E(n) = E(f) = f, \qquad (4.30)$$

because the deterministic function f has $E(f) = f$. Hence, noise reduction schemes try to reconstruct $E(g)$ from various assumptions about f as follows.

- Linear filtering assumes f to be locally constant. E is then estimated by averaging over a local neighborhood.
- Median filtering assumes that noise is normally distributed, f is locally constant, except for the edges, the signal at the edges is higher than the noise, and the edges are locally straight.
- Diffusion filtering assumes that f is locally constant, except at the edges, and that the properties of the edges and noise can be differentiated by amplitude or frequency.

- Bayesian image restoration requires f to be locally smooth, except for the edges. It further requires that in some local neighborhood edge pixels are not the majority of all pixels in that neighborhood.

Since most of the assumptions are not true everywhere in the image, filtering results in the various filter-specific artefacts.

4.3.1 Noise Reduction by Linear Filtering

If f is constant in some neighborhood around (i, j), $E(i, j)$ can be estimated by averaging over this neighborhood. The operation can be carried out in the spatial domain as a convolution with a *mean* (sometimes called *boxcar filter*) of size s:

$$f(i, j) \approx [g * c_{\text{boxcar},s}](i, j), \tag{4.31}$$

where "$*$" stands for the convolution operation. The convolution kernel $c_{\text{boxcar},s}$ is a square matrix of size $s \times s$ with s being odd and the filter being centered:

$$c_{\text{boxcar},s} = \frac{1}{s^2} \begin{pmatrix} 1 & 1 & \dots & 1 \\ 1 & & \dots & 1 \\ \dots & & & \dots \\ & & 1 & 1 \end{pmatrix}. \tag{4.32}$$

The estimate of $E(g(i, j))$ improves with the size of s, but the likelihood that f is constant in this neighborhood for all locations (i, j) decreases, leading to increased blurring at the edges.

Several other linear filters also deliver an estimate of $E(g)$. The *binomial filter* is a convolution kernel $c_{\text{binom},b}$ whose one-dimensional version contains the binomial coefficients of order b. A 2D kernel can be computed from convolving two 1D filters. A 1D filter of order b is created from the repetitive convolution of a 1D filter of order 1:

$$c_{\text{binom},b}^{1D} = \frac{1}{2^b} c_{\text{binom},b-1}^{1D} * c_{\text{binom},1}^{1D}, \quad \text{with } c_{\text{binom},1}^{1D} = [1 \quad 1]. \tag{4.33}$$

The 2D filter $c_{\text{binom},b}$ is computed by $c_{\text{binom},b} = c_{\text{binom},1}^{1D} \times (c_{\text{binom},1}^{1D})^{\text{T}}$, where T denotes the transpose of a matrix. The analysis of the binomial filter in frequency space shows that it produces fewer artefacts than the boxcar filter (see Fig. 4.13). It also emphasizes pixels in the neighborhood that are closer to the center pixel when estimating $E(g)$. This strategy is reasonable as the likelihood of f having the same value than $f(i, j)$ decreases with the distance of a pixel to the center location (i, j).

With higher order, the binomial filter approaches a *Gaussian filter*. A Gaussian with a given standard deviation σ can be used for noise filtering as well. The infinite support of the Gaussian function

$$c_{\text{Gauss},\sigma}(x) = \frac{1}{\sigma\sqrt{2\pi}} \exp\left(-\frac{x^2}{2\sigma^2}\right) \tag{4.34}$$

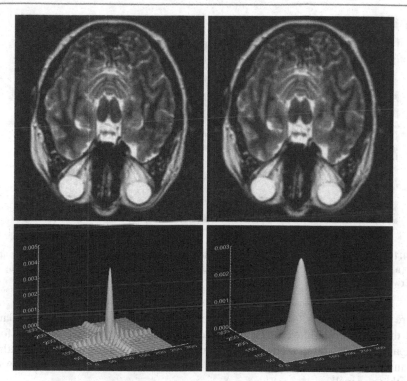

Fig. 4.13 If high frequency attenuation in frequency space by neighborhood averaging (*left*) or a binomial filter (*right*) is comparable, the results look very similar. However, attenuation in frequency space is highly anisotropic (*lower left*) while this is not the case for the binomial filter. It may cause anisotropic enhancement of edges which may be a source of problems for subsequent boundary detection steps

has to be transformed into a finite support region with some window size $|x| < x_{max}$. Selecting $|x_{max}| > 3\sigma$ ensures that the values $x > x_{max}$ are sufficiently close to zero to avoid significant changes in the result. After cutting the function it has to be normalized. Two-dimensional Gaussian kernels are created by multiplying a 1D kernel with its 1D transpose.

The separability of the Gaussian and also that of the Binomial filters reduces computational costs when filter sizes are large. Instead of explicitly creating a 2D filter of size $s \times s$ and convolving the image with this filter, noise reduction is done by subsequent convolution with the two 1D filters. The computational costs per pixel are $O(s)$ instead of $O(s^2)$.

Filtering may be carried out by multiplication in the frequency domain. Noise in the frequency domain is modeled as a random process whose expected value for the amplitude is either constant (so-called white noise) or much slower decreasing with frequency than the amplitude of the signal (colored noise). In either case, noise dominates the high frequency range and noise reduction consists of applying a low pass filter. The ideal low pass filter with cut-off frequency w_{max}, however, produces

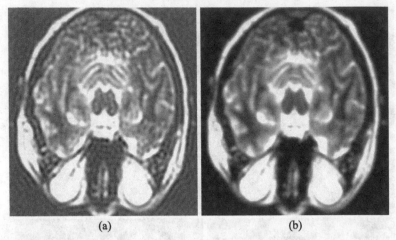

(a)   (b)

Fig. 4.14 Filtering in frequency space with an ideal low pass filter produces severe ringing arte-facts (**a**) that can be avoided by a filter using gradual attenuation of high frequencies such as the Butterworth filter (**b**)

severe ringing artefacts.[4] Examples for filters that do not cause ringing are the Gaussian, the Butterworth filter, the Hamming, or the Hann windows (see Fig. 4.14 for a comparison of two filters). The latter two are often used for noise and artefact reduction in tomographic image reconstruction, but are useful for additional a posteriori smoothing as well.

The Gaussian for filtering in frequency space corresponds to a Gaussian in the spatial domain with inverted standard deviation. The *Butterworth filter* attenuates noise proportional to frequency with cut-off frequency w_{max}:

$$C_{Butterworth, \omega_{max}}(u, v) = \frac{1}{1 + ((u^2 + v^2)/\omega_{max}^2)^k}, \tag{4.35}$$

where k regulates the steepness of the damping function at ω_{max}. The Hamming and Hann windows with cut-off frequency w_{max} are two similar filter functions. They are defined by

$$C_{Ha, \omega_{max}}(u, v) = \begin{cases} \alpha - (1 - \alpha) \cos\left(\frac{\sqrt{u^2 + v^2}}{\omega_{max}} \pi\right), & \text{if } u^2 + v^2 < \omega_{max}^2, \\ 0, & \text{otherwise.} \end{cases} \tag{4.36}$$

The filter is called a *Hamming* window if $\alpha = 0.53836$. For $\alpha = 0.5$ it is called the *Hann* window.

Low pass filtering in frequency space has similar effects as approximating $E(g)$ in the spatial domain in that both methods blur the edges. The reason is the same. The Fourier transform F of an image f containing an ideal step edge is a func-

---

[4]The reason for this is easily seen when the filter is transformed into the spatial domain in order to form the corresponding convolution kernel. The result is a sinc function which obviously causes the repetitions of edges after filtering, which is called ringing.

tion with infinite support, i.e., there exists no cut-off frequency w_{max} for which $F(u, v) = 0$ if $u^2 + v^2 > \omega_{max}^2$.

If the SNR is high and the noise is white, selecting a proper w_{max}—or in spatial filtering selecting a proper filter size—is a compromise between the loss of signal at edges due to blurring and the overall improvement of the SNR.

Noise reduction in medical images may be difficult because often spatial resolution must not be reduced. Small structures or structures with a very convoluted surface must still be visible after noise removal. If, e.g., voxels in an MR brain image have an edge length of 1.0 mm, it may be expected that small gyrii are recognizable which are only a few millimeters apart. The assumption of a constant image function f over an area of several pixels for smoothing by linear filtering is violated in such regions. Smoothing makes detail less visible or may even make it to disappear.

Smoothing either requires a sufficiently high object-dependent contrast in the input image, a low level of spatial detail, or a combination of both. High contrast images are, for instance, MR soft tissue images, CT bone images, contrast-enhanced CT or MR angiograms, or some nuclear images. CT soft tissue images are difficult to smooth because of the low contrast between tissues. The same is true for ultrasound images because of the high ratio of low frequency noise and artefacts. Noise removal in nuclear images, such as SPECT, may also be inappropriate since—despite a good contrast—it may further reduce the already low spatial resolution.

Linear filtering will generally produce poor results if the SNR is low or if the ratio of low frequency noise is high. Successful noise reduction in such cases requires an edge model as an integral part of the smoothing process. Such methods are called *edge-preserving smoothing*.

4.3.2 Edge-Preserving Smoothing: Median Filtering

A *median filter* is a nonlinear rank order filter that selects the result at some location (i, j) from an ordered list of values. The values are taken from pixels in the neighborhood of (i, j). A filter is a median filter if the median rank is selected from the list. A 3×3 median filter would thus sort nine pixel values—the pixels in an 8-neighborhood of (i, j) plus (i, j) itself—and select the one ranked at position five. The neighborhood is usually square-shaped covering an odd number of pixels (e.g., 3×3, 5×5, or 7×7 neighborhoods).

The result of a median filter approaches the expected value with increasing filter size if Gaussian noise can be assumed. Under such conditions, the median filter has similar noise reduction capabilities as the linear filters presented in Sect. 4.3. However, there is more to the median filter. If the neighborhood region of a median filter contains an edge, it preserves the edge under the following conditions (compare results in Fig. 4.15).

- The edge is straight within the neighborhood region.
- The signal difference of the two regions incident to the edge exceeds the noise amplitude.
- The signal is locally constant within each of the two regions.

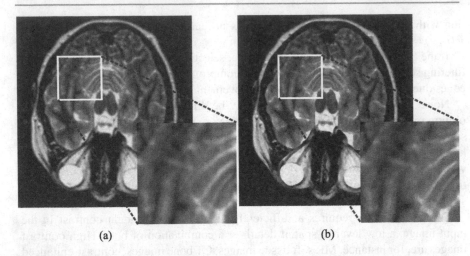

(a)   (b)

Fig. 4.15 Comparison between boxcar filter (**a**) and median filter (**b**) of the same size. It can be seen in the enlarged part that the median filter preserves sharp edges while the boxcar filter produces blur

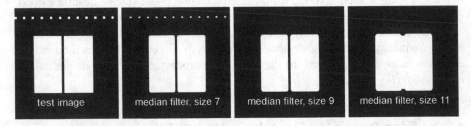

Fig. 4.16 Median filtering on a simple test image. Corners are rounded by filters of any size, since there exists no neighborhood size in which the boundary is locally straight at corners. Object details are removed if the filter size is larger than the detail

Under these conditions it can be shown that the filter result for a pixel (i, j) in some region r_1 at an edge separating r_1 from r_2 will always be chosen from r_1.

Although the filter is edge-preserving at such edges, it does not reduce noise since the probability distribution of pixels $p \in r_1 \cup r_2$ is certainly not Gaussian. In summary, the median filter is noise-reducing in neighborhoods with a constant value and edge-preserving at the edges.

The median filter does not work properly if the conditions listed above do not hold (see Fig. 4.16). Some of the problems that may arise are as follows.

1. Noise reduction improves with the size of the filter under the condition that the function f is constant in this region. The usual compromise is that the neighborhood region is as large as possible while f may still be assumed to be constant. An extreme case is given if the size of a region is a single pixel. Median filtering will remove the pixel. If it were noise (such as in impulse noise), this is a wanted behavior, but otherwise the structure would just vanish.

2. Boundaries are rarely straight. Again, the neighborhood size will be a compromise resulting in a neighborhood region just as large so that the boundary is (approximately) straight. At sharp corners where no neighborhood with straight boundary exists, median filtering removes the corners.

3. The SNR at edges separating regions r_1 and r_2 may not be high enough to ensure that the noise amplitude is always lower than the signal difference between r_1 and r_2. Filtering a pixel in r_1 may lead to the selection of a pixel from r_2. The course of the boundary would change. This is particularly unwanted because the median filter tends to enhance the contrast between any two regions. The new boundary is visually more pleasing than the noisy boundary before filtering, but it is the wrong boundary nonetheless.

4. More than one edge may exist within the region covered by the filter. In such a case, neighboring structures may be merged. This, again, is a serious alteration of the image.

All this can happen in medical images. Conditions 1, 2, and 4 are often violated because the image depicts structures or boundary details that are smaller than the filter size (consider again the detailed structure of the cortex surface in MR brain images). Condition 3 is often violated in CT soft tissue images as the contrast between different tissues is small compared to the noise level.

The median filter—or any other edge-preserving filter—should be used with care. It may remove or alter edges that do not follow the (implicit) edge model. It can result in difficulties for later human or computer vision tasks relying on a faithful depiction of edges. This is especially true when the user is not aware of the implicit edge model.

4.3.3 Edge-Preserving Smoothing: Diffusion Filtering

The median filter has two disadvantages: It does not remove noise at edges even if the edge follows the implicit edge model, and it may alter edges in a random fashion that does not follow the edge model. Diffusion filtering is an alternative that enables smoothing at edges. It may also accommodate a wide range of edge models.

Diffusion filtering uses the diffusion of a liquid or gaseous material as a model for noise reduction. Using homogeneous and inhomogeneous diffusion for data filtering was first proposed by Perona and Malik (1990) and has since become very popular for edge-preserving smoothing. The popularity is probably due to the relative simplicity of the concepts, the intuitive behavior of a diffusion process, and a fairly simple implementation.

For applying a diffusion process as a filter, image intensity is taken as material density. Noise is taken as density variation and diffusion is carried out iteratively. After an infinite number of iterations, *homogeneous diffusion* (Fig. 4.17a) levels any density inhomogeneity resulting in a noise-free image without edges.

Diffusion across edges should be inhibited for edge enhancement. Since the boundaries are unknown (otherwise edge-preserving smoothing would be trivial), the edge response from edge enhancement is used to indicate the potential bound-

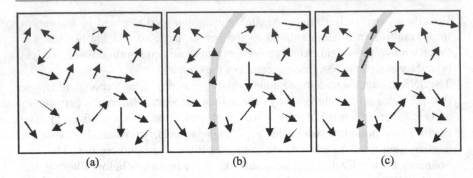

$$(a) \qquad\qquad\qquad (b) \qquad\qquad\qquad (c)$$

Fig. 4.17 (a) Homogeneous diffusion is only dependent on the density gradient, (b) inhomogeneous diffusion decrease at edges, (c) anisotropic diffusion decrease at edge in edge normal direction

ary locations. *Inhomogeneous diffusion* (Fig. 4.17b) treats such boundary locations as a semi-permeable material. The process will still level densities (i.e., image intensities), but the process will be slower at potential edge locations. It will not be prohibited, however, because the gradient response may also be caused by noise. Hence, noise removal should stop after a number of iterations to prevent leveling the intensity difference between objects. The stopping criterion depends on the image characteristics and on the parameters of the diffusion equation.

Preserving boundaries may be improved if, instead of restricting any kind of diffusion at edges, it is only restricted across the edges. This is called *anisotropic diffusion* (Fig. 4.17c). Allowing diffusion parallel to an edge enables noise removal by smoothing while inhibiting diffusion across an edge. Gradient direction is used as a discriminative feature between noise and the edges. The gradients between adjacent edge pixels tend to have similar directions while this is not true for the gradients of adjacent noise pixels. Diffusion in regions with noise pixels will be in random directions supporting homogenization while it will be directed in boundary regions supporting contrast enhancement.

All three diffusion types can be described by the diffusion equation introduced in Sect. 2.2.8 on MR diffusion imaging. Diffusion in a 2D scene at some location (x, y) causes a flux $\mathbf{j}$ according to Fick's law

$$\mathbf{j}(x, y) = -\mathbf{D}(x, y) \times \nabla \mathbf{u}(x, y) = -\mathbf{D}(x, y) \times \begin{pmatrix} \dfrac{\partial f(x, y)}{\partial x} \\ \dfrac{\partial f(x, y)}{\partial y} \end{pmatrix}. \qquad (4.37)$$

The type of diffusion is described by the diffusion tensor $\mathbf{D}$. It specifies for the density gradient $\nabla \mathbf{u}$ how much diffusion takes place in any direction.

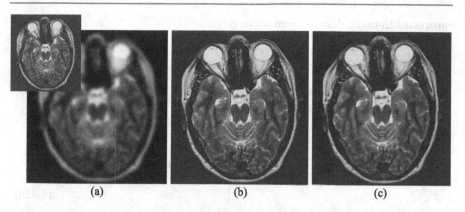

Fig. 4.18 Comparison of the different types of diffusion: (**a**) homogeneous diffusion, (**b**) inhomogeneous diffusion, (**c**) anisotropic inhomogeneous diffusion

Homogeneous diffusion is independent of the strength and direction of the gradient (see Fig. 4.18a). The diffusion tensor is the product of a diffusion coefficient ε_0 and the identity matrix

$$\mathbf{D}(x, y) = \varepsilon_0 \begin{pmatrix} 1 & 0 \\ 0 & 1 \end{pmatrix}. \tag{4.38}$$

Inhomogeneous diffusion depends on the gradient strength (see Fig. 4.18b). Perona and Malik, who presented diffusion filtering, suggested

$$\mathbf{D}(x, y) = \begin{pmatrix} \varepsilon(\|\nabla \mathbf{u}(x, y)\|^2) & 0 \\ 0 & \varepsilon(\|\nabla \mathbf{u}(x, y)\|^2) \end{pmatrix} \tag{4.39}$$

with

$$\varepsilon(\|\nabla \mathbf{u}(x, y)\|^2) = \varepsilon_0 \frac{\lambda^2}{\|\nabla \mathbf{u}(x, y)\|^2 + \lambda^2}. \tag{4.40}$$

Inhomogeneous diffusion depends on the location (x, y) and decreases with increasing gradient length $\|\nabla \mathbf{u}\|$. The parameter λ governs the influence of gradient length to diffusion. With λ approaching infinity, inhomogeneous diffusion turns into homogeneous diffusion.

The tensor is still a diagonal matrix imposing no constraints of the diffusion direction based on $\nabla \mathbf{u}$. This changes for anisotropic diffusion, where the diffusion tensor at each location (x, y) is chosen such that diffusion in the gradient direction is reduced while diffusion perpendicular to the gradient is not affected (see Fig. 4.18c for an example). As was already mentioned in Sect. 2.2.8, the amount of anisotropic diffusion is given by the eigen decomposition of $\mathbf{D}$. The desired result for edge-preserving anisotropic diffusion is an eigenvector of which the eigenvalue decreases with increasing gradient $\nabla \mathbf{u}$ and another eigenvector perpendicular to $\nabla \mathbf{u}$ of which the eigenvalue does not depend on the strength of $\nabla \mathbf{u}$. Hence, the tensor is constructed from the desired eigen decomposition

$$\mathbf{D}(x, y) = \begin{pmatrix} e_{1,1}(x, y) & e_{2,1}(x, y) \\ e_{1,2}(x, y) & e_{2,2}(x, y) \end{pmatrix} \begin{pmatrix} \lambda(x, y)_1 & 0 \\ 0 & \lambda_2(x, y) \end{pmatrix}$$

$$\times \begin{pmatrix} e_{1,1}(x, y) & e_{1,2}(x, y) \\ e_{2,1}(x, y) & e_{2,2}(x, y) \end{pmatrix}, \tag{4.41}$$

with

$$\begin{bmatrix} e_{1,1}(x, y) & e_{1,2}(x, y) \end{bmatrix} = \frac{\nabla u(x, y)}{\|\nabla u(x, y)\|}, \qquad \lambda_1(x, y) = \varepsilon \big(\|\nabla u(x, y)\|^2 \big),$$

$$\tag{4.42a}$$

$$\begin{bmatrix} e_{2,1}(x, y) & e_{2,2}(x, y) \end{bmatrix} = \begin{bmatrix} e_{1,2}(x, y) & -e_{1,1}(x, y) \end{bmatrix}, \qquad \lambda_2(x, y) = 1.$$

$$\tag{4.42b}$$

Computing the diffusion requires solving a differential equation. It can be done analytically for homogeneous diffusion. Homogeneous diffusion at some time t equals the convolution of the image with a Gaussian with variance depending on t.

The other two diffusion types are more interesting for edge-preserving smoothing. Here, diffusion is computed iteratively, assuming constant diffusion over fixed (small) time intervals. The image $f(x, y)$ is assumed to be the density distribution $u(x, y, 0)$ at time t_0. Given the density at time t_i, the density at time t_{i+1} is computed as

$$u(x, y, t_{i+1}) = u(x, y, t_i) + (t_{i+1} - t_i) \frac{\partial u(x, y, t_i)}{\partial t}, \tag{4.43}$$

where $\frac{\partial u(x, y, t_i)}{\partial t}$ indicates the change of density due to diffusion. It can be computed from the divergence of the flux

$$\frac{\partial u(x, y, t)}{\partial t} = -\operatorname{div} \mathbf{j}(x, y, t) \quad \text{with } \operatorname{div} \mathbf{j} = \left(\frac{\partial j_x(x, y, t)}{\partial x} + \frac{\partial j_y(x, y, t)}{\partial y} \right). \tag{4.44}$$

Although it may look complex at first sight, implementation is straightforward. After specifying the appropriate diffusion tensor, an iterative scheme for updating the density according to (4.43) is implemented using the divergence of flux of (4.44).

Some care has to be spent on selecting appropriate parameters. The difference between time steps is critical, as it governs the approximation accuracy of solving an initial value problem by finite differences. However, if the step size is too small, noise reduction will progress slowly.

Selecting ε_0 influences the maximum diffusion per time step. Again, a small value causes slow progress, but if the value is too high diffusion may cause oscillation of density values.

Finally, λ restricts diffusion at edges. An ideal value of λ would cause edge contrast to increase faster than contrast decreases due to diffusion. However, λ also influences the behavior within regions. For a low SNR image there may be no value that is globally valid everywhere in the image.

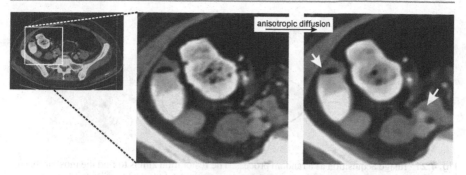

Fig. 4.19 Diffusion filtering in a CT body image. While noise is reduced and contrast is enhanced, small structures start to disappear and at some locations (indicated by *arrows*), the course of the boundary starts to change

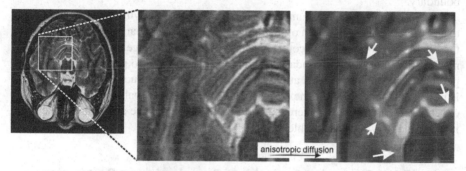

Fig. 4.20 Diffusion filtering in an MR brain image. Since structures are much smaller than in the CT image, the removal and change of boundaries due to diffusion is much more prominent than in the application depicted in Fig. 4.19

Discrimination between boundaries and noise can be enhanced if gradient approximation is different for computing ε and for computing the flux due to density variations. The gradient in (4.49) could be replaced by some gradient $\nabla \mathbf{g}(x, y)$, which is intended to measure the likeness of a pixel to be a part of a boundary. This boundary gradient $\nabla \mathbf{g}(x, y)$ can be, for instance, approximated by applying a Gaussian kernel with some variance σ^2 to the density image before computing the differences. The noise gradient $\nabla \mathbf{u}(x, y)$ would still be computed without Gaussian smoothing. Details that are smaller than the variance of the Gaussian are then treated as noise and would be diffused with time, whereas larger details are treated as boundaries inhibiting diffusion.

Using anisotropic diffusion for noise removal is often preferred to inhomogeneous diffusion because the resulting images look more pleasing to the observer. It should be noticed, however, that anisotropic diffusion may produce smooth but false boundaries if the true boundary contains details that are not recognized by the edge model (compare Figs. 4.19 and 4.20). Sometimes it is better to use an isotropic method that either leaves the noise unchanged or carries out a homoge-

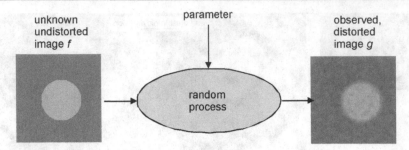

Fig. 4.21 Image acquisition as a random process. The restoration aim is to find the most probable undistorted image given the observation and the parameter of the a priori knowledge

neous smoothing. Both effects are more easily recognized as an artefact than a false boundary.

If kept going for a large number of iterations, diffusion will almost always lead to a complete homogenization of the image. It rarely can be parameterized such that the likeness to boundary, i.e., contrast, everywhere in the image increases faster than noise is dissolved at the boundaries. Hence, it is important to provide content- and parameter-specific thresholds at which diffusion stops. As such, diffusion filtering is not a suitable tool for the inexperienced user and will probably play a major role only in a research context where expert knowledge on the use and consequences of its application will be accessible.

4.3.4 Edge-Preserving Smoothing: Bayesian Image Restoration

Linear filtering assumes existing prior knowledge about the noise, but nothing about the image. Restoration in a probabilistic framework is able to incorporate smoothness constraints into the method. For this purpose, the image characteristics are assumed to be representable by a Markov random field (MRF, see Sect. 14.1).

Determining an unknown image function f from some observation g—which does not necessarily have to be an image, but must be associated with the image in some known fashion—given some probabilistic knowledge about the nature of the mapping from f to g is a powerful tool based on a simple concept (see Fig. 4.21). Its application fields in image processing are image reconstruction—e.g., in the reconstruction of nuclear images (see Sect. 2.4.2)—noise removal, segmentation, and classification.

For simplifying the notation, we assume that the pixels of an image are ordered as a vector. A vector $\mathbf{f}$ shall be restored from an observed vector $\mathbf{g}$. An individual pixel in the vector will be represented by f_i and g_i, respectively.

Noise reduction in a Bayesian framework searches for an image $\mathbf{f}$ that maximizes the conditional probability of observing a noisy image $\mathbf{g}$, given that the true image is $\mathbf{f}$. In Bayesian notation, we have

$$P(\mathbf{f}|\mathbf{g}) \propto P(\mathbf{g}|\mathbf{f}) \cdot P(\mathbf{f}). \tag{4.45}$$

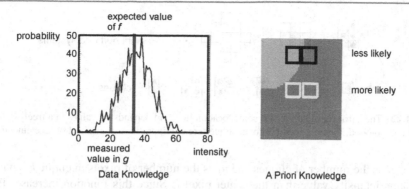

Fig. 4.22 Data knowledge and a priori domain knowledge about the images to be restored are the two components that define the probability of **f** having caused an observation **g**

The term $P(\mathbf{g}|\mathbf{f})$ is the data term since it describes the dependency of the observation on the unknown undistorted data **f**. The term $P(\mathbf{f})$ comprises domain knowledge about **f** independent of an observation (e.g., that in most images neighboring scene elements have similar values, see Fig. 4.22).

The conditional probability of observing **g** given the image **f** is characterized by the type of noise. For the following, we assume zero-mean Gaussian noise with covariance matrix Σ:

$$P(\mathbf{g}|\mathbf{f}) = \frac{1}{Z_1} \exp\left[-\frac{1}{2}\left((\mathbf{f} - \mathbf{g})^T \Sigma (\mathbf{f} - \mathbf{g}) \right) \right]. \tag{4.46}$$

The factor Z_1 is the normalizing constant of the Gaussian distribution. If it is assumed that the probabilities of the individual pixels are independent of each other and that they all have the same variance σ^2, the above equation simplifies to

$$P(\mathbf{g}|\mathbf{f}) = \frac{1}{Z_1} \exp\left[-\sum_{i=0}^{N-1} \frac{(f_i - g_i)^q}{2\sigma^2} \right]. \tag{4.47}$$

The a priori probability $P(\mathbf{f})$ is modeled as an MRF among elements of the image **f**. The probability of an MRF is

$$P(\mathbf{f}) = \frac{1}{Z_2} \exp\left(-U(\omega) \right), \tag{4.48}$$

where Z_2 is a normalization constant and $U(\omega)$ is the clique potential of all cliques in a neighborhood system. The neighborhood is defined as the spatial adjacency and the cliques are possible configurations of scene elements in the neighborhood (see Fig. 4.23). The clique potentials are designed such that they enforce smoothness in the image. An example for clique energies has been given by Besag (1986),

$$U(\omega) = \beta \sum_{k=0}^{K-1} u_{ik}, \tag{4.49}$$

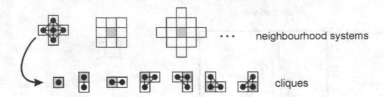

Fig. 4.23 The a priori probability for some location in a grid depends on values in a freely definable neighborhood. Given a neighborhood, cliques are configurations of a subset of its elements

where K is the number of cliques and u_k is the number of pixels in clique k having the same intensity value than the center pixel i. Since this function increases the potential only for equal values, it will lead to strong edges.

If we now use (4.46) and take into account that the Markovian property ensures the independence of $P(\mathbf{f})$ outside some neighborhood, we arrive at (omitting the normalization factors)

$$P(\mathbf{f}|\mathbf{g}) \propto \exp\left(-\frac{1}{2}(\mathbf{f} - \mathbf{g})\, \Sigma\, (\mathbf{f} - \mathbf{g})^T\right) \cdot \exp(-U(\omega))$$

$$= \prod_{i=0}^{N-1} \exp\left(-\frac{(f_i - g_i)^2}{2\sigma^2}\right) \cdot \exp\left(-\beta \sum_{k=0}^{K-1} u_{i,k}\right)$$

$$= \prod_{i=0}^{N-1} \exp\left(-\frac{(f_i - g_i)^2}{2\sigma^2} - \beta \sum_{k=0}^{K-1} u_{i,k}\right)$$

$$= \exp\left(-\sum_{i=0}^{N-1} \left(\frac{(f_i - g_i)^2}{2\sigma^2} - \beta \sum_{k=0}^{K-1} u_{i,k}\right)\right). \tag{4.50}$$

The maximization of $P(\mathbf{f}|\mathbf{g})$ means minimizing the exponent

$$\sum_{i=0}^{N-1} \left(\frac{(f_i - g_i)^2}{2\sigma^2} - \beta \sum_{k=0}^{K-1} u_{i,k}\right). \tag{4.51}$$

Finding the optimal estimate for $\mathbf{f}$ given the observation $\mathbf{g}$ is difficult as the number of configurations increases exponentially. Various techniques such as simulated annealing (Geman and Geman 1984), ICM (Besag 1986), or mean-field annealing (Zhang 1992) will be discussed in Sect. 14.1.

When Geman and Geman (1984) presented MRF Bayesian image restoration, the application example was a kind of relabeling of homogeneous regions. The definition of clique potentials and the optimization technique was geared toward the restoration of a true labeling from a small set of labels. The greedy method of Besag (1986) was much more appropriate for dealing with a large number of potential labels (i.e., a large number of possible intensities). However, the clique potentials defined by Geman and Geman (1984) already included an edge component supporting the creation of edges between homogeneously labeled regions. The a priori

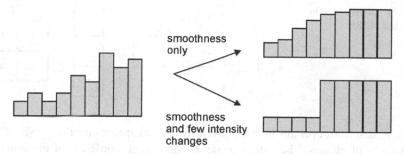

Fig. 4.24 If only similarity is required, the restored image will be blurred. The constraint from (4.55) also enforces as few intensity changes as possible, which enhances edges as well

model consists of two components. One essentially smoothes the data while the other supports the creation of label discontinuities at the region boundaries based on some line model.

Later approaches integrated the discontinuity condition parameter-free into the a priori model. In Geman and Reynolds (1992), the authors proposed a constraint that enforced the smoothness of some function with the values known at some locations by producing the smallest possible number of intensity changes (see Fig. 4.24). The function defining the a priori probability of the MRF is

$$\phi(u) = \frac{-1}{1 + |u|^\beta}. \tag{4.52}$$

This function is strictly concave for $0 < \beta < 2$ (in their experiments, the authors used $\beta = 1$) and it can be shown that for some 1D function f with values $f(x_1) = a$ and $f(x_2) = b$ with $x_1 < x_2$ and $a < b$ the result of minimizing $\int_{x_1}^{x_2} \phi(u)\,du$ is a function that is constant between x_1 and x_2, except for one location where f jumps from a to b. This is the opposite behavior to the use of interpolation functions such as $\phi(u) = u^2$, which would cause f to decrease gradually from x_1 to x_2. The behavior resulting from applying (4.52) achieves smoothness of data by maximizing the area of constant values while it enhances the edges at the same time.

The two components of the logarithm of $P(\mathbf{f}|\mathbf{g}) \propto P(\mathbf{g}|\mathbf{f}) \cdot P(\mathbf{f})$ for two cliques finding first-order discontinuities, which consist of pairs of horizontally and vertically adjacent pixels, are now

$$\ln P(\mathbf{g}|\mathbf{f}) : \lambda \sum_{i=0}^{MN-1} (g_i - Kf_i)^2 \tag{4.53}$$

and

$$\ln P(\mathbf{f}) : \sum_{c=1}^{C} \phi\left(\frac{\mathbf{f}_s^{(c)} - \mathbf{f}_t^{(c)}}{\Delta}\right), \tag{4.54}$$

Fig. 4.25 Cliques used in
(4.56) and (4.58)

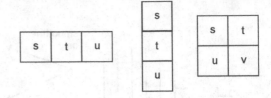

where K describes operator blurring given by a point spread function (PSF). C is the number of cliques. The indices s and t stand for a reordering of elements in f such that $f_{s,i}^{(c)}$ and $f_{t,i}^{(c)}$ contain the two members of a clique c. The term to be minimized

$$f = \arg\min_{f} \sum_{c=1}^{C} \phi\left(\frac{\mathbf{f}_s^{(c)} - \mathbf{f}_t^{(c)}}{\Delta}\right) + \lambda \sum_{i=0}^{MN-1} (g_i - Kf_i)^2, \qquad (4.55)$$

is not differentiable because of ϕ. For optimization, Geman and Reynolds (1992) suggested using simulated annealing. As the number of values that a pixel in f may take is large and the images may be large as well, two shortcuts to the optimization are provided.

- At each iteration, a value at some site i is chosen from a range of values determined by the intensities of the four neighbors of f and from the value of g at site i. The authors reported no visible degradation if using a range of six values reducing the total number of states from 256 to 25 (4×6 plus the value of g_i). Although this probably has to be adopted to suit a larger range when dealing with medical images with a range of originally 4096 values, it does reduce the cost by a factor of 10.
- Annealing is not started with some random values for f, but with a good guess (which could be a smoothed version of g which essentially is the maximum likelihood estimate for g without considering the Markovian prior).

It is noted that using cliques of pixels in the horizontal and vertical directions may bias the result against the diagonal edges. An extension to diagonal neighborhoods was published later (Hurn and Jennison 1996).

Reducing noise based on the assumption that the image is locally constant may be overly restrictive, as most scenes may contain some smooth intensity variation within the bounded regions. Hence, Geman and Reynolds (1992) extended the a priori term defining a second- and third-order versions of ϕ that used the first- and second-order derivatives of f instead f itself.

For the first-order derivative, three different cliques are defined: two cliques with three members s, t, u organized horizontally or vertically, respectively, and one clique with four members s, t, u, v organized in a square with the length of two pixels (see Fig. 4.25). The function ϕ_2 is defined as

$$\phi_2\left(\frac{\mathbf{f}_s^{(c)} - 2\mathbf{f}_t^{(c)} + \mathbf{f}_u^{(3)}}{\Delta}\right) \quad \text{and} \quad \phi_2\left(\frac{\mathbf{f}_s^{(c)} - \mathbf{f}_t^{(c)} - \mathbf{f}_u^{(3)} + \mathbf{f}_v^{(3)}}{\Delta}\right), \qquad (4.56)$$

depending on whether the clique consists of three or four members. For the second-order derivative, four cliques are defined. Two of the cliques have four members organized horizontally with

$$\phi_3\left(\frac{\mathbf{f}_s^{(c)} - 3\mathbf{f}_t^{(c)} + 3\mathbf{f}_u^{(3)} - \mathbf{f}_v^{(4)}}{\Delta}\right). \tag{4.57}$$

The other two cliques have two rows s_1, s_2, s_3 and t_1, t_2, t_3 of pixels organized either horizontally or vertically. The term is

$$\phi_3\left(\frac{\mathbf{f}_{s1}^{(c)} - 2\mathbf{f}_{s2}^{(c)} + 3\mathbf{f}_{s3}^{(3)} - (\mathbf{f}_{t1}^{(4)} - 2\mathbf{f}_{t2}^{(4)} + \mathbf{f}_{t3}^{(4)})}{\Delta}\right). \tag{4.58}$$

Edge-preserving smoothing using the Bayesian approach requires that noise can be differentiated from edges based on local attributes, which requires a fairly good SNR. In the original paper, a mean SNR of approximately 15 to 20 has been used and restoration was able to restore the image in the presence of large blur artefacts. Higher noise may be accommodated when blurring is excluded.

It was observed by the authors that using the second- or third-order constraints may lead to step artefacts because these constraints only approximate an intensity step edge.

A better result is achieved from the consecutive application of constraints. The measured image is used as an estimate for first-order discontinuity. The result serves as the initial estimate for a model allowing continuous shading using the second-order constraint. This result is subjected to the third constraint resulting in smooth surfaces. The parameters λ and Δ need to be chosen carefully. Geman and Reynolds (1992) investigated restoration of a horizontal or vertical step edge for first-, second-, and third-order discontinuity. They showed that λ and Δ are dependent on each other and that, given Δ, the parameterization of λ depends on the noise characteristics and on the order of the constraint.

Noise removal using Bayesian restoration has been used occasionally (Hu and Dennis 1991; Johnson et al. 1991; Garnier et al. 1995). It does play a more important role in image segmentation where the noise model is included into the segmentation task. The applications are tumor enhancement, detection, and segmentation in mammography and radiography (Li et al. 1995; Baydush and Floyd 2000), in MRI (Bouman and Shapiro 1994; Marroquín et al. 2002; Al-Zubi et al. 2002), or in CT. Hence, we will return to the subject in Chap. 7.

Using MRFs in a Bayesian framework for edge-preserving smoothing is an elegant approach to solve the inverse problem to regain the original image from a distorted image given knowledge about the attributes of noise and edges. Correct parameterization requires some understanding about the underlying methodology. As a tool, it should be preconfigured if it cannot be assured that expert knowledge is available. Similar to diffusion filtering, artefacts caused from parameterization errors may be difficult to interpret.

4.4   Concluding Remarks

The successful application of image enhancement methods require that information content can be separated a priori from any artefactual influences. Enhancement techniques attempt to extract this information or to suppress the artefacts. Since the definition of information content will be different for every image and for every possible request for information from an image, enhancement methods are a compromise that trades generality for the accuracy of this definition. Although most methods are parameterizable to accommodate the enhancement of different kinds of images, the user should be aware of the extent to which he or she can adapt the method to some image class by changing parameters.

Whether the application of a method makes sense and how parameters should be set is generally easy to decide if the method itself is simple (such as linear contrast enhancement or linear filtering). The efficient application of advanced methods such as diffusion filtering or Bayesian image restoration requires a good understanding of the various aspects and components of the method. Otherwise, a visually pleasing result may hide a degradation of the original information content.

Image enhancement is often a preprocessing step to segmentation. It is easier to find a segment boundary if it is clearly distinct in the image. There is a danger in this if edge-preserving smoothing has been applied. Since it is possible that false boundaries are created, segmentation results may be wrong as well. It can get difficult to detect the source of this problem when the enhanced image is sent to the segmenter without anybody checking the correctness of the enhancement step.

4.5   Exercises

- Name a difference in the goals of an enhancement technique applied to support the human perception of an image as opposed to enhancement to support computer-assisted analysis.
- What contrast measure captures the local contrast at object boundaries?
- Name at least two problems when equating the perceived contrast with global contrast.
- What kind of images do not profit from contrast enhancement by histogram equalization? What is the disadvantage when using adaptive histogram equalization instead?
- Why is histogram equalization not useful as preprocessing for an automatic image analysis method such as an automatic segmentation?
- What would filter masks for a Sobel filter look like if the partial differentials are approximated along the diagonal directions? How could the gradient be computed from the response of two such filters?
- How could linear filtering be used to sharpen edges? Would this be useful as preprocessing for a subsequent automatic image analysis? Explain why or why not.
- Why is it useful to combine a Laplace filter with a smoothing filter (such as a Gaussian)?

- Name the disadvantages of using a mean filter instead of a binomial filter.
- Why will the integral of all linear smoothing filters always sum up to unity?
- What kind of image degradation will always happen when using a linear low-pass filter?
- What kind of artefacts will be produced by median filtering? Under what conditions?
- Explain why the median filter will not reduce noise at edges.
- How will the results of isotropic and anisotropic diffusion filtering differ from each other?
- How and where is the anisotropy of diffusion encoded in the diffusion process?
- Why will any diffusion filtering result in a completely homogeneous image provided that diffusion has been carried out long enough?
- What kind of artefact can be created by anisotropic diffusion that seriously affects the perception of image content? Explain why this is inherent to the diffusion procedure.
- What conditions need to be met so that a stochastic process is a Markov random field?
- What domain knowledge is represented by the a priori probability of an MRF?
- Why is it so difficult to find the optimal images given an observation if the observed values are an instantiation of an MRF?
- What is the role of a clique in an MRF and how does it relate to the representation of domain knowledge?

References

Al-Zubi S, Toennies KD, Bodammer N, Hinrichs H (2002) Fusing Markov random fields with anatomical knowledge and shape based analysis to segment multiple sclerosis white matter lesions in magnetic resonance images of the brain. Proc SPIE 4684:206–215 (Medical imaging 2002)

Baydush AH, Floyd CE (2000) Improved image quality in digital mammography with image processing. Med Phys 27(7):1503–1508

Besag J (1986) On the statistical analysis of dirty pictures. J R Stat Soc B (Methodol) 48(3):259–302

Bouman CA, Shapiro M (1994) A multiscale random field model for Bayesian image segmentation. IEEE Trans Image Process 3(2):162–177

Garnier SJ, Bilbro GL, Gault JW, Snyder WE (1995) Magnetic resonance image restoration. J Math Imaging Vis 5(1):7–19

Geman S, Geman D (1984) Stochastic relaxation, Gibbs distributions, and the Bayesian restoration of images. IEEE Trans Pattern Anal Mach Intell 6(6):721–741

Geman D, Reynolds G (1992) Constrained restoration and the recovery of discontinuities. IEEE Trans Pattern Anal Mach Intell 14(3):367–383

Hu Y, Dennis TJ (1991) MAP estimation in image restoration by a local search enhanced genetic algorithm. In: 6th intl conf digital processing of signals in communications, pp 123–128

Hurn M, Jennison C (1996) An extension of Geman's and Reynold's approach to constrained restoration and the recovery of discontinuities. IEEE Trans Pattern Anal Mach Intell 18(6):657–662

Johnson VE, Wong WH, Hu X, Chen, CT (1991) Image restoration using Gibbs priors: boundary modeling, treatment of blurring, and selection of hyperparameters. IEEE Trans Pattern Anal Mach Intell 13(5):413–425

Li HD, Kallergi M, Clarke LP, Jain VK, Clark RA (1995) Markov random field for tumor detection in digital mammography. IEEE Trans Med Imaging 14(3):565–576

Marroquin JL, Vemuri BC, Botello S, Calderon E, Fernandez-Bouzas A (2002) An accurate and efficient Bayesian method for automatic segmentation of brain MRI. IEEE Trans Med Imaging 21(8):934–945

Peli E (1990) Contrast in complex images. J Opt Soc Am A 7(10):2032–2040

Perona P, Malik J (1990) Scale-space and edge detection using anisotropic diffusion. IEEE Trans Pattern Anal Mach Intell 12(7):629–639

Raya SP, Udupa JK (1990) Shape-based interpolation of multidimensional objects. IEEE Trans Med Imaging 9(1):32–42

Zhang J (1992) The mean field theory in EM procedures for Markov random fields. IEEE Trans Signal Process 40(10):2570–2583

Feature Detection

5

Abstract

Data-based features in images such as key point locations or potential parts of object boundaries can be extracted from local image characteristics. Boundary parts are generated from the results of an edge enhancement step while key point locations are local extrema of some local object property. Features may also be computed from samples of an object's boundary or interior.

Potential object boundary parts are used for detecting or delineating objects in images. Key points may, in some simple cases, also be used to detect objects. In most cases, however, object characteristics are too complex to be captured by the attributes of a key point. They can be important attributes nonetheless. Key points define an object-dependent reference system in which they may be used to map objects of the same class onto each other.

Concepts, notions and definitions introduced in this chapter

> Edge tracking
> Canny edge detector
> Hough transform for lines
> SIFT and SURF features, MSER features, local shape context, HOG features, gist and saliency

Image analysis aims at reducing information to a subset that is relevant to some analysis question. An example would be volumetry where the user wants a single number (the volume of a certain organ or pathological structure) from the image sequence. Other examples are the detection of metastases or the delineation of an organ boundary for radiotherapeutic treatment planning. Information reduction often happens gradually with information being reduced until the desired result is extracted from the data. The first level of reduction computes local features that are assumed to pertain to objects of interest. Examples for local features are edges, blobs, or ridges in the image. Such features carry more information than a pixel,

K.D. Toennies, *Guide to Medical Image Analysis*,
Advances in Computer Vision and Pattern Recognition,
DOI 10.1007/978-1-4471-2751-2_5, © Springer-Verlag London Limited 2012

as they represent a first differentiation between the object attributes and influences from image acquisition.

There are a number of reasons to apply a feature detection step in medical image analysis. In cases where the object of interest is simple, its attributes may be captured directly by the feature detector. This then leads to object detection. More often it is a preprocessing step. Feature locations and attributes may serve as an object-specific reference if the same object is captured by different images that shall be compared. While the content of the images may be different (e.g., if one of the images is CT and the other MRI), the object features such as edges or corners should be extractable in both images. Features may also help to define a region of interest that shall be further inspected. A blob detector, for instance, could find potential regions of interest that may comprise the blob-like lymph nodes. Further processing will then be restricted to these regions. Features may also help to guide a segmentation process in cases where the data are noisy or of low contrast. Edge features, for instance, could be generated that support segmentation if noisy data would produce too many spurious responses from applying a simple gradient operator. Finally, features may also be used to characterize deviations from an assumed norm of an anatomic structure. As an example, features to enhance tubular structures may highlight the potential sites of aneurisms in the vascular system since they deviate from the normal, tube-like shape of vessels.

The description of a feature is richer than that of a pixel. It comprises at least the feature location in image space and the feature type (e.g., edge or corner) and some measure of strength of the feature response at that location. It may include other information such as scale (e.g., size of a blob) or orientation (e.g., the direction of an edge).

5.1   Edge Tracking

Structures are meant to be detectable by a change of appearance between it and the background. Furthermore, the shape given by a structure's outline may be an important characteristic to differentiate it from other objects or to specify object-specific locations. Hence, edges are relevant features for several types of analysis tasks.

Edges can be those of intensity but may also separate different textures. The following section will deal with intensity edges. Most of the techniques can be applied to textures as well, provided that the texture measure can be mapped on a single scalar value.[1] Texture edges are then edges of this scalar value.

The detection of intensity edges uses the output of an edge enhancement step. Edge strength is given by the length of the intensity gradient. The edge location is given by the zero crossings of a Laplace operator (see Fig. 5.1). However, a large gradient does not automatically mean that there is an edge. Finding salient edges in an image can be difficult. Saliency can be based on many different attributes ranging

---

[1]This can be difficult, however, since texture measures are estimated from a local neighborhood that is assumed to have the same texture. This is not true at texture boundaries.

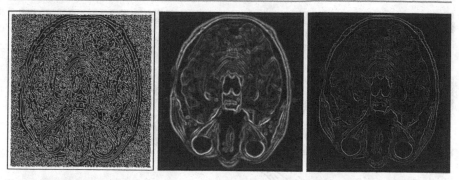

Fig. 5.1 Zero crossings computed from applying an LoG operator (**a**) may be combined with information about edge strength from a gradient operator (**b**) to find edge locations and rate their importance based on edge strength (**c**)

from local smoothness and continuity constraints to high-level domain knowledge. Hence, edge detection is still an open problem in the general field of image analysis. An extensive survey of past and recent techniques can be found in Papari and Petkov (2011).

For edge detection in medical images, various, rather simple assumptions are used to separate edges from noise.

- The gradient for edges is often stronger than that caused by noise.
- The edge direction varies slowly along the edge.
- The edge strength varies slowly along the edge.

These assumptions are too simple to detect all edges defining an object boundary. They are, however, sufficient since edges resulting from a tracking step are usually not the final result. Rather, these edges initialize some top-down analysis step to find boundaries of an organ, pathological process, or other structure of interest.

The *Canny edge operator* (Canny 1986) takes into account all three assumptions. It consists of an edge-enhancement step and an edge tracking step. Edge enhancement is carried out by taking the maximum response from several one-dimensional edge filters because—under an idealized edge model—the optimal response for an edge is created by a one-dimensional smoothing differential operator orthogonal to the yet unknown edge direction. The local maximum of the gradient length then specifies the edge location. In most applications, this step is replaced by a two-dimensional gradient operator (e.g., the derivatives of the Gaussian) combined with a nonmaximum suppression step that reduces the edge response to a single pixel in the gradient direction. Nonmaximum suppression can be done by computing zero-crossings of the second derivative.

Edge tracking is done by hysteresis thresholding. Two thresholds, t_1 and t_2 with $t_1 > t_2$, are defined and applied to the gradient length $|\mathbf{g}|$. If $|\mathbf{g}| > t_1$ for some pixel, this pixel always belongs to an edge. Pixels with $|\mathbf{g}| > t_2$ are edge pixels if they are adjacent to other edge pixels. The algorithm proceeds as follows (see also Fig. 5.2).

- Select the next pixel with $|\mathbf{g}| > t_1$ that is not yet assigned to an edge and assign it to a new edge.
- Track the edge as long as the adjacent pixels are found with $|\mathbf{g}| > t_2$.

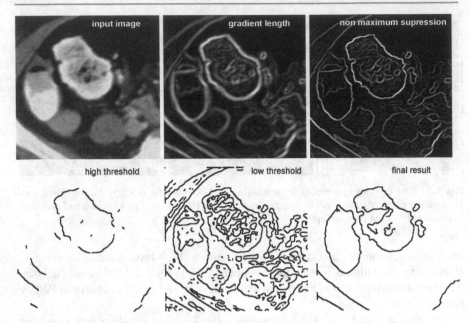

Fig. 5.2 The different steps of the Canny Edge Operator (the result from non-maximum suppression has been dilated for better visibility)

This process is repeated until no further pixels with $|\mathbf{g}| > t_1$ are found. The method finds connected edge segments. At intersections, it will track only one of the continuing curves. The other curve will be found as well if at least one of its edge pixels has a gradient larger than t_1. The value for t_1 should be high enough to make sure that none of the starting pixels is a noise pixel. However, since the continuation of an edge is only found between neighboring pixels, the threshold t_2 should be low so as not to hinder tracking (see the effect of different selections for t_1 and t_2 depicted in Fig. 5.3).

The Canny edge detector (or similar tracking approaches) will create edges as a subset of all edge locations with a certain strength. Since the locations to be considered for an edge are local maxima of the gradient length, edges may be false if noise has distorted the course of the edge. Low-pass filtering before computing the gradient prevents some of these erroneous responses, but it may also lead to false local maxima locations if smoothing causes the nearby edges to fuse.

Multiresolution edge detection and multiresolution edge tracking are two ways to get around this. In *multiresolution edge detection*, the gradient response is calculated at different scales. For each location, an optimal scale is chosen to compute the response. Hence, instead of deciding on a single scale for the complete image—as it is done when selecting the variance in Gaussian smoothing—a different scale is selected for each location. The wavelet decomposition of an image into localized frequency components is a good way to arrive at such a multiscale edge response. Mallat and Zhong (1992) have presented the appropriate wavelet transform. While wavelets provide for an (almost) redundancy-free representation

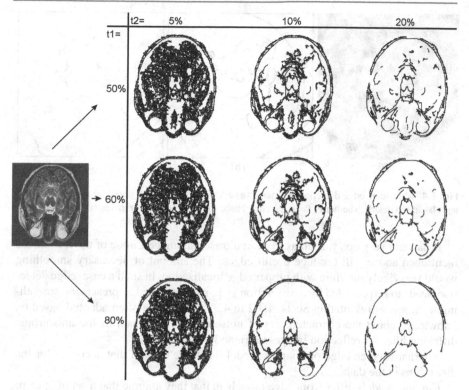

Fig. 5.3 Different choices for the two thresholds of the Canny Edge Detector lead to different results. Thresholds are given as percentage of the strongest gradient in the image

of scale and frequency components, redundant decomposition schemes such as using a sequence of Gaussians with different variances could be applied as well (a good survey on these techniques including multiresolution tracking techniques is given in Basu 2002).

In *multiresolution edge tracking*, edges are searched at different scales. The process commences with the lowest resolution and then proceeds to the next higher resolution (see Fig. 5.4). At the higher resolution, edge locations from the previous resolution level are used to initiate the search for edges on the current level. In Williams and Shah (1990), e.g., three different scales are used by convolving the image with three different Gaussians with standard deviations σ, $\sqrt{2}\sigma$, and 2σ and computing gradients on each resolution level. The basic resolution σ has to be determined based on the expected resolution and noise in the image. Edges are found in the lowest-resolution image and are confirmed on the next higher resolution. The detected edge locations on the current resolution image replace edges from the lower resolution if they are close to an already found edge and have a similar direction. This way, edge detection on the coarser resolution suppresses spurious edges while at the same time allowing for corrections of accidentally fused edges or of an overly smoothed course of an edge.

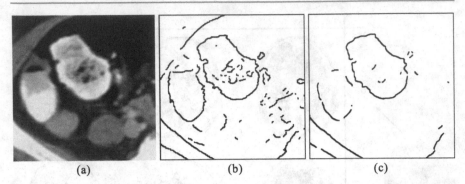

Fig. 5.4 Multiscale edge detection on image (**a**) allows to detect edge detail on a high scale image (**b**) and to decide whether to keep the edge based on a low resolution image (**c**)

If data are very noisy, such as, e.g., in ultrasound images, none of the techniques mentioned above will produce useful edges. The amount of necessary smoothing would very likely interfere with proper edge localization. In such a case, edge detection needs to be preceded by a restoration step, such as the edge-preserving smoothing techniques presented in Sects. 4.3.2 to 4.3.4. Filters are often adapted based on knowledge about the characteristics of noise or artefacts, such as the anisotropic diffusion filter for reflection images in Yu and Acton (2002).

Alternatively, an edge or contour model has to be created that accounts for the distortions in the data.

Contour models differ from edge models in that they assume that a set of open or closed contours are searched in the image in a top-down fashion while edge models generate edges in a bottom-up fashion based on a (possibly very elaborate) model of what an edge is in this particular image. Contour models will be discussed in Chap. 9 (Active Contours and Active Surfaces).

An *edge model* is usually just a local template that is convolved with the image. The template represents the ideal edge. The response to the match can be exploited to determine edge locations as well as a measure of confidence for the edge to be present (see, e.g., Meer and Georgescu 2001). For ultrasound images, an example for such a template model would be that of a stick model presented by Czerwinski et al. (1993) who argued that the boundaries in an ultrasound are not visible as intensity changes but as reflection lines at tissue boundaries. Hence, they matched a line model with the image. The expected response for a location being part of an edge is then a threshold that is derived from known noise characteristics in the ultrasound images (Czerwinski et al. 1994).

5.2   Hough Transform

The *Hough transform* computes edge features by comparing image evidence with a very specific edge model. Given an image containing edge information of an unknown number of edges of a known kind, the Hough transform finds instances of this kind.

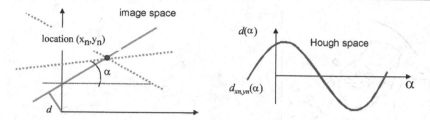

Fig. 5.5 Each edge point (x_n, y_n) in image space is represented by a curve in Hough space. The curve describes all parameter combinations $\alpha, d(\alpha)$ for lines passing through (x_n, y_n)

The Hough transform is a voting scheme that was first presented to find straight lines in images and then was extended to find arbitrary kinds of boundaries. Each location of a potential boundary—e.g., each location where the gradient length exceeds some threshold—votes for reference points in parameter space that are associated to certain shapes. Parameter combinations that receive the most votes describe likely object instances.

Being a voting system, the Hough transform keeps its ability to predict structure locations even if some votes are missing because of occlusion or a missing signal. The method is robust with respect to noise or artefactual edges that do not follow the edge model. Small variations from the predicted shape are tolerated.

The Hough transform can be defined for any dimension, but is most often applied in 2D because the number of parameters (i.e., the dimensionality of parameter space in which voting takes place) increases fast with the increasing dimension of the images.

The transform for finding straight lines was presented in Hough (1962). A line in 2D space $\mathbf{x} = (x_1 \; x_2)$ can be defined by the following variant of the line equation

$$d(\alpha) = x_i \cos(\alpha) + y_i \sin(\alpha), \tag{5.1}$$

where α is the angle and $d(\alpha)$ the distance to the origin of a line passing through a point $(x_i \; y_i)$. The Hough transform for a given potential boundary point $(x_i \; y_i)$ computes $d(\alpha)$. This point votes for all locations in parameter space $(d(\alpha), \alpha)$ for which (5.1) is true (see Fig. 5.5). The parameter space is digitized into bins in which votes accumulate (called *accumulator cells*). The number of votes for a potential boundary point in an image depends on its probability of being part of a boundary. It could be, for instance, a function of the gradient length.

The lines in the image are those for which corresponding accumulator cells are local maxima and have received a sufficiently high number of votes. The QoF (quality of fit) measure is a threshold on the number of votes (see Fig. 5.6 for an example).

A number of strategies increase the computation speed of the Hough transform and can be applied to most of its variants.

• The order in which votes are cast does not matter, which makes the method inherently parallelizable.

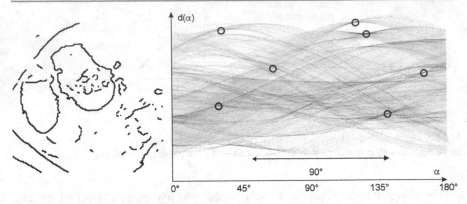

Fig. 5.6 Example of applying the Hough transform on an edge image. The predominance of edges at angles 45° and 135° with respect to the x-axis is visible as local maxima in Hough space

- If gradient directions in the edge images are reliable, the number of votes may be reduced by letting every edge point only vote for those solutions of (5.1) for which α is almost perpendicular to the gradient direction.
- If edge points are selected randomly from the image, the intermediate results of the voting process may already be a good estimate for the final outcome.

There are also some strategies for increasing the robustness of the Hough transform with respect to noise, artefacts, and shape variation.

- A multiscale strategy may be applied by computing an initial Hough transform only for large accumulator cells. The result is used as a prediction for ranges of parameters in Hough space that represent potential lines. The accumulation of votes at higher resolution is reduced to these ranges.
- Vote distribution in parameter space may be smoothed to take variation due to noise and artefacts into account.

The voting strategy of the Hough transform is not restricted to the search of straight line segments. Any boundary structure that can be represented by a small set of parameters can be found. Hence, the Hough transform is suitable to represent shape information for searching object instances instead of object features in the image. This will be detailed in Chap. 11.

5.3 Corners

Corners in an image indicate specific locations pertaining to an object. Such locations are important if objects of the same kind are to be compared or if the same object shall be compared in different images (e.g., comparing brain data of a patient from CT and PET). Another reason to identify specific locations is to classify an unknown object by its characteristic outline as given by the corner point locations.

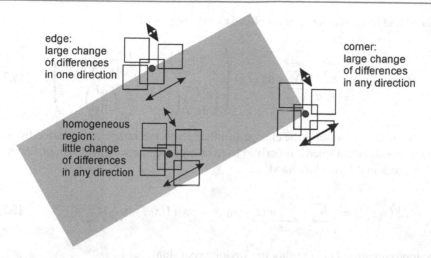

edge:
large change
of differences
in one direction

corner:
large change
of differences
in any direction

homogeneous
region:
little change
of differences
in any direction

Fig. 5.7 The Harris corner detector measures changes of intensity of a region around a point. A corner causes significant changes for displacement in arbitrary direction, an edge only if displaced orthogonal to it

The identification of a characteristic location will always require further knowledge (e.g., anatomical knowledge about configuration or appearance), but the minimum requirement is that this location is identifiable as a specific point. This is what a *corner detector* does.

Corners belong to a class of local features that can be computed from images, but represent attributes of depicted objects. This is of interest in many fields of computer vision. For more details the reader is pointed to a survey about feature detectors in Tuytelaars and Mikolajczyk (2007) who discussed the purpose, requirements, methods, and applications of local image features. The characteristic that is exploited for most corner detectors is that the so-called aperture problem does not exist for a corner.

The *aperture problem* states that for at least one direction the appearance of the image in a small window does not change if the window is moved in this direction. In homogeneous regions this is true for arbitrary directions. At edges it is true for the direction along the edge. For corners this is not true for any direction.

The *Harris corner detector* (Harris and Stephens 1988) is based on this assumption and has been shown to have a good performance (Schmid et al. 2000). The detector computes a quantity for a location $(x \ y)$ that depends on averaged intensity variations in arbitrary directions around $(x \ y)$. If this variation is high in almost all directions a point of interest is found (see sketch in Fig. 5.7). The neighborhood across which this variation is averaged constitutes the scale of the corner detector. A second scale parameter is that of the image, given by the amount of smoothing prior to compute the intensity variation between pixel locations.

The corner feature is computed from the eigenvalue of the *Harris matrix*. It consists of the partial derivatives, weighted with some function w of the image function $I(x, y)$ in a neighborhood k around a direction $(x_0 \ y_0)$ in which the image is displaced and then subtracted. It is defined as follows:

$$H(x_0, y_0) = \sum_{x=x_0-k}^{x_0+k} \sum_{y=y_0-k}^{y_0+k} w(x, y) \begin{pmatrix} \left(\dfrac{\partial I}{\partial x}\right)^2 & \left(\dfrac{\partial I}{\partial x}\right)\left(\dfrac{\partial I}{\partial y}\right) \\ \left(\dfrac{\partial I}{\partial x}\right)\left(\dfrac{\partial I}{\partial y}\right) & \left(\dfrac{\partial I}{\partial y}\right)^2 \end{pmatrix}. \tag{5.2}$$

This matrix represents the change of intensity, if the image were shifted by $\pm k$ and then subtracted since it is derived from computing the weighted sum of squared differences in this neighborhood

$$S(x_0, y_0) = \sum_{x=x_0-k}^{x_0+k} \sum_{y_0-k}^{y_0+k} w(x - x_0, y - y_0)\big(I(x_0, y_0) - I(x, y)\big)^2 \tag{5.3}$$

by approximating $I(x, y)$ using the Taylor expansion

$$I(x, y) = I(x_0, y_0) + (x_0 - x)\frac{\partial I(x_0, y_0)}{\partial x} + (y_0 - y)\frac{\partial I(x_0, y_0)}{\partial y} \tag{5.4}$$

around (x_0, y_0), which results in

$$S(x_0, y_0) = \sum_{x=x_0-k}^{x_0+k} \sum_{y_0-k}^{y_0+k} w(x - x_0, y - y_0)\left((x - x_0)\frac{\partial I(x, y)}{\partial x} + (y - y_0)\frac{\partial I(x, y)}{\partial y}\right)^2. \tag{5.5}$$

Setting

$$\mathbf{H}_p = w(x - x_0, y - y_0) \begin{pmatrix} \left(\dfrac{\partial I}{\partial x}\right)^2 & \left(\dfrac{\partial I}{\partial x}\right)\left(\dfrac{\partial I}{\partial y}\right) \\ \left(\dfrac{\partial I}{\partial x}\right)\left(\dfrac{\partial I}{\partial y}\right) & \left(\dfrac{\partial I}{\partial y}\right)^2 \end{pmatrix} \tag{5.6}$$

and substituting $u = x_0 - x$ and $v = y_0 - y$ this can be written as

$$S(x_0, y_0) = \sum_{x=x_0-k}^{x_0+k} \sum_{y=y_0-k}^{y_0+k} (u \quad v)\mathbf{H}_p(u \quad v)^{\mathrm{T}} = (u \quad v)\mathbf{H}(u \quad v)^{\mathrm{T}}. \tag{5.7}$$

If the point in question is a corner, this difference should be large for arbitrary directions $(x_0 \quad y_0)$. Hence, the two eigenvalues of $\mathbf{H}$ should be large. If just one eigenvalue is large, an edge has been found since there exists one specific direction (the corresponding eigenvector) in which the difference is large. Hence, three different cases can be derived from inspecting the eigenvalues λ_1 and λ_2 of $\mathbf{H}$.

• A corner has been found if λ_1 and λ_2 are large.
• An edge has been found if either λ_1 or λ_2 is large.
• The region is locally homogeneous if λ_1 and λ_2 are low.

   The detection is not scale-invariant, however. The scale of the response is given
by two parameters. The first is the amount of smoothing that is part of the approximation of the partial derivatives and the second is the window size over which the
Harris matrix is averaged. The corner detector can be made rotation-invariant by
using a rotationally symmetric window function w (e.g., a Gaussian).

   Another popular corner detector that performed well in comparison tests is *SU-
SAN* (Smallest Univalue Segment Assimilating Nucleus; Smith and Brady 1997).
The operator assumes

- that a point of interest has a different intensity than locations in a prespecified
  neighborhood,
- that this difference is larger than a threshold value g,
- that this point of interest is a local maximum of this difference.

First an intensity-gradient-based response in some neighborhood N is computed
as follows:

$$R(x, y) = \sum_{(u,v)\in N} \exp\left(-\frac{[I(x, y) - I(u, v)]^6}{t}\right). \tag{5.8}$$

   The exponent has been found experimentally. The value of t governs the strength
with which the intensity difference is influencing R. The higher the average intensity difference is in N the lower is the response. To compute the final response
S_{SUSAN}, R is inverted and thresholded with g

$$S_{SUSAN} = \begin{cases} g - R(x, y), & \text{if } g - R(x, y) > 0, \\ 0, & \text{otherwise.} \end{cases} \tag{5.9}$$

   The value of S_{SUSAN} is a local maximum if (x, y) is a corner or a single point.
The operator is faster to compute than the Harris corner detector, but was found to
be more sensitive to noise.

5.4 Blobs

Blobs are circular structures in the images. *Blob detection* either detects such structures (e.g., in counting microorganisms in cell microscopy) or highlights blobs as
important features of an object to be detected (e.g., in the detection of lung nodules; Coppini et al. 2003; Schilham et al. 2003). Formally speaking, a blob is a local
maximum or minimum of a radially symmetric intensity distribution.

   Blobs are characterized by their size and location. If the size is known, blobs
can be enhanced by a matched filter of the same size and shape. The *Laplacian of
Gaussian* with standard deviation σ according to the blob size is often used

$$LoG(x, y) = -\frac{1}{\pi\sigma^4}\left(1 - \frac{x^2 + y^2}{\sigma^2}\right)\exp\left(-\frac{x^2 + y^2}{\sigma^2}\right). \tag{5.10}$$

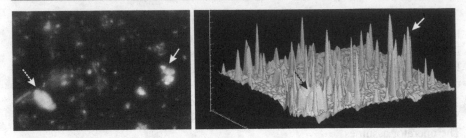

Fig. 5.8 Result of a blob detection on a microscopy with blob-like microorganisms. Locations of organisms are the local maxima of the detector response map. The large and bright *structure on the lower left* (see *arrow*) produces a small response, because only the (barely visible) blobs in this structure are of the expected blob size. The blob *conglomerate on the right* (see *arrow*) is nicely resolved into its constituent blobs

Alternatively, the *Difference of Gaussians* (DoG) filter may be used. The response of a DoG filter is computed by subtracting the filter response of the image with two Gaussians with different standard deviation from each other.

Potential blob sites are the local maxima (or minima, if the blob is darker than the background) of the convolution result (see Fig. 5.8 for an example). Blobs of size σ are detected by thresholding the result. If finding a suitable threshold is difficult, blob responses may be ordered by the strength of the response and the threshold is defined by selecting the n most prominent blobs.

Since the scale and hence the size of the blob in image coordinates is not known, blob detection can be extended to a scale-invariant detection including σ as a parameter in $LoG(x, y, \sigma)$. To make the response independent of the size of the blob, the function needs to be normalized with σ yielding

$$LoG_{\mathrm{norm}}(x, y, \sigma) = -\frac{\sigma}{\pi \sigma^4}\left(1 - \frac{x^2 + y^2}{\sigma^2}\right)\exp\left(-\frac{x^2 + y^2}{\sigma^2}\right). \qquad (5.11)$$

The local minima or maxima in this space represent the blob location and the size of the blob.

A different approach is to use the determinant of the *Hessian matrix*. It evaluates the differential properties of the point-like shape of blobs. The Hessian is the matrix of partial derivatives of a function. For a 2D image $I(x, y)$ it is

$$\mathbf{H} = \begin{pmatrix} \dfrac{\partial I^2}{\partial^2 x} & \dfrac{\partial I}{\partial x}\dfrac{\partial I}{\partial y} \\[2mm] \dfrac{\partial I}{\partial x}\dfrac{\partial I}{\partial y} & \dfrac{\partial I^2}{\partial^2 y} \end{pmatrix}. \qquad (5.12)$$

Its determinant $\det(\mathbf{H})$ should be large if the image intensity peaks at some location (i.e., if this location is a blob). Hence, blob detection consists of detecting local maxima of the determinant. Again, the detector can be made scale-invariant by including the scale parameter into the function and by searching for local maxima in space and scale. Since the value of the determinant decreases with increasing blob size, the response is normalized by the blob size σ

$$Blob_{\text{Hessian}}(x, y) = \sigma^2 \det(\mathbf{H}(x, y)). \tag{5.13}$$

A different approach is to use the shape of a blob directly by applying a kind of watershed transform (Lindeberg 1993). If a blob is a local maximum (or minimum), the pixels surrounding the blob center should have lower (or higher) values. A standard watershed transform on such an image would segment the image into regions of which blobs that are darker than the background are a subset. The watershed transform treats intensity values as heights in a 3D landscape and computes watersheds by flooding the landscape. Flooding starts from local minima in the image (the sources in the landscape). A watershed is found when flooding water from different sources meets (for details on the watershed transform see Roerdink and Meijster 2001 or Sect. 6.4 in the segmentation chapter).

To separate blobs from the background, flooding stops if an intensity level is reached beyond which everything counts as background. Blobs that are brighter than the background can be found as well by inverting the procedure (i.e., by flooding from the brightest pixel and again stopping at some threshold intensity).

5.5 SIFT and SURF Features

The *scale-invariant feature transform* (SIFT) was developed by Lowe (1999, 2004), and patented by the University of British Columbia. SIFT generates and uses features to detect and identify objects in images. Local features are identified and represented in a descriptor. Objects are identified by comparing expected feature configurations with all possible subsets of configurations from features detected in an image. The object is detected if a sufficiently large correspondence has been found. The method proceeds in several steps:
- key point generation,
- key point reduction,
- feature computation,
- key point matching.

In *key point generation*, rotation- and scale-invariant features are generated by searching for the local extrema of a multiscale blob detector based on a multiscale Difference of Gaussian (DoG, see previous section and Fig. 5.9). The detector is insensitive with respect to noise by determining an optimal smoothing for each scale. This is done by computing a sequence of Gaussian smoothings $S(\sigma_i)$ with standard deviations $\sigma_i = \sigma_1, \sigma_2, \ldots, \sigma_n$ and computing a sequence of DoG $D(\sigma_i) = S(\sigma_i) - S(\sigma_{i-1}), i = 2, n$ (see Fig. 5.10). A local extremum is maximal or minimal not only in scale, but also along the range of different smoothing scales σ_i.

Key point generation will create numerous responses from noise and artefacts. In *key point reduction*, the contrast at local extrema is used to remove low contrast blob locations (Lowe 1999).

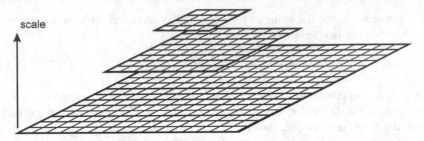

Fig. 5.9 Key point responses are computed at different scales of an image pyramid. Potential key points are local extrema in scale space

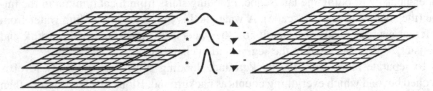

Fig. 5.10 Additionally to being an extremum in scale space it also has to be an extremum for differently smoothing DoG filters

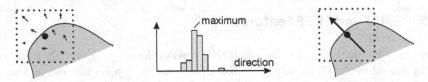

Fig. 5.11 Key point orientation is computed from a histogram of binned gradient directions in the vicinity of the key point

Responses are also removed if contrast is high, but the localization is unstable. This is the case along edges where the average contrast may be high because the feature is prominent across the edge but the localization accuracy is low because the feature strength varies little along the edge. The selection criterion to remove edge responses uses corner detection schemes such as local curvature or the determinant of the Hessian (see previous section). In Lowe (2004), an improved version of this step was presented where the feature response function was interpolated and the attributes of the interpolated function were used to remove unstable feature locations.

In *feature computation*, orientation attributes are determined and stored for each remaining key point. A histogram of gradient directions is computed for locations in the neighborhood of a key point (see Fig. 5.11). Gradient directions are computed at the scale that was determined for the key point in the first step. The maximum of this histogram indicates the local key point orientation. A threshold of 80% of this maximum is set and it is tested whether any other local maximum in the histogram exceeds this threshold. If it is the case, multiple key points with the same location but different orientations are created. The key point orientation is then used to compute

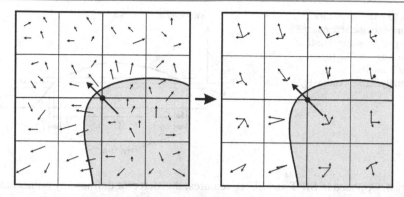

Fig. 5.12 The feature vector for a key point consists of binned histograms of normalized, relative gradient directions with respect to the key point orientation. Hence, key points are represented by a kind of rotation-invariant texture features

rotation-invariant features. A local window at the feature scale is defined around the point location. Gradients within this window are weighted with a Gaussian. Then, local gradient histograms in subwindows around the key point location are used as key point features (see Fig. 5.12). The features are organized in a feature vector that is then normalized to make the feature independent from intensity variation. Hence, the feature vector describes the relative gradient length distribution for different gradient directions in the vicinity of the key point.

Key point features can then be used for *matching* model key points with the key points extracted from the image. Although the objective for developing the SIFT procedure was to identify objects by key features, its main application in medical image analysis is to support feature-based registration algorithms (for registration methods see Chap. 10). Registration finds a transformation to map two images of the same object onto each other. The reason for using SIFT features is that it can be assumed that this mapping will only be successful if a sufficiently large number of features corresponds in the two images. A registration is particularly easy if this correspondence is given by sets of pairs of corresponding feature locations. Since most medical image registration problems are 3D, the SIFT features have been extended to 3D as well (Allaire et al. 2008).

A faster variant to SIFT is SURF (*speeded-up robust features*; Bay et al. 2006). It uses essentially the same mechanism, except for the fact that the slow convolutions in SIFT are replaced by faster approximations. The methodology is patented in the United States and is claimed by the author of not only being faster but also more robust than the SIFT features.

5.6   MSER Features

Locations, such as the center of gravity, generated from *maximally stable extremal regions* (MSER) were presented by Matas et al. (2002). The key concept of this approach is to separate an image into local homogeneous regions with maximum

Fig. 5.13 The instability measure rates the size change of a region for some threshold variation against the region size. It is minimal for a maximally stable extremal region

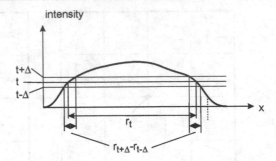

contrast. Opposed to SIFT and SURF features, this detector defines key points based on intensity and not on gradients.

The definition for an MSER can be found in Matas et al. (2002). It can be described informally as follows.

- A region r_t is any connected set of scene elements $\mathbf{s}$ with intensity $f(\mathbf{s}) > t$, where t is an arbitrary threshold.
- An instability measure $s_\Delta(r_t, t)$ (see Fig. 5.13) rates the size change of r_t when the threshold is varied by some value Δ

$$s_\Delta(r_t, t) = |r_{t+\Delta} - r_{t-\Delta}|/|r_t|, \tag{5.14}$$

where $|\cdot|$ indicates computing the volume of the respective region.

- A region r_t is maximally stable if $s_\Delta(r_t, t)$ is minimum for t.

Centers of maximally stable extremal regions serve as key points and features of the regions can be used as key point attributes. Compared to the computation of SIFT features the generation of MSER features is very fast ($O(n \log n)$ with n being the number of scene elements, see Matas et al. 2002). Several ways for an even more efficient computation have been proposed (Donoser and Bischof 2006a; Nistér and Stewénius 2008).

Although MSER has been first presented for 2D applications it easily extends to 3D since the definition does not depend on the dimension of the scene. Maximally stable regions in 3D have been used for the segmentation of medical images (Donoser and Bischof 2006b). Since MSER features have been applied in feature-based correspondence analysis for stereo vision (Matas et al. 2002), they could be used for registration as well although we are currently not aware of such an application in medical image analysis. In Forssen and Lowe (2007), MSER were combined with SIFT features. SIFT features were computed at the locations of a maximally stable extremal region and provided a richer description than the original features.

5.7   Key-Point-Independent Features

The features mentioned so far are meant to characterize key point locations at boundaries or in regions in an image. However, features may also be generated from sampling the boundary or a region-of-interest. Two popular examples will be described in the following.

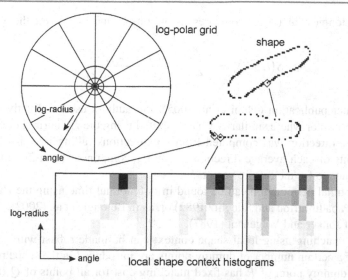

Fig. 5.14 Local shape context is represented by 2D histograms for points that contain frequency of occurrences of other points. The histogram is binned in a log-polar grid. It can be seen that shape contexts of similar point locations result in similar histograms

Local shape context (Belongie et al. 2002) describes an object by boundary features that need not be—and in most case will not be—key points. The purpose of using local shape context is to be able to match two structures based on the shape context information. Local shape context is defined on boundary points that stem from sampling boundaries of an object-of-interest that are generated by an edge detection procedure such as the Canny edge detector. The boundary needs not to be closed. However, edge detection of two similar objects should result in similar sets of boundary parts. Sampling may be arbitrary, but in the absence of further knowledge it should generate point locations distributed evenly over the boundary parts.

A structure is then represented by a sequence of points $P = \{p_1, \ldots, p_N\}$. For each point, shape context is computed by comparing its position to the position of all other points. It results in a set of direction vectors $D_i = \{d_{i,1}, \ldots, d_{i,N-1}\}$, where each direction is a vector from p_i to some other point p_j, $j \neq i$. The directions are binned in a log-polar coordinate system. In Belongie et al. (2002), five distance ranges and 12 sectors were used to determine the bin size. The histogram now gives the number of occurrences of other points with respect to the p_i per bin (see Fig. 5.14). The feature is translation-invariant as it defines the context with respect to the location of p_i. It can be made scale-invariant by normalizing the distances with the average distance of all points p_j to p_i. If necessary, it can be made rotation-invariant by computing the histogram based on a coordinate system that is fixed to the tangent direction at p_i.

Given the shape context for every point p_i of P, a match to points q_j of some other figure Q is computed by finding a permutation $j = \pi(i)$ such that the sum of local similarities $S(\pi) = \sum_{i=0,N} S(i, \pi(i))$ is maximal. The local similarity measure of Belongie et al. (2002) compares histograms h_i and $h_{\pi(i)}$ using the X^2 metric

$$S(i, \pi(i)) = \frac{1}{2} \sum_{k=1}^{K} \frac{(h_i(k) - h_{\pi(i)}(k))^2}{h_i(k) + h_{\pi(i)}(k)}. \tag{5.15}$$

In a later publication (Moni et al. 2005), the authors used a slightly different feature descriptor where similarity was computed using the L_2-norm. For each bin, an average direction was computed from all directions falling into this bin. The components of each average direction (x- and y-component for a 2D image) are concatenated to for the feature vector.

The optimal permutation can be found in polynomial time using the Hungarian method (Papadimitriou and Stieglitz 1982) or, as in Belongie et al. (2002), the faster method of Jonker and Volgenant (1987).

Shape matching using local shape context can be made robust with respect to outliers if a certain number of dummy points are introduced in the shape representation. A dummy point of P has fixed matching cost for all points of Q (and vice versa for dummy points of Q). If the similarity of all points in P to a point q_j in Q is worse than the matching cost for the dummy point then q_j is matched to the next free dummy point. Hence, a fixed number of points in P and Q are allowed to have no counterpart.

Given the match, a transformation between the two scenes that contain P and Q can be interpolated so that not only P and Q, but also the two scenes are registered with respect to each other (for further details on registration see Chap. 10).

Although shape context does not attempt to find key points it still requires parts of object boundaries to be found. This may be unwanted if a boundary is difficult to detect because of insufficient image contrast or artefacts. The *histogram of gradients* (HOG) (Dalal and Triggs 2005) is a feature detector that does not rely on boundaries as it samples a dense gradient texture map and uses this to generate the features. Hence, HOG features are always computed from a gridded region of interest that is assumed be mostly occupied by the structure to be analyzed.

A HOG cell is defined at each gridline intersection. The authors suggest two types of cells. R-HOG cells have a rectangular shape while C-HOG cells have a circular shape. Gradients are computed for each pixel. Each pixel within a cell votes for a direction in a binned histogram of gradient directions. The vote is weighted with the strength of the gradient.

To make the response insensitive to intensity variation, cells are grouped into larger blocks. The gradient strength is normalized with the average gradient in this block.

The authors used the HOG *features* for accurately detecting pedestrians in images using cell sizes of 4×4 to 12×12 pixels and block sizes of 1×1 to 4×4 cells with the best results with block sizes between 2×2 and 3×3 and cell sizes between 6×6 and 8×8. They reported that the method was most successful when using the simplest gradient operator and no smoothing of the data, although this may be different when using HOG features on medical images with its higher noise levels.

5.8 Saliency and Gist

Saliency and gist are image features, which are different to the features discussed above that pertain to structures in the image. Image features are not immediately useful for the analysis of objects. However, as they characterize the image, they may be used to guide image analysis in application such as a feature-based search in an image data base.

Saliency is an attribute that guides the attention of human vision to certain locations in the image. Focusing on certain parts in an image is an integral part of the perception process of a human operator who searches, recognizes, and categorizes structures in an image as it allows the operator to single out subsets of the image and focus on attributes of this subset. A salient location in an image is a region where features differ significantly from features in the vicinity. Since saliency is a concept of biologically inspired computer vision, features are those perceived at early stages of visual perception. Examples are image intensity, image color, and local orientation. A biologically plausible method for computing saliency has been presented by Itti et al. (1998). Several other methods exist as well.

Computer vision techniques use saliency in the same manner for quickly directing attention to subparts of an image which may contain objects that are searched. Such rapid scene analysis is seldom the goal when working with medical images, but the distribution, extent, and properties of salient locations characterize images in a way that can be useful for search and comparison tasks between images. This is even more so considering the fact that occlusion problems—which change such configuration—do not occur if the images are 3D.

The *gist* of an image is an overall categorization of an image (e.g., by characterizing an image as a CT image of a head depicting a subdural hemorage). In human vision, deriving the gist of an image allows to pick a constraining category for further analysis. Being able to compute the gist of an image can substantially speed up image analysis as it reduces the number of possible explanations for depicted objects. Since gist summarizes information from all parts of the image to come up with an overall categorization, methods to compute gist are integrations from feature values everywhere in the image. Computer-based methods to compute gist sometimes assign to rather broad categories (Torralba et al. 2003), but combining gist and saliency computation has been shown to provide differentiation between quite similar but different categories (Siagian and Itti 2007).

Using gist features will probably be of little use for analyzing medical images where the gist is usually known. As with the case of saliency, gist features may help in the automatic categorization of images in a data basis of medical images. Here, meta-information may describe the gist of the image only in the context of the clinical or research question that gave rise to the production of the image.

5.9 Bag of Features

When features such as the ones discussed above will be used to detect objects they need to be combined to some kind of a superstructure since the semantic of a single feature is usually insufficient for representing the object characteristics. A simple

way to arrive at a higher level semantic is to just collect features (points, edges, textures) from a region that shall be recognized. Feature collection is done by picking
regularly or randomly distributed patches from the region and computing feature
attributes in these region (Nowak et al. 2006).

Each patch is assumed to be a "visual word" making up the visual sentence describing the image. It is a *bag of features* that represents the (main) meaning of the
region from which the features are taken. Since the content of the bag is not spatially ordered, the representation is invariant with respect to translation and, if the
feature values are invariant to rotation or scale, invariant with respect to these two
transformations as well.

The feature values of the different elements in the bag will all be different and
their frequency of occurrence will characterize the region recognition is possible,
if the expected feature occurrences for different objects has been trained from the
examples.

The bag of feature approach is attractive for search in image data bases and has
been successfully applied to solve content-based image retrieval tasks for medical
images by Caicedo et al. (2009) and Wang et al. (2011).

5.10 Concluding Remarks

Feature detection is an intermediate step for generating semantics from an image. Computing such features changes the attribute representation from an image-
centered to an object-centered reference system. Since features are defined on image
attributes, this has to be taken with a grain of salt, however. Feature computation often assumes that object attributes can be defined based on local image attributes in
an invariant fashion. In reality, object attributes visible in an image may well be
different for the same type of object.

Feature computation always consists of two parts. First, attributes are computed
and then a criterion is applied to find locations where attributes are assumed to be
relevant. The latter should be applied with care as well. Since the definition of feature attributes will not exactly separate object features from image artefacts, setting
a strong relevancy criterion might remove the necessary object features. This can be
critical if the subsequent steps are automatic so that input to a later analysis module is not verified by user input (a search for an object boundary may fail if the
edge-tracking step removed too many of the potential boundary parts).

5.11 Exercises

- What is the purpose of the two thresholds used in edge tracking by the Canny
  edge detector? What guidelines should be followed when setting the thresholds?
- Name situations or problems for which edge tracking is a useful preprocessing
  step.
- What would happen if the size of the accumulator cells of the Hough transform
  were made smaller? Under what circumstance would it be an advantage?

- Describe the steps of finding lines by the Hough transform?
- Explain strategies to speed up the Hough transform. Why is the Hough transform generally advantageous in a real-time environment?
- What are the underlying assumptions for a corner detector?
- What features of the Harris matrix are used for corner detection? How are they used for corner detection?
- What is the difference of the features used by the SUSAN corner detector compared to the Harris corner detector?
- What filters can be used for blob detection?
- How is the blob detector made scale-invariant?
- Describe an algorithmic sketch for detecting blobs of unknown size in an image. What kind of prior information is needed to parametrize the method?
- Describe the steps that lead to SIFT key points.
- How are the SIFT features made rotation-invariant?
- What kind of features represent a SIFT key point?
- How are the SIFT made (approximately) invariant to illumination changes? Under what circumstance is invariance with respect to intensity changes no longer given? Why?
- Describe the condition that needs to be met for a point being the center of an MSER (maximally stable extremal region).
- Why can it be expected that MSER centers do not (not even approximately) coincide with SIFT key points?
- What are the potential applications of using SIFT key points or MSER centers in a medical image analysis method? What would be their purpose?
- What differences are between SIFT features and shape context features?
- Explain the strategy by which shape context is made insensitive to feature points that cannot be matched.

References

Allaire S, Kim JJ, Breen SL, Jaffray DA, Pekar V (2008) Full orientation invariance and improved feature selectivity of 3D SIFT with application to medical image analysis. In: IEEE computer vision and pattern recognition workshops, CVPRW'08, pp 1–8

Basu M (2002) Gaussian-based edge-detection methods—a survey. IEEE Trans Syst Man Cybern, Part C, Appl Rev 32(3):252–259

Bay H, Tuytelaars T, van Gool L (2006) SURF: Speeded up robust features. In: Europ conf computer vision ECCV 2006. LNCS, vol 3951, pp 404–417

Belongie S, Malik J, Puzicha J (2002) Shape matching and object recognition using shape contexts. IEEE Trans Pattern Anal Mach Intell 24(4):509–521

Caicedo JC, Cruz A, FA Gonzalez (2009) Histopathology image classification using bag of features and kernel functions. In: Artificial intelligence in medicine. LNCS, vol 5651, pp 126–135

Canny J (1986) A computational approach to edge detection. IEEE Trans Pattern Anal Mach Intell 8(6):679–698

Coppini G, Diciotti S, Falchini M, Villari N, Valli G (2003) Neural networks for computer-aided diagnosis: detection of lung nodules in chest radiograms. IEEE Trans Inf Technol Biomed 7(4):344–357

Czerwinski RN, Jones DL, O'Brien WD (1993) An approach to boundary detection in ultrasound imaging. In: Proc IEEE ultrasonics symposium, Baltimore

Czerwinski RN, Jones DL, O'Brien WD (1994) Edge detection in ultrasound speckle noise. In: Proc IEEE intl conf on image processing, Austin, pp 304–308

Dalal N, Triggs B (2005) Histograms of oriented gradients for human detection. In: IEEE comp soc conf computer vision and pattern recognition (CVPR'05), vol 1, pp 886–893

Donoser M, Bischof H (2006a) Efficient maximally stable extremal region (MSER) tracking. In: Proc conf computer vision and pattern recognition (CVPR), pp 553–560

Donoser M, Bischof H (2006b) 3d segmentation by maximally stable volumes (MSVs). In: Proc conf intl conf pattern recognition (ICPR), pp 63–66

Forssen PE, Lowe DG (2007) Shape descriptors for maximally stable extremal regions. In: IEEE 11th intl conf computer vision (ICCV), pp 1–8

Harris C, Stephens M (1988) A combined corner and edge detector. In: Alvey vision conference, pp 147–151

Hough PVC (1962) Method and means for recognizing complex pattern. US patent no 3.069.654

Itti L, Koch C, Niebur E (1998) A model of saliency-based visual attention for rapid scene analysis. IEEE Trans Pattern Anal Mach Intell 20(11):1254–1259

Jonker R, Volgenant A (1987) A shortest augmenting path algorithm for dense and sparse linear assignment problems. Computing 38:325–340

Lindeberg T (1993) Detecting salient blob-like image structures and their scales with a scale-space primal sketch: a method for focus-of-attention. Int J Comput Vis 11(3):283–318

Lowe DG (1999) Object recognition from local scale-invariant features. In: Intl conf computer vision ICCV 1999, vol 2, pp 1150–1157

Lowe DG (2004) Distinctive image features from scale-invariant keypoints. Int J Comput Vis 60(2):91–110

Mallat S, Zhong S (1992) Characterization of signals from multiscale edges. IEEE Trans Pattern Anal Mach Intell 14(7):710–732

Matas J, Chum O, Urba M, Pajdla T (2002) Robust wide baseline stereo from maximally stable extremal regions. In: Proc of British machine vision conference, pp 384–396

Meer P, Georgescu B (2001) Edge detection with embedded confidence. IEEE Trans Pattern Anal Mach Intell 23(12):1351–1365

Moni G, Belongie S, Malik J (2005) Efficient shape matching using shape contexts. IEEE Trans Pattern Anal Mach Intell 27(11):1832–1837

Nistér D, Stewénius H (2008) Linear time maximally stable extremal regions. In: Proc Europ conf computer vision ECCV 2008. LNCS, vol 5303, pp 183–196

Nowak E, Jurie F, Triggs B (2006) Sampling strategies for bag-of-features image classification. In: Europ conf computer vision ECCV 2006. LNCS, vol 3954, pp 490–503

Papadimitriou C, Stieglitz K (1982) Combinatorial optimization: algorithms and complexity. Prentice Hall, New York

Papari G, Petkov N (2011) Edge and line oriented contour detection: state of the art. Image Vis Comput 29:79–103

Roerdink JBTM, Meijster A (2001) The watershed transform: definitions, algorithms and parallelization strategies. Fundam Inform 41:187–228

Schilham AMR, van Ginneken B, Loog M (2003) Multi-scale nodule detection in chest radiographs. In: Medical image computing and computer-assisted intervention—MICCAI 2003. LNCS, vol 2878, pp 602–609

Schmid C, Mohr R, Bauckhage C (2000) Evaluation of interest point detectors. Int J Comput Vis 37(2):151–172

Siagian C, Itti L (2007) Rapid biologically-inspired scene classification using features shared with visual attention. IEEE Trans Pattern Anal Mach Intell 27(2):300–312

Smith SM, Brady JM (1997) SUSAN—a new approach to low level image processing. Int J Comput Vis 23(1):45–78

Torralba A, Murphy KP, Freeman WT, Rubin MA (2003) Context-based vision system for place and object recognition. In: IEEE intl conf computer vision (ICCV), pp 1023–1029

Tuytelaars T, Mikolajczyk K (2007) Local invariant feature detectors: a survey. Found Trends Comput Graph Vis 3(3):177–280

Wang J, Li Y, Zhang Y, Wang C, Xie H, Chen G, Gao X (2011) Bag-of-features based medical image retrieval via multiple assignment and visual words weighting. IEEE Trans Med Imag 30(11):1996–2011

Williams DJ, Shah M (1990) Edge contours using multiple scales. Comput Vis Graph Image Process 51:256–274

Yu Y, Acton ST (2002) Speckle reducing anisotropic diffusion. IEEE Trans Image Process 11:1260–1270

Segmentation: Principles and Basic Techniques 6

Abstract

The purpose of image segmentation is to generate pixel agglomerations from an image that constitute parts of the depicted objects. In medical imaging, segmentation often refers to the delineation of specific structures. Hence, it includes parts of classification as well. Segmentation strategies in medical imaging combine data knowledge with domain knowledge to arrive at the result. Data knowledge refers to assumptions about continuity, homogeneity, and local smoothness of image features within segments. Domain knowledge represents information about the objects to be delineated.

In this chapter, basic strategies for integrating the two types of knowledge into the segmentation process will be discussed. We will also describe basic segmentation methods that are popular in medical image analysis.

Concepts, notions and definitions introduced in this chapter

> Data features: intensity and texture
> The role of homogeneity, smoothness, and continuity in segmentation
> Using object localization and appearance as domain knowledge
> The role of interaction
> Basic segmentation techniques: thresholding, region merging techniques, region growing, watershed transform, live wire

The quantitative analysis of a medical image requires objects or object features in the image to be identified and delineated. First, the image is segmented into regions that are possible candidates of objects. This is followed by assigning meaning to these regions. For analyzing a digital photograph, this *segmentation* task would group pixels to regions that may belong to (parts of) objects based on the attributes of these regions. Hence, the segmentation of images is similar to creating phonemes in speech or detecting syllables in a written text as it creates basic semantic entities from images.

K.D. Toennies, *Guide to Medical Image Analysis*,
Advances in Computer Vision and Pattern Recognition,
DOI 10.1007/978-1-4471-2751-2_6, © Springer-Verlag London Limited 2012

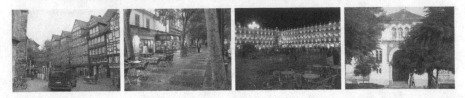

Fig. 6.1 Finding a general solution for a segmentation task would be very difficult even if only the houses depicted in the four examples would need to be segmented correctly

However, it is difficult to apply domain knowledge about objects in an image to segmentation. The purpose of segmentation is to create semantic entities in the first place. Ideally, object-independent criteria help to partition an image into segments. After segmentation, every pixel is assigned to exactly one segment since every location in an image carries just one meaning.

There is a problem with this. The appearances of objects in some image—consider a picture of a landscape with a house in the foreground, some trees and mountains in the background—may be very different within and between object classes (see, e.g., Fig. 6.1). A house may consist of visible surfaces of homogeneous color requiring a homogeneity criterion on color, a tree may be characterized by its natural texture and color, which requires the texture to be included in the criterion, and the depiction of the mountains in the background is mostly characterized by intensity and the faded color of distant objects. A uniform segmentation criterion for all of these objects will be difficult to find. Regions found by a simple criterion such as homogeneous color may segment some regions correctly but may fail in other regions.

For the *segmentation of medical images*, the situation is somewhat less grave, as a medical image represents (ideally) the measurement of a diagnostically relevant entity that is measured in the same way everywhere in the body. Consider CT, for instance, where x-ray attenuation is measured on the normalized Hounsfield scale. Attenuation should not vary with location but only with density and atomic number.

External influences such as shading or object-specific signal degradation still add an object- or location-dependent component to the measured and reconstructed signal. Furthermore, measured values are not unique for a specific object class. Hence, data-driven segmentation will almost always result in a collection of regions that in some cases will separate an object of interest into several segments and in other cases will fuse different objects into a single segment.

6.1   Segmentation Strategies

There are several ways to deal with the missing information without sacrificing the assumption that a low-level segmentation criterion is valid everywhere in the image.
- *Foreground segmentation* (Fig. 6.2) focuses on a single object in the image. Segmentation criteria create a good partitioning of foreground objects, whereas the quality of partitioning the background is irrelevant. Later analysis is carried out

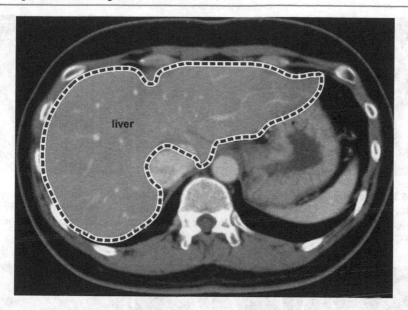

Fig. 6.2 If only the liver needs to be separated from the CT, a segmentation would be successful irrespective of any errors in regions outside the liver. A foreground segmentation that only incorporates information as to what differentiates liver from all other tissues would be sufficient

solely on foreground segments. The strategy requires some model knowledge to be applied after segmentation for separating foreground segments from the background. A simple way to introduce model knowledge would be to let the user point out foreground segments.

- *Hierarchical segmentation* (Fig. 6.3) applies a multiresolution concept for gradual refinement. A first segmentation creates segments that are smaller than the smallest object. It is assumed that a common criterion (in most cases a homogeneity criterion) can be found at this scale. The result is sometimes called *oversegmentation*. At the next level, some of these segments are merged into larger segments according to domain knowledge about object appearance. The successful application of this strategy requires that meaningful segments can be defined by a common criterion at a single but unknown scale. This scale is found by analyzing levels of the segmentation hierarchy.

- *Multilayer segmentation* (Fig. 6.4) is another multiresolution technique. It is assumed that a common segmentation criterion exists but that its scale may vary throughout the image (like a structured texture of objects in a photograph of which the scale varies with the distance of the object to the camera). Segmentation is carried out at different scales producing layers of segments. Later analysis will have to estimate local scales and patch segments according to it. It is more general than the previous strategy as the scale of a criterion often varies for different structures in an image. The analysis of segments is more difficult because an appropriate scale for every segment has to be established independently from other segments.

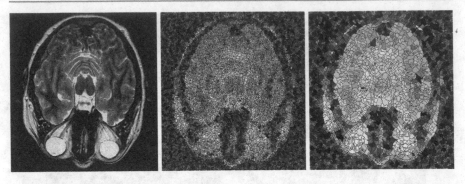

Fig. 6.3 In hierarchical segmentation, the first segmentation step provides little more than super-pixels. Two examples from segmenting (**a**) can be seen in (**b**) and (**c**), where slightly different homogeneity constraints lead to different sizes. The next hierarchy level attempts to combine superpixels to higher semantic units

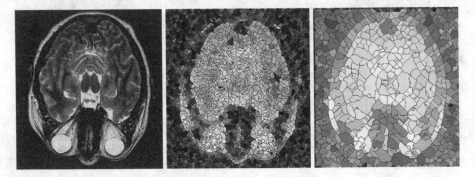

Fig. 6.4 In multilayer segmentation, segmentations at different levels of resolution are created and evaluated in parallel. In this example, the boundary between gray matter and CSF is captured quite well in the low resolution segmentation, while the boundary between fat and bone is captured better in the high resolution image

In medical imaging, different semantics stem from the intentional choice of the acquisition technique. The pixel value in a medical image is much more directly related to the diagnostic question than a pixel value of a photograph to the meaning of some outdoor scene. The acquisition technique has been chosen for the very reason that it is known to offer insight into some diagnostic question. This domain knowledge can be incorporated into the segmentation process. It becomes especially apparent for slice images. In some images, such as x-ray CT, function value, and membership to an organ class are related (see Fig. 6.5 and the Hounsfield Table 2.1 in Chap. 2). A segmentation criterion on pixel values may be sufficient for assigning class membership to a segment. Hence, segmentation and classification may mix in medical image analysis.

The search for occurrences of a specific structure by segmentation causes fore-ground segmentation to be more frequent in medical image analysis than in other image analysis tasks. Since it may involve a detection task, a model-driven approach

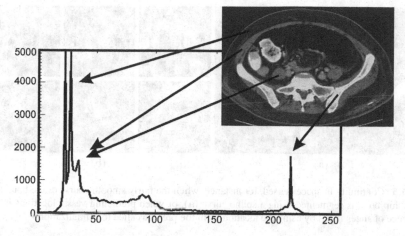

Fig. 6.5 In medical imaging there is often a much more direct relationship between pixel intensity and semantics compared to photographic pictures (although it is by no means a unique mapping)

then discriminates the structure from the background. Model knowledge may be integrated into the algorithm or supplemented interactively. Popular segmentation techniques, such as the various region growing techniques, the application of implicit or explicit active contours and surfaces, or active shape models use such a model-driven approach.

The use of domain knowledge from the acquisition technique and the reduction of segmentation to the search of foreground objects helps to solve the segmentation problem to an extent which exceeds the support of segmentation in general image processing. Furthermore, segmentation is often carried out in slice images with the consequence that occlusion does not have to be dealt with. On the other hand, the computer-assisted analysis of medical images is virtually impossible without segmentation.

6.2   Data Knowledge

Continuity in space and time are the two main data properties that are used for segmentation. An observable object is assumed to stand out in an image by some homogeneous intensity or texture in a region. Segmentation based on spatial continuity partitions a 2D or 3D image such that homogeneity within segments is larger than between the adjacent segments. It assumes that the course of the segment boundary does not change abruptly (see, e.g., Fig. 6.6a).

Temporal continuity can be used in the same fashion by treating time as the fourth dimension. Often, temporal continuity is exploited by computing a segmentation result at one time step and using it to constrain or initialize the segmentation at the next time step.

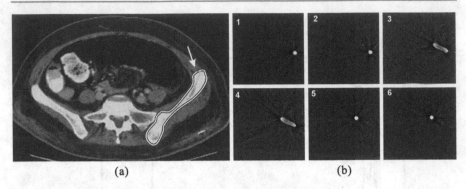

(a)   (b)

Fig. 6.6 Continuity in space is used, for instance, when the fairly smooth course of the boundary of the hip bone is segmented using a spline curve (**a**), or when predicting vessel locations in the sequence of slices in (**b**) by using the location from the previous slice for initialization

The strategy is sometimes applied as well for segmenting a sequence of 2D images of a 3D scene. Segmentation is carried out in a 2D slice. The result is then propagated into the next slice to initialize the segmentation in this slice (see Fig. 6.6b).

The propagation of segmentation constraints along the time axis or a spatial axis makes the result dependent on the initial segmentation. A developer should make sure that this initialization is a good as possible. This may be achieved by the following.

- Letting the user flip through slices or time steps for selecting the best starting point. Segmentation is then carried out from this initialization in both directions along the time or spatial axes.
- Starting the segmentation from several initialization points and selecting the best-rated segmentation from this. It requires a quality measure for segmentation results.
- Letting the process go several times back and forth through the data, improving the segmentation until a stable state of segmentation is reached.

Carrying out n-dimensional segmentation by imposing continuity constraints between adjacent segmentations in $(n - 1)$-dimensional space reduces the subsequent segmentation to a registration task if a 1-to-1 correspondence exists between segments in adjacent segmentations (see Fig. 6.6b). The task is simpler than registration in general since continuity assumptions predict that the corresponding segments are close to each other and have a similar shape. Such a situation often arises in 4D segmentation, where objects neither vanish nor are created between time steps. It is sometimes true for 3D segmentation from 2D slices as well, although this is not guaranteed. However, even if topology changes between slices, segments on the previous slice can be used to constrain the possible locations of an unknown number of segments with the same label in the current slice.

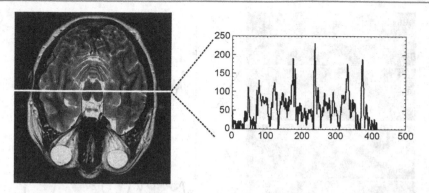

Fig. 6.7 Although contrast between tissues is good the image contains a substantial amount of noise that can be seen in a plot of intensities of one line in the image

6.2.1   Homogeneity of Intensity

Spatial and temporal continuity can be characterized by homogeneous local appearance. This refers in the simplest case to the homogeneity of intensity which is given by the intensity variance within a segment. Other approximations such as computing the difference between the brightest and the darkest pixels of a segment can be used as well.

Pixel or voxel intensities of a structure of interest often vary little throughout the segment. In consequence, intensity-based segmentation schemes are quite popular. However, a number of artefacts have to be accounted for. The best-known is noise. Segmentation in a noisy environment is more difficult than it seems since noise reduction capabilities of the human visual system are quite effective. A human may see a visible difference between neighboring segments long before homogeneity-based segmentation would separate the segments (see Fig. 6.7).

Noise is often modeled as Gaussian with zero mean value and a variance according to the SNR. Noise may be reduced during preprocessing, but this may cause small details to be removed (see Fig. 6.8). Noise reduction may be included into segmentation as well (e.g., by applying a multiresolution strategy). A multiresolution approach such as a *Gaussian pyramid* creates a sequence of images at different resolutions by repeated low-pass filtering and subsampling. Segmentation is carried out at a low resolution because of the noise-reducing effects of the low-pass filter. Low-pass filtering also reduces the boundary detail and may remove small segments. Hence, the segmentation of a low-resolution image is transferred to the next higher resolution by applying the expanded operation of the Gaussian pyramid to the segmentation (which is essentially an interpolation). The expanded result constrains segmentation at the higher resolution in much the same way as the spatial constraints imposed in the sequential segmentation of temporal sequences (see Fig. 6.9).

Shading is another artefact that sometimes influences intensity-based segmentation. It usually stems from image acquisition. Examples are shading in an MRI due to field inhomogeneities or shading in ultrasound images due to acoustical shad-

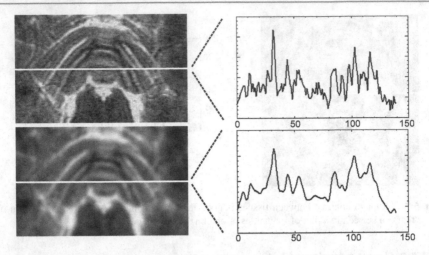

Fig. 6.8 Noise reduction prior to segmentation may cause loss of detail which is most critical if small structures are to be extracted by segmentation

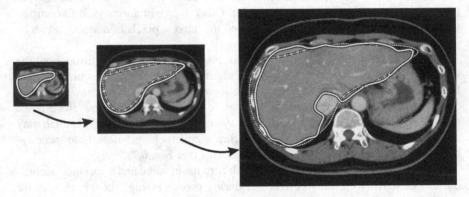

Fig. 6.9 Applying a multi-resolution strategy to segmentation: segmentation in a low resolution image is used as initialization on the next higher resolution

ows. If the shading effects are less pronounced than segment homogeneity, they can be removed during preprocessing. Multiple sclerosis lesion segmentation in MRI presented in Chap. 1, for instance, estimates shading based on a segmentation of white matter. White matter is highly contrasted against the background and thus easy to segment without shading correction. As white matter should have constant intensity, any intensity variation is attributed to shading, which is then extrapolated for every location in the image. Alternatively, intensity-based segmentation may be carried out locally if intensity variation per unit distance is smaller than the contrast between segments. The image is partitioned into subregions and segmentation is carried out separately for every subregion.

Some of the problems from shading can be resolved when resorting to boundary criteria instead of region criteria. If a segment is contrasted against neighboring segments, high intensity gradients indicate the boundaries between segments. Boundaries are either localized by tracking zero crossings of the second derivative of the intensity function or by computing local maxima of the gradient length. Gradient-based segmentation is simplest if the gradient length (i.e., the intensity difference between adjacent segments) is approximately equal throughout the image or if all nonzero gradient lengths are caused by segment boundaries. The former is rarely the case and the latter is never the case since images are not noise-free. Hence, many edge-based segmentation schemes include a significance threshold on the gradient strength that needs to be exceeded for a pixel to be accepted as part of the segment boundary. It may remove parts of the true boundary that fall below the significance threshold. This information has to be added as part of the domain knowledge for creating a segmentation (e.g., by requiring closed boundaries or by enforcing a shape prior).

Compared to region-based segmentation, a major disadvantage of edge-based segmentation is the sensitivity to noise. Hence, noise reduction as part of gradient computation is mandatory. Using a multiresolution strategy such as in region-based segmentation is possible. It requires registering boundaries from the expanded images with the edges in the original image.

6.2.2 Homogeneity of Texture

Continuity may refer to the texture of structures. Textures are difficult to define, as they are a kind of microstructure in a structured world (samples from the Brodatz textures in Fig. 6.10 show some of the variety of different textures). Just where an entity stops being a structure and starts to be a microstructure is a matter of viewpoint. The fabric of a curtain, for instance, may be called a texture, but at close inspection a thread of the fabric may be a structure itself having a texture from its constituting filaments.

Textures have two properties in common.

1. A texture has a repeating pattern. It may be an exact repetition as in manufactured surfaces or a repetition with a random component as in many textures of natural objects.
2. The computation of texture features requires a texture-specific minimal size of the window in which all scene elements belong to the same texture.

Deterministic texture patterns on an object are usually found on manufactured objects. The representation of such textures is by their constituting, deterministic texture elements (texels). In medical imaging applications, textures on objects are caused by the structure of the organs imaged. Constituting elements certainly exist but they are usually much smaller than the imaging resolution. Visible textures are caused from the interaction between the measured signal and these structures. The textures can be described statistically in the spatial or the frequency domain.

It has been shown that three properties are necessary for differentiating adjacent regions by texture.

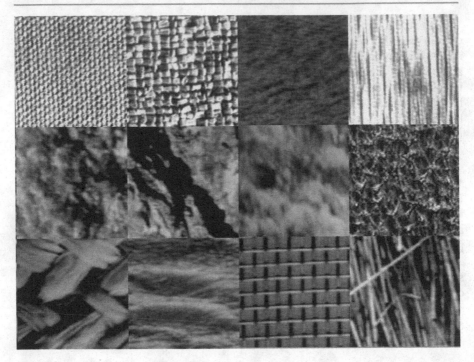

Fig. 6.10 Samples from the Brodatz textures. It can be seen that it will be difficult to define feature sets that capture the characteristics of all these textures

1. Texture *orientation* can best be explained in frequency space. Textures possessing one or more pronounced orientations will have most of the energy in frequency space in sectors along those orientations.
2. Texture *periodicity* relates to the smallest region necessary to represent all properties of a texture.
3. Texture *complexity* relates to the composition of it. A texture that is composed of basic elements of the same size is less complex than one that consists of basic elements of different sizes. A texture that consists of white noise is less complex than one consisting of colored noise.

Textures of distinguishable, adjacent segments need to be different in at least one of the three aspects.

Segmentation by texture plays a minor role in medical image analysis, as most properties from differently textured organs are too subtle to be exploited. Examples for exemptions are as follows.

- MRI, where artefacts from tissue-specific magnetic field inhomogeneities contribute to noise.
- Ultrasound, where tissue-specific refraction artefacts influence the signal.
- Photographic images of the skin, where, e.g., scars exhibit macroscopic textures.
- Microscopic images, where cell textures can be spatially resolved.

A multitude of different texture measures exists, but in view of the rather limited use of texture as a feature we will list just some that are exemplary for different ways of measuring the statistical properties of texture.

- *Haralick's features* of the co-occurrence matrix measure second-order statistical attributes of the gray level co-occurrence matrix (GLCM). GLCM features were presented in Haralick et al. (1973). Later experiments confirmed that second-order statistical features are important for object discrimination (Julesz 1975, 1981).
- *Spectral features* are created from integrating amplitudes over a partitioning of the texture representation in the frequency domain. They are a direct measure of the orientation and periodicity of a texture in the frequency or spatial domain (e.g., He and Wang 1991). Gabór filters are a specific variant of this as they combine spatial and frequency characteristics by a bank of differently oriented, windowed frequency transforms (Grigorescu et al. 2002).
- *Law's filter masks* are a set of orthogonal convolution kernels to measure the periodicity and orientation of textures in the spatial domain.

The attributes of textures can be determined in many ways and some research has been devoted to estimate the quality of such features (e.g., du Buf et al. 1990 who presented a framework for testing textures). A comparative study for determining the discriminative power of 15 types of texture measures including the above-mentioned three measures in Wagner (1999), which was carried out on six very different types of textures ranging from the Brodatz textures to textures in microscopic cell images, found no significant difference between the measures. It was found, however, that different measures excelled in the six classes. This corroborates a strategy of carefully selecting a texture measure based on the characteristics of the texture to be differentiated.

The reliability of a computed texture feature depends on the size of the region from which it is computed. This is apparent for Haralick's GLCM features. The measure of co-occurrence in some neighborhood of a pixel is just an estimate whose reliability depends on neighborhood size. The dependency on neighborhood size exists for other texture measures as well because the texture of a pixel is always defined by intensity variation in some neighborhood. Hence, regions from which textures are computed should be large. However, texture-based segmentation implicitly assumes that an image contains at least two different textures to be separated. Texture computation at unknown segment boundaries becomes unreliable if pixels of more than one segment contribute to the texture measure. This would point to selecting the smallest possible neighborhood for texture computation.

There are three strategies to deal with this problem.

1. Texture measures are chosen that require only a small number of pixels for computing reliable features. Unreliability at segment boundaries is neglected or may even be used as a characteristic for finding a boundary. An example is Lorigo et al. (1998) who segmented MR knee images by a geodesic active contour, which used local variance as a textural feature.

2. Segmentation is carried out iteratively. At initialization, the neighborhood around a pixel of a given texture is assumed to contain only pixels of that texture. At a second step, regions for texture computation are refined using edge information

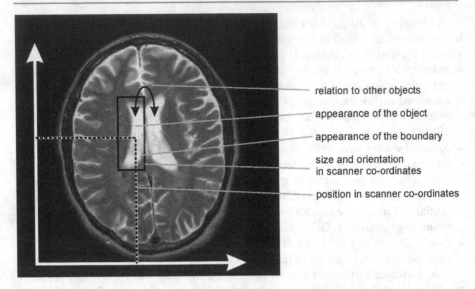

relation to other objects

appearance of the object

appearance of the boundary

size and orientation
in scanner co-ordinates

position in scanner co-ordinates

Fig. 6.11 Different kinds of domain knowledge can be used to guide an analysis process

from the first step. An example is the work of Pitiot et al. (2002) on MR images. They used features of the co-occurrence matrix and estimated segment boundaries using Gabòr filters. Another example for iterative segmentation is the work of Reyes-Aldasoro and Bhalerao (2003) who used spectral features and combined them with a multiresolution approach.

3. Segmentation is carried out in a multiresolution framework. Low-reliability results computed at a low resolution initialize the segmentation at higher resolution. This requires that textures be computed at different levels of resolution and that resolution-dependent reliability can be computed. An example is the work of Muzzolini et al. (1993) on texture-based segmentation of ultrasound images.

It has already been mentioned that texture-based segmentation includes components of classification. Texture-based classification without segmentation is more widespread in medical image analysis than texture-based segmentation. In classification, a sample region with homogeneous texture is already computed. The problem of computing regions with homogeneous texture does not exist.

6.3   Domain Knowledge About the Objects

Detecting an object requires additional information about what to segment. While the underlying model in data-driven segmentation is simple (homogeneity of intensity or texture), further knowledge may be entered through an explicit description of the properties of boundaries in a segmentation or about a foreground object. Domain knowledge consists of information about (see Fig. 6.11) the following:

1. the appearance of boundaries between segments,
2. the location of an object within an image,

3. the orientation and size of the object with respect to the scanner coordinate system,
4. spatial relationships (location, orientation, or relative sizes) of the object with respect to other objects in the image,
5. the shape and appearance of the object.

Most of the attributes relate to foreground segmentation where an object shall be separated from the background. Just what information is used depends on the specific segmentation task. To be useful, domain knowledge for describing a foreground object should be

- *discriminative*, i.e., the object and background must have different properties with respect to the feature;
- *generalizable*, i.e., the property must be true for all possible instances of the object of interest in all possible images within the field of intended use;
- efficiently *computable* with sufficient reliability.

The efficiency of computation is not mandatory, but domain knowledge should not contain unnecessary information. If, for instance, bone segmentation in CT images using a simple threshold for discriminating bone from the less dense background materials delivers sufficient accuracy, it is not efficient to require an additional shape model for describing a specific type of bone.

6.3.1   Representing Domain Knowledge

Domain knowledge may be introduced to a segmentation method via an adjustable model that is included in the segmentation method or interactively at run-time. Using incorporated domain knowledge allows predicting the behavior of the method for a given data set.

If a method operates fully automatically based on data and a priori information, the failure on the part of the model indicates that the domain knowledge does not conform to the reality in the data. Validation will determine whether and to what extent segmentation errors may be attributed to incomplete or wrong assumptions about the objects. It will thus support improving a segmentation method by improving the descriptive power of the incorporated domain knowledge. This is not true if knowledge is introduced interactively since human behavior cannot be exactly predicted.

Validation will be discussed further in Chap. 13, but it should be noted that the consequences of validation will be different if domain knowledge is supplied interactively as compared to automatic segmentation using an incorporated model.

Each of the five types of domain knowledge listed above can be represented by the following.

- A *parameterized description* such as the representation of a segment orientation by a vector in scanner space.
- A *sampled description* such as the representation of shape by a sequence of boundary points.
- An *implicit description* such as the representation of a shape by a function on image domain describing its boundary.

A parameterized description reduces a property to a set of parameters. The parameters can usually be represented with arbitrary precision. Other aspects corresponding to the same property are excluded. Describing the shape of an approximately oval object by the center as well as the length and orientation of its two major axes, for instance, fails to represent any deviation of the true object from the elliptical shape.

The properties described by samples require a sufficiently high sampling rate. The almost oval shape in the example above could be described by a finite number of boundary points. The number and distribution of these points determines the accuracy with which actual shapes are described.

The properties described implicitly as a function of the image domain require a number of base functions on this domain, which can be combined to describe the object boundary. The description accuracy depends on the number and complexity of the base functions.

The property values of any of the descriptions may be combined in a property vector describing the expected features of a segment.

6.3.2 Variability of Model Attributes

Domain knowledge about objects in images describes the properties of a class of objects. Incorporating it into a segmentation method has to include known variation among instances of a class. Variation is specified by a range of permissible property values in the property vector. Information about acceptable variance within a class may be obtained from expert information or from training.

The reliability of expert information depends on the expert and on the kind of knowledge. Many implicit knowledge representations use simple assumptions about the local smoothness of object boundaries which can be readily assumed for most structures occurring in medical imaging. Apart from a few parameters governing the influence of intensities or their derivatives on the model, no further information has to be introduced prior to applying a model-driven segmentation technique. The strategy may have limited success in the case of artefacts or an insufficient relationship between image information and object appearance. Nonetheless, a very popular segmentation paradigm is based on the implicit representation of local domain knowledge. An implicit representation, called *level set representation*, integrates many aspects of low-level knowledge about segments in a common concept and will be detailed in Chap. 9 on active contours and surfaces.

High-level knowledge characterizing class membership and the variation of shape and appearance of an object is more difficult to acquire. An expert (a radiologist, a surgeon, etc.) certainly has vast experience about the possible appearances of structures that are of interest to him or her. This experience by far surpasses the capabilities of the computer-based representation of it. However, the expert uses the knowledge as needed and may never have to express it a priori in an unambiguous fashion.

The type of domain knowledge also influences the ease with which a description may be created. It is, for instance, easy to establish the average size and position of the heart in x-ray CT. It is much more difficult to describe its expected shape and shape variation.

Resorting to training solves some of the problems mentioned above. Training samples are usually taken from the same kind of images that are to be segmented later. The transfer from human knowledge to the representation of domain knowledge in a segmentation method takes place when a human operator prepares the training samples.

Training is time-consuming and may also suffer from lack of samples. If, e.g., the property vector of the parameterized description of oval shapes contains just five elements (x- and y-coordinates of the center, angle of the long axis with respect to the x-axis, lengths of long and short axes), training the expected value and variance in this 5D space from, say, 25 samples would not be very reliable. Asserting reliability gets worse if the size of the property vector increases.

Automated training may facilitate the acquisition of training samples. Still, a sufficient number of images must exist for training. Furthermore, an analysis module is needed to retrieve property values from these images. Developing the analysis module may require so much domain knowledge about the objects to be segmented that it solves the segmentation problem altogether. Automatic training from segmentation with an adjustable model component can still make sense because it may be used as a learning component, which causes performance to improve with continuous training.

Segmentation employs such descriptive a priori information by producing segments whose properties resemble properties as predicted by the model. Probability is sometimes computed using a Bayesian formulation where the domain knowledge is part of the a priori model. Often, probability is used much more informally and segments are chosen with properties that are in some defined way closest to an average appearance predicted by the model.

6.3.3   The Use of Interaction

The interactive incorporation of domain knowledge has the advantage of being flexible because an expert user decides about the necessary input at segmentation time. If the system responds immediately to interaction, knowledge incorporation at runtime also delivers cues about potential input errors.

Interactive input may happen directly on the image or it may be an adjustment of segmentation parameters. The former is attractive to most users as it allows them to directly interact with the medium that they want to segment. However, the interaction on the image can be tedious if

- it is required for a prolonged time,
- interaction devices are inappropriate,
- the relation between interaction and consequence for the result is not intuitive.

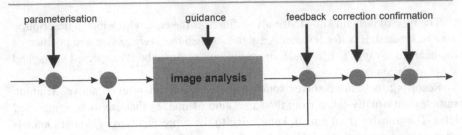

Fig. 6.12 The five different kinds of interaction that may happen during image analysis

This may affect the quality of segmentation or reduce the acceptance of the method. If tiresome interaction cannot be avoided, small input errors need to be tolerated and corrected automatically while large errors should be detected. Depicting structures instead of requiring their delineation is to be preferred because the depiction is less sensitive to input errors than delineation. If delineation is necessary, the cues from the image—often delineation should follow high gradient curves—and from the underlying assumption about the depicted object—the boundaries are often smooth and not ragged—should be used to detect and correct potential errors.

Interaction by parameter setting is often more robust with respect to erroneous interaction, but the effects on the segmentation are less intuitive. A way to cope with the semantic gap between the abstract parameter setting and its effect is to produce an immediate result. The user learns the dependencies between parameter settings and segmentation result from immediate experience.

In any case, an explanation of the mode of operation of a parameter should be available on request by the user. The seemingly complex behavior of parameter adjustment should be described by example and be available to the user as well (e.g., in a documentation or an online tutorial).

Interaction in a segmentation algorithm may come in one of five varieties (see Fig. 6.12).

1. In a priori *parameterization* the user is requested to enter parameter values of an adjustable segmentation algorithm. Once parameters are set—such as indicating the location of an object of interest or setting thresholds of the expected intensity range of the object—the segmentation algorithm proceeds automatically until it produces the result.
2. Through segmentation *guidance* the user supports the segmentation until a satisfactory result is generated. An example would be the entering of boundary points in a user-guided delineation of an organ boundary.
3. *Feedback* happens after segmentation has been carried out. The user varies parameters or changes the way of guidance to improve the quality of the result. An example is the threshold variation in threshold segmentation. Feedback requires the recomputation of the segmentation.
4. *Correction* changes the segmentation result according to user expectation. An example would be the removal of parts of a segment that do not belong to the object of interest. Correction usually implies positive confirmation.
5. *Confirmation* is the process by which the user accepts or rejects a result.

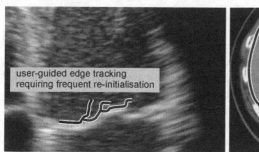 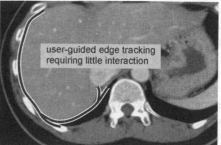

Fig. 6.13 It depends on the image (and information and artefacts contained in it) whether a certain interaction component is useful and efficient or not

Parameterization is often required. Adapting parameters will be successful in applications that follow the underlying assumptions of the segmentation method and which can be characterized by a proper parameter setting. The limitation of parameterization is that interactively added knowledge can only specify but not extend or counteract the knowledge implemented in the segmentation method.

Using guiding interaction is more powerful but at the cost of reduced control about the result. A very general and very simple segmentation tool using guidance would draw a boundary of a foreground object according to interactive mouse input from the user. This method would be able to segment any object that the user recognizes in the image. It also puts the burden of retrieving and using domain knowledge on the user.

Guidance may also counteract an inappropriate segmentation model. One could imagine, for instance, guiding an edge-tracking method in an ultrasound image. Since most of the high gradients stem from noise and artefacts the user will constantly have to correct tracking errors that are due to the false hypothesis of high gradients being mainly caused by object boundaries (see Fig. 6.13).

However, a similar edge tracking could be very suitable for some CT image with its high contrast. Tracking will only occasionally loose the boundary. It may be easier to let the user enter the information on the spot instead of providing a model that covers those rare cases. Hence, guidance can be an efficient and effective means to support segmentation if its use is justifiable. It should not be an excuse for a poor model of domain knowledge.

Feedback differs from guidance in that is does not interfere with the segmentation process itself but offers the user the chance to repeat the segmentation with refined parameters. It is less susceptible to misuse in the case of an inappropriate segmentation method because feedback cannot change the segmentation model.[1] The advantageous use of feedback requires the expert to understand the underlying

---

[1] If the model is mainly based on its parameterization and requires frequent feedback, it again would indicate a poor design of the segmentation model. This should not happen in practice, because in such case the success of segmentation would vary substantially with different parameter settings making segmentation time-consuming and awkward to use.

a priori model of the segmentation method. The expert, who knows what a successful segmentation should look like, can then decide based on current results how parameterization should be changed.

Receiving feedback can be a frustrating experience, however, if the change of parameter values leads to unexpected behavior because the consequences of the segmentation result are not intuitive. Sometimes, understanding about proper parameterization can be gained by observing the behavior of a segmentation algorithm even if the correspondence between the segmentation result and parameter setting is not straightforward. Gaining experience from the feedback of the method improves with the speed with which the results are computed.

Interaction through correction is another powerful tool because discrepancies between the expected and computed results can be removed. However, correcting segmentation results hints at deficiencies of the incorporated domain knowledge. An example for interaction through correction is the combination of thresholding with subsequent correction because object intensity does not differ everywhere from the background intensity.

The use of correction should be limited to cases where the inclusion of the missing domain knowledge is inefficient because costs exceed benefits. Correction that is required regularly for creating a valid segmentation indicates an inappropriate segmentation method.

Interaction by confirmation does not extend the bandwidth of the applications of a given segmentation method directly. It may be used, however, to adapt a segmentation method to some application. Every time that a user accepts or rejects a result new information is given. Some segmentation algorithms are able to profit from confirmation by adapting the automatic parameter setting accordingly. Confirmation also assures that the final decision as to whether a segmentation result is correct belongs to the expert user.

6.4   Interactive Segmentation

The algorithmically simplest way of segmentation is to completely rely on user guidance to outline the boundary of a foreground structure. Employing some input device such as a mouse, a trackball, or an electronic stylus on a graphical tablet, the user traces the boundary on a rendition of a 2D scene. The method can be applied to arbitrary 2D scenes assuming that the user has all the necessary domain knowledge. Interactive segment delineation by an expert often provides a reference for a semi-automatic or automatic segmentation scheme. The underlying assumption is that a domain expert provides proper model knowledge.

The main problem of interactive segmentation is that it can neither be guaranteed that a user really possesses all the necessary information for a perfect segmentation of an image nor that this information is applied correctly during segmentation. Interactive segmentation as a validation tool hence requires some modeling of human error when segmenting an image. As no analytical model of this kind exists, it is estimated from an assumed error distribution based on the input from several different observers.

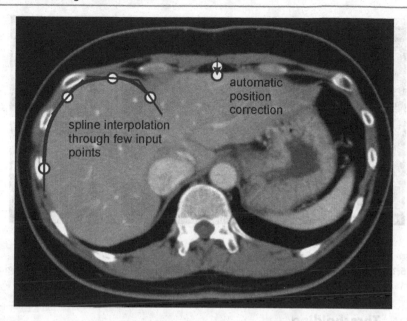

Fig. 6.14 Interactive delineation is supported if the user has only to click at few boundary points and if positions selected by user input are automatically corrected by displacing them towards the position with locally highest gradient

If interactive delineation is used in routine segmentation, these accuracy problems may occur as well. Delineating boundaries in data is tedious and time-consuming. The performance of a user depends on individual experience, on stress, on tiredness, and similar factors. Hence, interaction is often supported by low-level techniques borrowed from image enhancement or data-driven segmentation. Examples are as follows.

- The boundaries to be delineated are highlighted by displaying the intensity gradient instead of the original image. Edge contrast is increased by noise removal techniques such as edge-preserving smoothing.
- Just a small number of boundary points are provided by the user (see Fig. 6.14). They are connected by automatically generated line segments (straight lines or curves).
- User input is corrected automatically by offsetting the boundary orthogonal to its tangent toward the nearest highest gradient (see Fig. 6.14).
- The user is allowed to correct a delineated boundary. This is most efficient if the boundary does not consist of a sequence of neighboring pixels, but of a sequence of points connected by curve segments. User correction of a single point then induces a corresponding correction of its two incident line segments.

Segmenting 3D data sets using interactive delineation requires the successive delineation on a sequence of 2D slices. The process can be simplified by projecting results from the previous slice to the current slice and letting the user correct it.

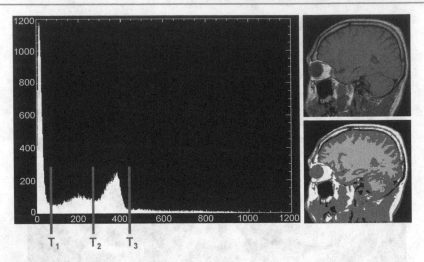

Fig. 6.15 Thresholding can be done interactively and separates the image into different regions. Valleys in the histogram indicate potentially useful threshold values

6.5   Thresholding

Medical images are made on purpose. Often, the object of interest stands out by having intensity values higher or lower than the background. Hence, thresholding is an often-used tool in segmenting medical images (a survey of early thresholding methods can be found in Sahoo et al. 1988). Segmentation s of an image f by threshold t at a pixel or voxel $\mathbf{v}$ is given by

$$s(\mathbf{v}) = \begin{cases} 1, & \text{if } f(\mathbf{v}) > t, \\ 0, & \text{otherwise.} \end{cases} \quad (6.1)$$

Thresholding produces a separation of image pixels into foreground pixels ($s = 1$) and background pixels ($s = 0$). If more than one threshold is chosen, separation into several different regions is possible as well (see Fig. 6.15).

Sometimes, the result already separates the object-of-interest from the background (e.g., if thresholding was used on contrast-enhanced images such as digital subtraction images). If not all foreground regions are part of the object-of-interest, a connected component analysis (CCA) follows, which labels all foreground regions. Regions forming the object-of-interest are then identified by the user.

Thresholding can be done interactively. The user selects a threshold and segmented structures are displayed. The threshold is varied until the segmented structure meets the expectations of the user. This kind of interaction should be avoided if it is difficult to display the segmentation result (e.g., if data are 3D or 4D) or if it can be expected that the result will include too much user-caused variation.

Automatic thresholding techniques attempt to use the underlying assumptions of thresholding. Since it is assumed that foreground pixels have a different value than background pixels, the histogram of the image should have two peaks (a so-called

Fig. 6.16 An iteration step of Otsu's method to find a threshold: The new threshold is halfway between the expected values of the two distributions separated by the old threshold

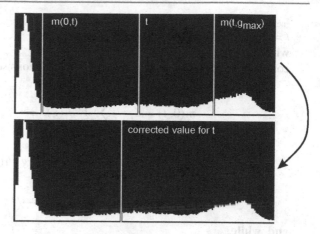

bimodal histogram). The threshold should be somewhere between the two peaks. Since distributions forming a bimodal histogram usually overlap, the threshold is found at a location between the peaks that produces the smallest number of wrong label assignments.

However, noise will cause the histogram to have several local maxima and minima. Otsu (1978) presented an iterative procedure to find an optimal threshold for a histogram h with bimodal distribution. It is based on the assumption that the distribution characteristics for foreground and background pixels are approximately equal except for their expected value. It finds a threshold based on an initial estimate t as average between these expected values (see Fig. 6.16 and the algorithmic sketch in Fig. 6.17).

The initial estimate for t is computed as the local minimum of a smoothed histogram. If the histogram is too noisy, a first estimate can be taken as $t = 0.5 \cdot g_{max}$. The method has been extended to separate more than two classes by applying it recursively on the foreground or background pixels (Cheriet et al. 1998).

A similar approach uses the fuzzy set theory to iteratively determine thresholds (Tobias and Seara 2002). The authors defined two subsets of gray values that belong to the foreground and the background and a third subset of gray values between the two of which membership is initially unknown. Gray values from this set are assigned fuzzy memberships that depend on the histogram of the foreground and background pixels and on that of the nonclassified region. The final threshold is then found at the location where the two fuzziness functions for foreground and background intersect.

Finding the threshold minimum can be difficult if the number of foreground pixels is small compared to the number of background pixels. The peak for foreground pixels is then in the range of noise variation and it may be impossible to determine. A solution for finding the threshold in such a case has been given by the algorithm of Zack et al. (1977) (see Fig. 6.18).

- Compute a line between the two local maxima of the two distributions.
- Compute the distance $d_L(h)$ for each entry h of the histogram to this line.

$t_{new} = \infty$,

$t = t_{init}$,

while $|t - t_{new}| >$ eps **do**

compute the expected values of the two distributions separated by t:

$$m(0, t) = \frac{1}{t+1} \sum_{g=0}^{t} g \cdot h(g),$$

$$m(t, g_{max}) = \frac{1}{g_{max} - t + 1} \sum_{g=t}^{g_{max}} g \cdot h(g),$$

$$t_{new} = 0.5 \cdot \big(m(0, t) + m(t, g_{max})\big)$$

end_while.

Fig. 6.17 Sketch of the loop of Otsu's algorithm to determine a threshold in a bimodal histogram given some initial threshold t_{init}

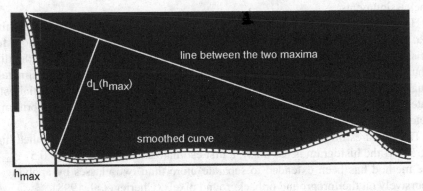

Fig. 6.18 The algorithm of Zack defines the threshold as the location where the distance of a curve through the histogram from a line through the two maxima is maximum

- Convolve d_L with a smoothing kernel to remove the effects from noise.
- The threshold is h_{max} for which $d_L(h_{max})$ is maximum.

The algorithm of Zack is a good, albeit heuristic, approximation of an optimal solution under a Bayesian assumption. Under this assumption, the histogram would be the combination of two probability distributions $P_f(\mathbf{v}|g)$ for $\mathbf{v}$ being a foreground pixel given its gray value g and $P_b(\mathbf{v}|g)$ for it being a background pixel weighed by their a priori probabilities (i.e., the two a posteriori distributions). The optimal threshold producing the smallest number of false classifications would then be the intersection of the two distributions. This is not always the minimum of the histogram. If the variance of one of the two distributions is smaller than that of the other, the algorithm of Zack moves the threshold toward the former, which is qual-

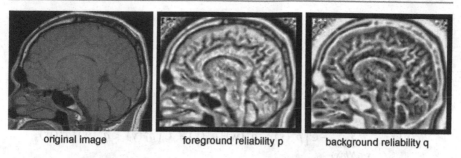

original image   foreground reliability p   background reliability q

Fig. 6.19 For relaxation labeling, initial foreground and background reliabilities are computed by evaluating the distance of each pixel intensity from the threshold

itatively similar to what happens for the optimal threshold under the Bayesian assumption.

Thresholding may not work, although the contrast between the foreground and background is seemingly high, if underlying shading distorts the image. This happens in MR imaging when the coil used for inducing the imaging signal does not produce a constant signal within the scene (see Hou 2006; Vovk et al. 2007 for reviews). Microscopy is another field where shading complicates the threshold-based segmentation (see Tomazevic et al. 2002 for a review). If shading correction is impossible during image generation, it can be done retrospectively if the knowledge exists at least in parts of the image to separate shading effects from other intensity variations.

Another adverse influence stems from noise. Mainly at segment boundaries, many of the pixels may be assigned to the wrong segment. A simple way to deal with this is a morphological postprocessing (opening or closing) to remove artefacts. Alternatively, Rosenfeld and Smith (1981) presented a variant of relaxation labeling which takes into account a measure of certainty of segment membership when correcting segment labels.

Initial reliabilities p and q are computed for each pixel $\mathbf{v}$ belonging to the foreground or background based on some threshold t (see Fig. 6.19):

$$p(\mathbf{v}) = \frac{1}{2} + \frac{1}{2}\frac{g(\mathbf{v}) - t}{g_{\max} - t}, \qquad (6.2)$$

$$q(\mathbf{v}) = \frac{1}{2} + \frac{1}{2}\frac{t - g(\mathbf{v})}{t - g_{\min}}. \qquad (6.3)$$

Reliability values are iteratively updated based on the foreground and background membership of surrounding elements $\mathbf{w}$. At some iteration k, support values S_f and S_b for $\mathbf{v}$ belonging to the foreground or background are then computed from the eight neighbor pixels $\mathbf{w} \in Nb(\mathbf{v})$

$$S_f(\mathbf{v}) = \frac{1}{8}\sum_{\mathbf{w} \in Nb(\mathbf{v})} C\big[p^k(\mathbf{v}) > q^k(\mathbf{w})\big]p^k(\mathbf{v}) - C\big(p^k(\mathbf{v}) < q^k(\mathbf{w})\big)q^k(\mathbf{w}), \quad (6.4)$$

Fig. 6.20 Example for
computing support values in
an 8-neighborhood

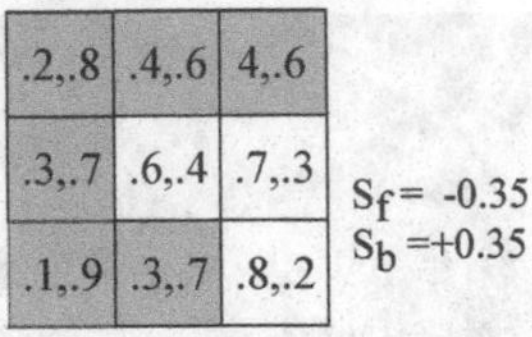

.2,.8	.4,.6	4,.6
.3,.7	.6,.4	.7,.3
.1,.9	.3,.7	.8,.2

$S_f = -0.35$
$S_b = +0.35$

$$S_b(\mathbf{v}) = \frac{1}{8} \sum_{\mathbf{w} \in Nb(\mathbf{v})} -C\left[p^k(\mathbf{v}) > q^k(\mathbf{w}) \right] p^k(\mathbf{v}) + C\left(p^k(\mathbf{v}) < q^k(\mathbf{w}) \right) q^k(\mathbf{w}),$$

$$(6.5)$$

where $C()$ is an indicator function that is 1 if the expression in the brackets is true
and 0 otherwise (see Fig. 6.20).

Given the support from neighboring pixels the segment membership reliabilities
are now updated:

$$p^{k+1}(\mathbf{v}) = \frac{p^k(\mathbf{v})[1 + S_f^k(\mathbf{v})]}{p^k(\mathbf{v})[1 + S_f^k(\mathbf{v})] + q^k(\mathbf{v})[1 + S_b^k(\mathbf{v})]}, \qquad (6.6)$$

$$q^{k+1}(\mathbf{v}) = \frac{q^k(\mathbf{v})[1 + S_b^k(\mathbf{v})]}{p^k(\mathbf{v})[1 + S_f^k(\mathbf{v})] + q^k(\mathbf{v})[1 + S_b^k(\mathbf{v})]}. \qquad (6.7)$$

This process continues until the change in reliability values falls below some
prespecified minimum.

Thresholding is more difficult if multichannel functions are to be segmented
since it requires the specification of a region in multidimensional feature space.
For more than two channels, the feature space needs to be projected on 2D space.
Thresholds are defined interactively in several different projections. Backprojection
of threshold boundaries from the different 2D spaces to the original feature space
produces the multidimensional region boundary. Interacting with such a system for
correcting the initial guesses of thresholds can be very demanding. Each projection restricts the set of definable threshold boundaries. Finding good thresholds will
require manipulation in the projections as well as manipulation of the projection
directions.[2]

Thresholding is a simple technique that is fast, easy to implement, and easy
to understand. It may be extended to separate several different classes in images
with multimodal histograms. Finding thresholds automatically may become unstable when it becomes difficult to find reliable criteria for differentiating between true
and false local maxima in the histogram.

---

[2]Thresholding is essentially a classification in feature space as it finds a decision boundary. If
the feature space is multi-dimensional, the user should resort to classification techniques that are
described in Chaps. 7 and 12.

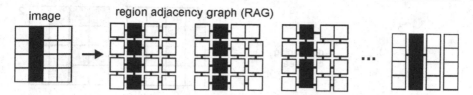

Fig. 6.21 Schematic view at the region merging process. At each iteration the two most similar regions are merged until such merging would violate the similarity criterion for pixels belonging to the same region

6.6   Homogeneity-Based Segmentation

Segmentation based on local intensity homogeneity does not require an absolute threshold but a local variance criterion that is valid for all pixels within a segment. The goal is to separate an image into the smallest number of segments so that for each of the segments this criterion is fulfilled. Examples for homogeneity criteria are the variance of pixel values, maximum deviation between pixel intensities, or the probability that all pixels belong to the same probability distribution.

Two basic segmentation algorithms for this are region merging and the split-and-merge algorithm. Both are not guaranteed to produce an optimal result, as they only ensure the homogeneity criterion and not that the smallest number of segments is found.

The following are the steps for computing a segmentation by *region merging* (see Fig. 6.21).

- Initially, each pixel is considered to be its own region.
- Map regions to a region adjacency graph (RAG) in which nodes represent regions and adjacent regions are connected by an edge.
- Compute the homogeneity value for each edge for a region that consists of the two regions connected by the edge.
- As long as there exists at least one edge of which the homogeneity value fulfills the homogeneity criterion,
  - merge the two most similar regions and
  - update the RAG accordingly.

The result is a segmentation where each region fulfills the homogeneity criterion. It is not necessarily optimal because the greedy strategy always merges the most similar regions without considering the influence of this merge with respect to adjacent regions. Region merging should be implemented using efficient data structures for accessing RAG nodes and for sorting elements after a merge step. Otherwise, the method will be slow because the naïve approach has a $O(N^2)$ computation cost with N being the initial number of regions (which can be very large if for instance 3D data sets are segmented). There are a number of strategies to get around this.

- Compute an oversegmented image on which region merging is to be carried out so that N is small.
- Use the fact that only few changes in the sorting order take place when two regions are merged and use an appropriate data structure.

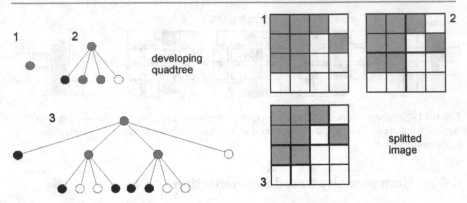

Fig. 6.22 During the first phase of the split-and-merge algorithm, regions are split into subregions until each subregion fulfills the homogeneity criterion. The split procedure is documented in a quadtree

- Change the selection order in a way that does not require a new sort after each merge.

All of these strategies have been used. Using an already partially segmented image is, for instance, done when combining region merging with a prior region splitting process by the *split-and-merge algorithm*. It starts with the complete image being a single region and keeps splitting the image until each region fulfills the homogeneity criterion. The split part has the following steps (see Fig. 6.22).

- Initially the complete image is a single region.
- As long as a region exists that does not fulfill the homogeneity criterion
  - split this region in four quarters (for a 2D image) or eight subvolumes (for a 3D volume) and
  - document the split in an appropriate data structure (quadtree or octtree).

If no further regions need to be split, the current segmentation is turned into a RAG on which a region merging is carried out to merge regions that were accidentally split. Even when using naïve representations and sorting techniques the combination with the split step will reduce the computation time substantially as splitting should result in much fewer regions then there are pixels or voxels in the image.

For computing initial regions, other segmentation techniques can be used as well. An example is the watershed transformation (WST) that is discussed in the next section. Although the WST criteria are different from the homogeneity criteria discussed here, the oversegmentation, which is usually the result of applying WST, results in homogeneous segments. Combining this with a merging step, hence, is more efficient than just using region merging alone.

In Haris et al. (1998), the method was sped up further by using a priority queue for keeping the ordered list of RAG edges. The gain in speed results from the fact that merging requires removing and adding only a few edges from the list instead of having to sort the whole list again. Another way to increase the performance of the merging process is to avoid resorting altogether (Nock and Nielsen 2004).

This is an approximate solution which is possible based on an external model about pixels belonging to the same region. The predicate for this criterion is computed and ordered only once and region merging proceeds by this order.

6.7   The Watershed Transform: Computing Zero-Crossings

Intensity edges defining segment boundaries are somewhat complementary to the homogeneity of intensity-defining segments. There is a difference, however. Intensity edges may still be discernable and can be used for separating segments even if intensity variation from shading makes definition of a homogeneity criterion impossible. On the other hand, relying on edge information is inherently less robust with respect to noise since computing derivatives of the intensity information also enhances noise. Hence, many edge-based segmentation schemes require that noise reduction takes place either in a preprocessing step or as part of the edge-based segmentation method.

The *watershed transform* (WST) is a popular way to use edge information as criterion to separate segments (an excellent review of WST techniques can be found in Roerdink and Meijster 2000). If the WST is carried out on the gradient lengths of the intensity gradient, it is equal to defining segment boundaries by the zero crossings of the Laplacian of the intensity function. For twice differentiable functions on a real domain the locations of the zero crossings are closed, non-overlapping boundaries. For images defined on a discrete domain this is only approximately true, but it is a very nice parameter-free way of image segmentation with the appeal that zero crossings have been shown to be important features for analysis by human vision (Marr and Hildreth 1980). The watershed transform to compute the segments is defined as follows.

- The scene is treated as a landscape in which function values (i.e., the gradient length) represent height.
- Each local minimum in this landscape is a sink.
- Watersheds in this landscape are boundaries in the terrain which separate regions that drain into different sinks.

Given this description, an image will decompose in as many segments as there are sinks. If the sinks are local minima of the gradient length, every local minimum, maximum, or saddle point in the original intensity image will be a center of a segment. If the image contains noise it will produce a severe over-segmentation. Using the WST for segmentation, therefore, requires either noise reduction before applying the WST, or noise reduction included into the WST, or intentional use as presegmentation to be further processed by some other process that merges WST segments.

Computing the watershed transform can be done by flooding where sinks are treated as sources (see Fig. 6.23 and the sketch of the algorithm in Fig. 6.24).

If noise in the image is not dealt with during preprocessing and if the number of segments shall be reduced, the WST can be applied in a hierarchical fashion (Beucher 1994). In this case, the segments of the first WST are superpixels for another WST. Gradients can be estimated by computing average intensity differences

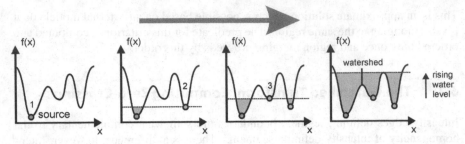

Fig. 6.23 The watershed transform can be carried out by flooding the scene from sources at local minima in the image

set the initial flood level for an image f to $l = \min_\mathbf{v}(f(v))$
while $l < \max_v(f(\mathbf{v}))$ **do**
    Detect all pixel $\mathbf{v}_l$ that are newly flooded at level l
    if a pixel $\mathbf{v}_l$ is connected to pixels which all have a segment label L **then**
            segment L is extended by $\mathbf{v}_l$.
    if a pixel $\mathbf{v}_l$ is not connected to any pixel that has a segment label **then**
            this is the first pixel of a new segment: label it L_{new}.
    if a pixel $\mathbf{v}_l$ is connected to at least two pixels with different labels **then**
            label the pixel W (for watershed)
    $l = l + 1$
end_while

Fig. 6.24 Sketch of the flooding algorithm for the watershed transform

to neighboring segments weighted by the size of the neighboring segments. The hierarchical WST reduces the number of segments, but it also increases the size of the watershed (super)pixels. It can be avoided when watersheds are not pixels but pixel boundaries. The waterfall algorithm of Beucher does exactly this. Different basins are merged if their watersheds are lower than those to surrounding basins. The hierarchy of merging basins can be used to assign a saliency measure to the segments (Najman and Schmitt 1996). Saliency is higher when a merge happens later.

It is not guaranteed that a hierarchical WST produces more meaningful segments than the original WST. The hierarchical WST transforms the segmentation into scale-space and the underlying assumption is that there is an optimal scale for the complete image. In reality, however, there is certainly an optimal scale for objects or parts of objects, but this scale varies within the image. Hence, for each object the optimal segment is found on a different scale. Unless the existence of an optimal scale can be predicted a priori, the only way to deal with this is to include expert knowledge into the segmentation that comprises information about the appropriate scale.

The watershed transform can be combined with user interaction by providing a picking component (Meyer and Beucher 1990; Vincent 1993). Oversegmentation from standard WST arises because the underlying model for segments (each local

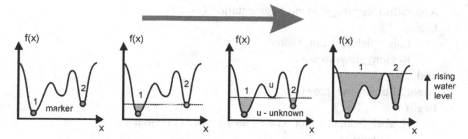

Fig. 6.25 Marker-based WST proceeds in a similar fashion than the original WST, except for the fact that flooding occurs only from marker positions. Regions that are not connected to a marker-labeled region receive a provisional label "unknown"

minimum in the map of gradient lengths is a segment) does not describe what is wanted (i.e., the separation of organs in a medical image). The *marker-based WST* (mWST) adds information about objects to be segmented by replacing local minima as a source for flooding by prespecified marker positions (see Fig. 6.25).

At least one marker needs to be placed into any foreground or background region to be differentiated. The watershed transform still increases the water level. However, regions that are not flooded from a marker position become a provisional label "unknown." If a region with this label merges with a marker-labeled region it receives the label from the latter. By providing markers the number of segments is predefined (it cannot be larger than the number of markers). A region may be represented by more than one marker if they have the same label. Marker positions can be set manually or may be computed by a detection process (e.g., Grau et al. 2004 where marker positions are computed from skeletonized probability maps).

6.8 Seeded Regions

Region growing combines data-driven constraints with interactively added domain knowledge (Zucker 1976). The user points out an object that needs to be separated from the background by specifying a seed point in the object. A homogeneity criterion characterizes the appearance of the region to be segmented. Region growing detects all pixels or voxels that can be reached from the seed point by paths of adjacent pixels or voxels for which the homogeneity criterion applies.

Pointing out a structure in an image is much easier than delineating its boundary. It requires the user to recognize at least one location that surely belongs to the foreground object. The underlying assumption is that the homogeneity criterion is independent of the seed point location so that different seed point locations deliver the same result (this assumption needs to be tested in a later validation).

In Fig. 6.26 a sketch of the region growing algorithm is given that is started on an image $f(\mathbf{x})$ with seed point $\mathbf{x}_{seed}$ and homogeneity predicate $hom(f(\mathbf{x}))$. The function "neighbor$(\mathbf{x}, i)$" is assumed to return the ith neighbor of $\mathbf{x}$.

Algorithm Region_growing_segmentation (xseed)
begin
    Label_field[] = not_visited
    Region_grow(xseed)
end
Algorithm Region_grow(x)
begin
    if label_field[x] = not_visited **and** hom($f(x)$) **then**
        begin
            label_field[x] = visited
            for $i = 1$, nbs **do**
                region_grow(neighbor(x, i))
        end
end

Fig. 6.26 A simple region growing algorithm

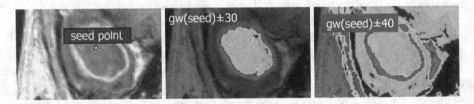

Fig. 6.27 Finding the best homogeneity criterion is often done by trial-and-error and can be difficult in region growing

Homogeneity needs to be computable for a single pixel or voxel. It is often the variance of the intensity function $f(\mathbf{x})$ around some expected value. This corresponds to the assumption that the foreground object can be separated by a lower and an upper threshold from the background.

It can be challenging to define the homogeneity criterion. Often, it is assumed that the intensity of the seed point corresponds to the expected value in the foreground region. The variance is entered by the user and is found by trial and error (see Fig. 6.27).

While finding a good homogeneity criterion can be done interactively in 2D, controlling results in 3D by visual feedback is much more difficult. Homogeneity may then be found automatically in a two-pass process assuming that the object is well contrasted against the background (Pohle and Toennies 2001). In the first pass, a seed point is set and homogeneity is computed based on an estimate of the expected value and variance. This estimate is based on the number of elements in the region already found and the current variance among these elements.

Initially, since the region has only a few elements, the variance is assumed to be underestimated and corrected accordingly. With continuing growth, the homogeneity criterion approaches current estimates of the expected value and variance of

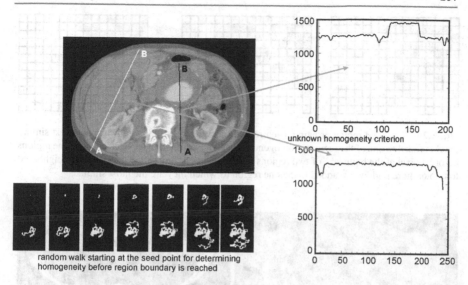

random walk starting at the seed point for determining
homogeneity before region boundary is reached

Fig. 6.28 The homogeneity criterion can be found in adaptive region growing by gathering information in a first path starting at the seed point. Region growing is then repeated with the same seed point when homogeneity has been determined

intensity. Growing terminates when no further scene elements can be included that follow the current estimate of the homogeneity criterion. The process is repeated with the same seed point, but with the homogeneity criterion computed in the first pass.

The algorithm is successful if the estimate of the region characteristics is reliable before the region boundary is encountered for the first time. Hence, the user is asked to place the seed point in the center of the foreground object. The neighborhood order in the for loop is changed at random producing a kind of random walk (see Fig. 6.28).

A variant to make the region growing process independent of parameters except for the seeds is *seeded region growing* that turns region growing into an mWST-like segmentation procedure (Adams and Bischof 1994). In seeded region growing the user specifies a number of seeds that separate the image in as many segments. Initially, each seed forms its own segment and the labels of all other pixels are unknown. Unlabeled neighbors of all labeled segments are ordered by some appropriate homogeneity criterion (e.g., intensity difference). The most similar unlabeled pixel is then selected to be labeled. If this pixel is adjacent to labeled pixels which all have the same label, it receives this label. Otherwise, it receives the label of the segment to which it is most similar (see Fig. 6.29).

It is often required that inclusion criteria for region growing depend on features at the seed location as this allows to implicit a definition of homogeneity by selecting just the right location for placing a seed. It does mean, however, that the results depend on the seed point location. If this is critical, *symmetric region growing* (Wan and Higgins 2003) may be used, which was shown by the authors to produce results

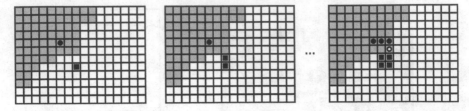

Fig. 6.29 In seeded region growing, each region receives a seed. Since always the most similar pixel is added to one of the regions, homogeneous sets of pixels will have been added to the regions before a pixel at the boundary of two regions is selected (e.g., the *white circle*). Pixels neighbored to two or more regions are added to the one region to which they are the most similar

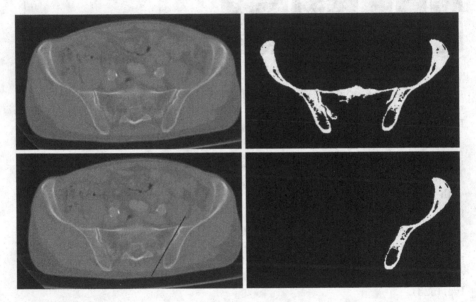

Fig. 6.30 Interactively adding an artificial boundary is a simple way to prevent region growing to leak into parts that do not belong to the object to be segmented

independent of the seed point location as long as the seed is placed into the segment. The algorithm requires a symmetric inclusion criterion (i.e., if this criterion allows a region to grow from some point A to some other point B, then the same criterion should allow growing from B to A).

Region growing sometimes leaks into the background because of noise, artefacts, or the approximating nature of the homogeneity criterion. Preventing leakage can be done either by interactively adding boundaries that must not be crossed by the growing process (see Fig. 6.30) or by using several seed points and creating the segment as the union of regions from these seed points. The former is suitable if—because of noise or other objects close by with a similar appearance—the leak happens only at a few isolated locations. The latter is appropriate when the image has a well con-

Fig. 6.31 The live wire
segmentation produces
boundary segments as
optimal paths between
user-specified start and end
points

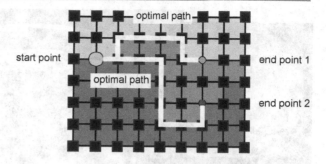

trasted foreground object with shading. Selecting several seed points then assumes
that the expected value of the intensity is at least locally constant.

6.9   Live Wire

If it is impossible to give a homogeneity criterion to separate an object from the
background, it may still be possible to define its boundary given interactive input.
There are a number of methods to do interactive edge tracking, but by far the most
popular in medical image analysis is the *live wire* method (Mortensen et al. 1992;
Barrett and Mortensen 1997; Falcão et al. 1998), also known as *intelligent scissors* (Mortensen and Barrett 1995). The concept is simple. The user selects a start
point on the boundary, then minimum cost paths according to some optimality criterion are computed to all other points and the user selects the most appropriate end
point among those (see Fig. 6.31). This becomes the start point for the next contour
segment. The procedure continues until the first boundary point is reached and the
boundary around the object of interest is closed.

The methodology is popular because interaction is easy and the response to interaction is fast. To understand the behavior of the live wire algorithm it is helpful
to know some of its details. Several components govern the behavior of a live wire
contour.

- The optimality criterion is a local criterion that can be evaluated at each pixel site
  and decreases with the increasing likelihood of this site being part of the contour.
- The distance between the start and end points indicates the maximum distance
  between sites where the optimality criterion overrides user input.
- Preprocessing separates artefactual influences from true edge information in the
  local optimality criterion.

Optimality is a combination of local pixel attributes and the boundary length. In
other words, in the absence of local attributes the optimal boundary between two
points is a straight line.

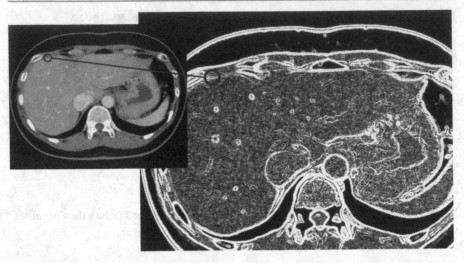

Fig. 6.32 Choosing maximal gradient length for live wire segmentation would not produce the desired result for segmenting the liver boundary. Using the gradient at the start point as training sample should be more successful

The image is turned into a graph by making nodes out of every pixel and by connecting two nodes by an edge if two pixels are neighbored (four- or eight-neighborhood). Nonnegative local costs are attributed to the nodes of the graph. An example for node costs $c(i, j)$ for a pixel (i, j) with function value $f(i, j)$ is

$$c(i, j) = \left(\left\|\nabla f(i, j)\right\| - \bar{g}\right)^2, \tag{6.8}$$

where $\bar{g}$ is the expected gradient length for pixels belonging to the boundary. This cost function assumes that the average strength $\bar{g}$ along the boundary is known and penalizes deviations from it.

Given the cost function for the nodes, the optimal boundary between (i_{start}, j_{start}) and (i_{end}, j_{end}) can be computed as the minimum cost path using Dijkstra's algorithm. This algorithm keeps a list of the active nodes and associated path costs for reaching this node. Initially, it contains only the start node of the path. The path cost is the node cost. Then, the node with the lowest path cost is selected and removed from the active node list. Path costs of nodes that are connected to the selected node by an edge are computed. These nodes are added to the active node list. The algorithm terminates when the end node is selected from the active node list. The minimum cost path is generated backtracking the path from the end node to the start node.

The value of $\bar{g}$ needs to be predefined. It could be the largest gradient in the image. In this case, a boundary with the strongest gradients is searched. It could be the gradient at the start point, which is then taken as a model for the boundary (see Fig. 6.32). It could also be computed in a training phase, where representative boundaries are delineated manually and an average gradient is computed along

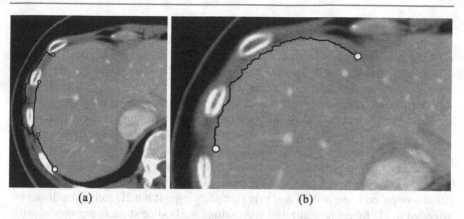

(a)   (b)

Fig. 6.33 Live wire is an interactive procedure. (a) After selecting a start point path, costs are computed for arbitrary end points and the user selects a point on the boundary where the minimum cost path still follows the object boundary. (b) Even if the path follows the boundary, noise in the image causes a rugged path instead of the expected smooth object boundary

these boundaries. The latter two solutions are especially useful when the optimal boundary does not contain the strongest edges in the image.

Given the cost function, optimal paths from the start pixels to all pixels can be computed at $O(N^2)$ costs, where N is the number of pixels. Backtracking from p_{end} can be done with cost $O(n)$, where n is the number of pixels along the boundary between p_{start} and p_{end}. Since n is small, this computation is possible in real time. Hence, after fixing the start point, path costs can be computed to every possible location in the image (the termination criterion is then that the list of active nodes is empty). The user may then move with the mouse over the image and the method will immediately produce the optimal boundary curve to the current mouse position (see Fig. 6.33). This makes interaction attractive as it allows the simple selection of appropriate start and end points for computing boundary sections.

The method has some features that a user should be aware of.

- The path costs are a combination of a local cost (usually dependent on the gradient) and the path length. The second of these may lead to unexpected behavior. A path may be preferred that consists of a small number of pixels although the gradients along the pixels do not resemble the expected gradient. An extreme case would be a start point that is also the endpoint of a boundary. The minimum coast path will always consist only of this point, no matter how well defined the boundary is.
- Delivering the shortest possible connection between the start and end points is a useful property in cases where part of the boundary is missing (i.e., not recognizable by a pronounced gradient). Noise, however, which is present in most medical images and which also leads to nonzero gradients, may cause the path to follow the noise pattern (see Fig. 6.33b). This happens even if the noise amplitude is so small that it is not visible to the user. Setting closely spaced boundary points in such regions can be a frustrating experience. It is better to let the user switch to an

alternative segmentation mode in low gradient regions (in the simplest case this would be just straight lines between boundary points).

• Using gradient characteristics of the start point for defining node costs can lead to unexpected results if the user has not placed the start point directly on the boundary. There are two ways to avoid this.
  – Start point selection may be followed by an automatic correction step that searches for a high gradient location in the vicinity of the start point location.
  – Alternatively, the user may be asked to select a model gradient from a choice of precomputed boundary gradients of different strengths.

Because of its simple and in most cases intuitive behavior, live wire segmentation is found in many software packages for medical workstations. Its main disadvantage is that—opposed to the mWST and to region growing—it is a 2D technique. It can be extended to 3D by using sequential processing. A 3D slice stack is segmented with results in previously segmented slices providing constraints for the segmentation in the current slice (Schenk et al. 2001). However, this makes only little use of the shape information orthogonal to the slice orientation.

The work of Falcão and Udupa (2000) takes 3D shape information into account by defining a two-pass procedure on a sequence of slices. In the first path, boundaries are generated using live wire on a number of slices orthogonal to the original slice direction. The intersections of these boundaries with the original slices are then starting points for a boundary search in the slices. Although it extends the method to 3D, the separation into two passes makes it less intuitive compared to the original live wire method.

6.10 Concluding Remarks

Segmentation in medical image analysis often attempts to delineate specific objects of interest. Hence, segmentation methods require additional domain knowledge. It can be included by the parameterization of a method. Since this may be too complex to be captured by a simple parameter estimation step, many of the basic segmentation techniques include an interactive component where a domain expert supplies missing information.

Basic segmentation techniques from general image analysis have been adapted accordingly, resulting in methods such as region growing or marker-based watershed transformation where the user points out the objects to be delineated. Other alternatives are the various live wire methods where the user directly indicates locations on the object boundary. While such interactively guided procedures can be very effective, its interaction should not be used to correct poorly applied model or data knowledge.

6.11 Exercises

• How can assumptions about continuity in time be used to support thresholding a time sequence of body CT images to segment the spine?

- How can 3D region growing based on a single seed point in a slice be realized? Discuss the potential problems of such an approach and give possible solutions for those problems.
- Give examples for the five types of interaction when used for a threshold segmentation of bone in CT images.
- What are the potential problems that could make homogeneity assumptions for intensity in a segment invalid?
- What is the difference between a hierarchical segmentation strategy and a multilayer segmentation strategy? What would an image look like where the latter would be preferred?
- What is the main problem when using the homogeneity constraint to guide a texture-based segmentation?
- Which of the segmentation methods presented in this chapter uses knowledge about the appearance of object boundaries as domain knowledge? How is it used in this method?
- How can knowledge about the location of an object be integrated into a threshold segmentation?
- Why is it necessary that domain knowledge must be generalizable?
- How could knowledge about the object size and acceptable size variance be gathered? How can it be used in threshold segmentation?
- Interactive boundary delineation of 3D data sets is tedious since it has to be repeated for every slice. What would be the appropriate means to support the user? Discuss the potential problems of the suggested method and how to deal with them.
- Discuss reasons for using Otsu's method for automatic threshold determination in threshold segmentation. What needs to be initialized and how is this done?
- What method could be used for threshold determination if the two local maxima of the bimodal distribution differ to a large degree? Why is that so?
- What is the reason for using relaxation labeling in threshold segmentation? What is the underlying assumption about the segments which must be true for relaxation labeling to succeed?
- How could a gradual refinement technique (hierarchical multiscale segmentation) be used to support segmentation by region merging? What would be the benefits of such a method?
- Explain why and under what circumstances segmentation by watershed transform is equal to segmentation by finding zero crossings of the second derivative in the image.
- How is the watershed transform extended to include a gradual refinement technique?
- Why is it not useful to maximize the sum of gradient lengths for a boundary as criterion in live wire segmentation?
- What are the potential problems that a user may encounter when using the live wire method for boundary delineation?
- How can the live wire approach be extended to 3D? Explain the kind of user interaction in this case.

References

Adams R, Bischof L (1994) Seeded region growing. IEEE Trans Pattern Anal Mach Intell 16(6):641–647

Barrett WA, Mortensen EN (1997) Interactive live-wire boundary extraction. Med Image Anal 1(4):331–341

Beucher S (1994) Watershed, hierarchical segmentation and waterfall algorithm. In: Serra J, Soille P (eds) Mathematical morphology and its application to image and signal processing. Kluwer Academic, Norwell, pp 69–76

Cheriet M, Said JN, Suen CY (1998) A recursive thresholding technique for image segmentation. IEEE Trans Image Process 7(6):918–921

du Buf JMH, Kardan M, Spann M (1990) Texture feature performance for image segmentation. Pattern Recognit 23(3–4):291–309

Falcão AX, Udupa JK, Samarasekera S, Sharma S, Hirsch BE, de A. Lotufo R (1998) User-steered image segmentation paradigms: live wire and live lane. Graph Models Image Process 60(4):233–260

Falcão AX, Udupa JK (2000) A 3D generalization of user-steered live-wire segmentation. Med Image Anal 4(4):389–402

Grau V, Mewes AUJ, Alcañiz M, Kikinis R, Warfield SK (2004) Improved watershed transform for medical image segmentation using prior information. IEEE Trans Med Imaging 23(4):447–458

Grigorescu SE, Petkov N, Kruizinga P (2002) Comparison of texture features based on Gabor filters. IEEE Trans Image Process 11(10):1160–1167

Haralick RM, Shanmugam K, Dinstein KI (1973) Textural features for image classification. IEEE Trans Syst Man Cybern 3(6):610–621

Haris K, Efstratiadis SN, Maglaveras N, Katsaggelos AK (1998) Hybrid image segmentation using watersheds and fast region merging. IEEE Trans Image Process 7(12):1684–1699

He DC, Wang L (1991) Texture features based on texture spectrum. Pattern Recognit 24(5):391–399

Herman GT, Carvalho BM (2001) Multiseeded segmentation using fuzzy connectedness. IEEE Trans Pattern Anal Mach Intell 23(5):460–474

Hou Z (2006) A review on MR image intensity inhomogeneity correction. Int J Biomed Imag 1–11. doi:10.1155/IJBI/2006/49515.

Julesz B (1975) Experiments in the visual perception of texture. Sci Am 232(4):34–43

Julesz B (1981) Textons, the elements of texture perception, and their interactions. Nature 290:91–97

Lorigo LM, Faugeras O, Grimson WEL, Keriven R, Kikinis R (1998) Segmentation of bone in clinical knee MRI using texture-based geodesic active contours. In: 1st intl conf medical image computing and computer-assisted intervention—MICCAI 1998. LNCS, vol 1496, pp 1195–1204

Marr D, Hildreth E (1980) Theory of edge detection. Proc R Soc Lond B 29, 207(1167):187–217

Meyer F, Beucher S (1990) Morphological segmentation. J Vis Commun Image Represent 1(1):21–46

Mortensen EN, Morse B, Barrett W, Udupa JK (1992) Adaptive boundary detection using 'live-wire' two-dimensional dynamic programming. In: Proc computers in cardiology, pp 635–638

Mortensen EN, Barrett WA (1995) Intelligent scissors for image composition. In: SIGGRAPH 95 (Proc 22nd intl conf), pp 191–198

Muzzolini R, Yang YH, Pierson R (1993) Multiresolution texture segmentation with application to diagnostic ultrasound images. IEEE Trans Med Imaging 12(1):108–123

Najman L, Schmitt M (1996) Geodesic saliency of watershed contours and hierarchical segmentation. IEEE Trans Pattern Anal Mach Intell 18(12):1163–1173

Nock R, Nielsen F (2004) Statistical region merging. IEEE Trans Pattern Anal Mach Intell 26(11):1452–1458

Otsu N (1978) A threshold selection method from grey-level histograms. IEEE Trans Syst Man Cybern SMC-8:62–66

Pitiot A, Toga AW, Ayache N, Thompson P (2002) Texture based MRI segmentation with a two-stage hybrid neuralclassifier. In: Proc intl joint conf neural networks (IJCNN'02), vol 3, pp 2053–2058

Pohle R, Toennies KD (2001) Segmentation of medical images using adaptive region growing. Proc SPIE 4322:1337–1346 (Medical imaging 2001)

Reyes-Aldasoro CC, Bhalerao A (2003) Volumetric texture description and discriminant feature selection for MRI. In: Information processing in medical imaging, IPMI 2003. LNCS, vol 2732, pp 282–293

Roerdink JBTM, Meijster A (2000) The watershed transform: definitions, algorithms and parallelization strategies. Fundam Inform 41:187–228

Rosenfeld A, Smith RC (1981) Thresholding using relaxation. IEEE Trans Pattern Anal Mach Intell 3(5):598–606

Sahoo PK, Soltani S, Wong AKC, Chen YC (1988) A survey of thresholding techniques. Comput Vis Graph Image Process 41(2):233–260

Schenk A, Prause GPM, Peitgen HO (2001) Local-cost computation for efficient segmentation of 3D objects with live wire. Proc SPIE 4322:1357–1364 (Medical imaging 2001)

Tobias OJ, Seara R (2002) Image segmentation by histogram thresholding using fuzzy sets. IEEE Trans Image Process 11(12):1457–1465

Tomazevic D, Likar B, Pernus F (2002) Comparative evaluation of retrospective shading correction methods. J Microsc 208(3):212–223

Vincent JL (1993) Morphological grayscale reconstruction in image analysis: applications and efficient algorithms. IEEE Trans Image Process 2:176–201

Vovk U, Pernus F, Likar B (2007) A review of methods for correction of intensity inhomogeneity in MRI. IEEE Trans Med Imaging 26(3):405–421

Wagner T (1999) Texture analysis. In: Jähne B, Haussecker H, Geisser P (eds) Handbook of computer vision and applications. Academic Press, San Diego, pp 275–308

Wan SY, Higgins WE (2003) Symmetric region growing. IEEE Trans Image Process 12(9):1007–1015

Zack G, Rogers W, Latt S (1977) Automatic measurement of sister chromatid exchange frequency. J Histochem Cytochem 25:741–753

Zucker SW (1976) Region growing: childhood and adolescence. Comput Graph Image Process 5(3):382–399

Segmentation in Feature Space

7

Abstract

Selection of an image acquisition technique is intentional in medical imaging. It can be assumed that pixel or voxel values in a medical image cover more semantics with respect to object class membership than intensity in a photograph. Hence, image segmentation can be done as classification in feature space where image intensities are the features.

The dimensionality of feature space is usually low and the number of samples characterizing object classes is high. Typical classifiers discussed in this chapter take this into account and estimate likelihood functions from samples. Classification is then done by computing a posteriori probabilities for each object class. Clustering in feature space will be discussed as well. Without requiring training, clustering may directly lead to a segmentation. Even if this is not the case, clustering may be used to reduce the workload for producing the training data.

Concepts, notions and definitions introduced in this chapter

> Classification of pixels and voxels
> Bayesian classification
> Computation of likelihood functions
> Kernel density estimators
> Gaussian mixture models
> Clustering in dense, low-dimensional feature spaces
> Association networks and Kohonen networks

Thresholding presented in the previous chapter is actually a solution of the segmentation problem as a classification task in feature space (see Fig. 7.1). In thresholding, scene elements are assigned to one of two classes—foreground or background—based on their intensity value. This assumes that some function exists that relates class membership probability to the intensity of the scene element. This is part of a Bayesian formulation of a classification problem. Solving segmentation in this

K.D. Toennies, *Guide to Medical Image Analysis*,
Advances in Computer Vision and Pattern Recognition,
DOI 10.1007/978-1-4471-2751-2_7, © Springer-Verlag London Limited 2012

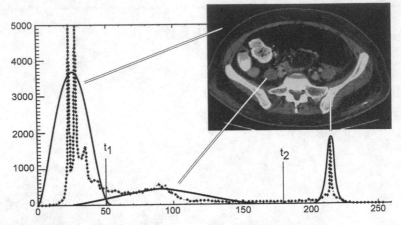

Fig. 7.1 Segmenting the image based on threshold implies underlying a posteriori probabilities for the different classes of which the histogram shows a non-normalized sum

way is adequate for many kinds of medical images where a relationship between measured intensity value and tissue type can be assumed. Methods to solve the classification task will be discussed in this chapter.

Segmentation is rather specific compared to other classification tasks. It makes some methods more appropriate than others. Typically, the dimension of the feature vector is low. It may consist of a single scalar (such as the image intensity in Fig. 7.1), of low-dimensional multichannel data (e.g., a triple of proton density, T_1, and T_2 relaxation in MRI imaging), or of a combination of intensity information with spatial information such as the coordinates of a scene element. Hence, the dimensionality of a feature vector is somewhere between 1 and 5. The number of samples is high since every scene element is a sample. The situation is almost opposite to a regular classification task, where few samples in high-dimensional feature space represent the probability density functions that are needed to estimate the a posteriori probability of an unknown sample. In segmentation, methods are preferred that rely on parameter estimation to compute the a posteriori probability of a scene element to belong to some object class.

If the number of features per scene element is high, classification techniques for sparse sample distributions in high-dimensional space need to be employed. These techniques will be discussed in Chap. 12.

7.1   Segmentation by Classification in Feature Space

Given an intensity $f(\mathbf{v})$ at some scene element $\mathbf{v}$ and two different classes—foreground fg and background bg—the optimal solution that minimizes the number of wrong decisions would be to assign the class with highest a posteriori probability $P(\mathbf{v} \in fg | f(\mathbf{v}))$ or $P(\mathbf{v} \in bg | f(\mathbf{v}))$, respectively, to $\mathbf{v}$. According to the Bayesian theorem the a posteriori probabilities can be computed from the a priori probabil-

Fig. 7.2 Sometimes the probability distributions intersect twice. Threshold t_1 is then disregarded, as it occurs at a location where probability for either of the two classes is low

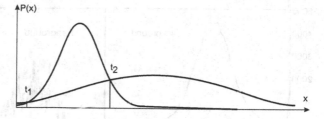

ities $P(\mathbf{v} \in fg)$ and $P(\mathbf{v} \in bg)$[1] and the likelihood functions $p(f(\mathbf{v})|\mathbf{v} \in fg)$ and $p(f(\mathbf{v})|\mathbf{v} \in bg)$:

$$P\big(\mathbf{v} \in fg | f(\mathbf{v})\big) = \frac{p(f(\mathbf{v})|\mathbf{v} \in fg)P(\mathbf{v} \in fg)}{P(\mathbf{v} \in fg)P(\mathbf{v} \in bg)}, \tag{7.1}$$

$$P\big(\mathbf{v} \in bg | f(\mathbf{v})\big) = \frac{p(f(\mathbf{v})|\mathbf{v} \in bg)P(\mathbf{v} \in bg)}{P(\mathbf{v} \in fg)P(\mathbf{v} \in bg)}. \tag{7.2}$$

The denominator is the same in both equations and can be omitted for finding the most likely class membership. Sometimes, the two a posteriori probabilities intersect only at one location. This is then the threshold value where the decision should switch from foreground to background. Otherwise, a priori probabilities and likelihood functions have to be evaluated for each value $f(\mathbf{v})$.

The two curves may intersect more than once (see Fig. 7.2). The extra intersection can be disregarded if it occurs at a location with low probability values. This would indicate a low reliability of the approximation of the true likelihood. It is, for instance, the case when Gaussian distributions with different mean and variance approximate the likelihood function. The second intersection of such distributions is usually out of the range of permissible values for $f(\mathbf{v})$. Even if it is within the range of values for $f(\mathbf{v})$, this intersection is assumed to be due to an inaccurate approximation of the likelihood function by the Gaussian function.

The a priori probability and likelihood function have to be generated from training data. It should be representative for the problem so that its feature values reflect the true likelihood function. If the appearance of the foreground and background may change for different patients (or even for the same patient if imaged several times), training data should come from several different image sequences. Individual variation of tissue characteristics, image artefacts that vary with different patients such as shading artifacts or weight-dependent contrast, or the use of imaging devices from different manufacturers or with different parameterization are reasons why such variation can be expected.

---

[1] The a priori probability is also called marginal probability, since P is marginalized over all possible feature values of $\mathbf{v}$.

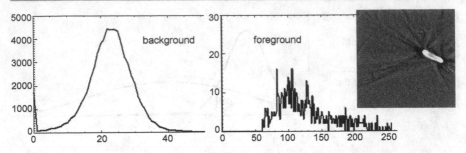

Fig. 7.3 Estimates for foreground and background probability can be generated from a representative sample. In the example above, vessels from 3D reconstructed DSA are to be separated from the background. It can be seen by inspection of the histograms that the background is well-approximated by a Gaussian while this is not true for the foreground

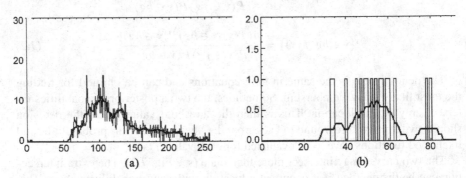

Fig. 7.4 (a) Noise in the sample data can be reduced by smoothing the histogram using a kernel density estimator. (b) The same technique can be used when the number of samples is too small for providing a reliable estimate for the probability distribution

7.1.1   Computing the Likelihood Function

Given classified training data, the estimate of the likelihood function for the two classes are normalized histograms h_{fg}^n and h_{bg}^n of the intensity values of scene elements belonging either to the foreground or the background. The histograms can be taken directly as likelihood functions (see Fig. 7.3) if the number of samples is high enough to cancel out the effects from noise.

Using a *kernel density estimator* (also known as *Parzen window*) helps to reduce unwanted effects from undersampling (see Fig. 7.4). It is based on the assumption that each sample value $f(\mathbf{v})$ is representative for a range of values in the vicinity of $f(\mathbf{v})$. Hence, $f(\mathbf{v})$ is assumed to be the mean of some unknown density function $d()$. A new estimate for the likelihood function is then computed by convolving the normalized histograms with the density functions d_{fg} and d_{bg}:

$$p() = h_{fg}^n * d_{fg}, \tag{7.3}$$

and

$$p() = h_{bg}^n * d_{bg}. \tag{7.4}$$

Since d_{fg} and d_{bg} are usually unknown, they are approximated by Gaussian distributions (based on the central limit theorem). The variance of the Gaussian is set based on the average sampling density in the normalized histograms and noise characteristics. If the number of histogram bins is small compared to the number of samples, a low variance should be chosen while a higher variance should be selected otherwise.

It is well possible that different variances are appropriate for foreground likelihood and background likelihood functions. The number of foreground samples from the training data may be much smaller than that of background samples. Furthermore, the range of intensity values in the foreground may be different to that in the background.

It may be necessary to constrain the likelihood function even further. If it is assumed that in a noise-free environment the foreground or the background has homogeneous intensity, the only reason for the variation of intensity values is noise. Noise is often assumed to be normally distributed with zero mean. The likelihood function is then a Gaussian with the mean value μ representing the expected foreground or background intensity and variance σ^2 representing measurement noise:

$$N(f; \mu, \sigma) = \frac{1}{\sqrt{2\pi}\sigma} \exp\left(-\frac{1}{2}\frac{(f-\mu)^2}{\sigma^2}\right). \tag{7.5}$$

A number of reasons may speak against using a Gaussian distribution (compare the distributions for the foreground and background in Fig. 7.3). The most notably non-Gaussian deviation is caused by the partial volume effect (PVE). If a bright foreground object is to be segmented from a dark background, some of the variation from the mean is not caused from normally distributed noise, but from the PVE between bright and dark scene elements. The intensity is no longer normally distributed and not even symmetric with respect to the mean. Another example is a projection image when using a contrast agent. In DSA imaging the ideal image should have a constant white background with vessels of varying degrees of black depending on the vessel thickness along the projection ray. Foreground variation from varying vessel thickness is non-Gaussian and a substantial cause for observed intensity variation.

Sometimes, it is known beforehand that the intensity distribution is actually a combination of several distributions. An example would be a foreground object that consists of different tissue types (see Fig. 7.5). The characteristic is captured by the normalized histogram with or without Parzen windowing. However, if the number of samples is too low for computing a reliable estimate without a model for the function, a *mixture of Gaussians* can be assumed with different means, variances, and a priori probabilities. It is a particularly appropriate model if the class that is to be described consists of a mixture of several substances with different appearance. The individual likelihood functions are allowed to overlap to a large extent since the classification of the substances is not the goal.

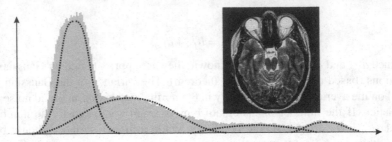

Fig. 7.5 Sometimes, the intensity distribution of a histogram has to be modeled as a mixture of several distributions with unknown parameters

A Gaussian mixture model Θ for one-dimensional distributions consists of a set of K Gaussian distributions $N(\mu_i, \sigma_i)$ with mean μ_i and standard deviation σ_i so that the probability of some event to have the value x_j is a weighted sum of the probabilities $N(\mu_i, \sigma_i)$:

$$P(x_j | \Theta) = \sum_{i=1}^{K} a_i N(x_j; \mu_i, \sigma_i). \qquad (7.6)$$

The weights a_i are the a priori probabilities for each distribution. For our application, the values x_j are the intensity values of the scene elements $\mathbf{v}$. The unknown mixture model needs to be estimated from samples. Obviously, the most fitting model for a set of sample values $X = \{x_j\}$ would be the one for which the probability $P(X|\Theta)$ is maximum, i.e.,

$$\Theta_{\max} = \arg\max_{\Theta} P(X|\Theta). \qquad (7.7)$$

There exists no analytical solution. However, a number of iterative techniques arrive at $\Theta_{\max}$ given some initial estimate. A popular approach is to use the *expectation maximization algorithm* (EM). Expectation maximization is an iterative procedure to estimate a maximum a posteriori solution such as the one in (7.6). A detailed look at this technique can be found in McLachlan and Krishnan (1996).

The application of the EM algorithm in this case requires the number K of Gaussians to be known. It consists of two steps, which are repeated until convergence is reached. In the E-step expectations y_{ij} of samples x_j belonging to distribution i are computed given the current estimates for μ_i, σ_i and a_i:

$$y_{ij} = \frac{a_i N(x_j; \mu_i, \sigma_i)}{\sum_{i=1}^{K} a_i N(x_j; \mu_i, \sigma_i)}. \qquad (7.8)$$

In the M-step, these expectations are used to compute new estimates. The new estimate for the a priori probability is simply the average of expectations for this class:

$$a_i' = \frac{1}{N} \sum_{j=1}^{N} y_{ij}. \qquad (7.9)$$

The estimates for the means and variances are then

$$\mu_i' = \frac{\sum_{j=1}^{N} y_{ij} x_j}{\sum_{j=1}^{N} y_{ij}}, \qquad (7.10)$$

and

$$\sigma_i' = \sqrt{\frac{\sum_{j=1}^{N} y_{ij} (x_j - \mu_i')^2}{\sum_{j=1}^{N} y_{ij}}}. \qquad (7.11)$$

The process converges to a local optimum. Since this may be far away from the global optimum, selecting good starting values is paramount. If these cannot be found easily, the search for the mixture model may be preceded by a clustering step (see Sect. 7.2) where K clusters are searched in the data. Cluster centers and within-class scatter are then the initial estimates for the mean and average deviation.

7.1.2 Multidimensional Feature Vectors

Computation does not change much if the feature is not a scalar but a vector. It is particularly easy if the features can be assumed to be independent of each other. The likelihood function for a feature vector $\mathbf{f}$ is then the product of the likelihood functions of the elements $f_1, \ldots, f_M$ of the vector:

$$p(\mathbf{f}|\mathbf{v} \in fg) = \prod_{m=1}^{M} p(f_m|\mathbf{v} \in fg). \qquad (7.12)$$

The estimation of the likelihood functions can be done individually in the same way as for scalar features.

The likelihood function becomes a function of M values if independence cannot be assumed and probabilities need to be estimated in multidimensional feature space (see Fig. 7.6). This is again not different to the case discussed in the previous section except for the density of samples. While in 1D the number of samples even from a single segmented image is high compared to the number of bins in the histograms, this changes dramatically if the feature vector has two, three, or more dimensions.

Let us assume that we have taken a single segmented slice with 512×512 pixels for training to illustrate this by an example. If 64.000 pixels of the total of 2^{18} pixels belong to the foreground and the intensity ranges from 0 to 4000, of which the foreground object occupies a range of 400 gray values, we have on average 160 samples (i.e., 64.000/400) per bin. Unless the image is very noisy, this would allow for using the sampled, normalized histogram directly as the likelihood function. However, if we had the same situation, but the image consisted of three channels (e.g., T_1, T_2, and proton density in MRI) where the foreground object spanned the range of 400 gray levels in each channel, the average number of samples would be down to 0.001 per bin, which is clearly insufficient even for applying a kernel

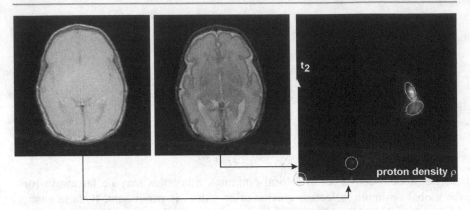

Fig. 7.6 Feature space becomes multi-dimensional if more than one feature describes the data

density estimator. Even if we used sequences from 50 patients with each sequence having 20 slices in which the foreground object is visible, the average number of samples would still be only one per bin.

Parametric distribution functions are therefore often used for estimating a multi-dimensional likelihood function. Based on the central limit theorem, a normal distribution is used as a model. Since features are not independent, the variances for each element of the feature vector have to be replaced by the covariances. The *covariance matrix* Σ for an M-dimensional feature vector consists of entries σ_{ij} that can be estimated from K sample features $\mathbf{f}^k$ by

$$\sigma_{ij} \approx \frac{1}{K-1} \sum_{k=1}^{K} (f_i^k - \mu_i)(f_j^k - \mu_j), \qquad (7.13)$$

where $\boldsymbol{\mu} = (\mu_1 \mu_2, \dots, \mu_M)$ is the estimated mean for features $\mathbf{f}^k$. For real-valued feature values the covariance matrix is symmetric and has the size K^2 for a K-dimensional feature vector (see Fig. 7.7). Given a 3D feature vector, in total nine parameters (three entries for the mean μ and six independent values of the 3×3 covariance matrix) have to be estimated. Hence, the 64.000 samples in this example would be more than sufficient.

The multidimensional normal distribution $N(\mathbf{f}; \boldsymbol{\mu}, \Sigma)$ for a feature vector $\mathbf{f}$ is then

$$N(\mathbf{f}; \boldsymbol{\mu}, \Sigma) = \frac{1}{\sqrt{(2\pi)^M \det(\Sigma)}} \exp\left(-\frac{1}{2}(\mathbf{f} - \boldsymbol{\mu})^{\mathrm{T}} \Sigma^{-1} (\mathbf{f} - \boldsymbol{\mu})\right), \qquad (7.14)$$

where Σ^{-1} denotes the inverse of Σ and $()^{\mathrm{T}}$ the transpose of a vector.

In principle, it is possible to compute a multidimensional threshold for a feature vector. Different methods will be presented in the chapter on classification since it is particularly appropriate when the sampling density is too sparse for computing reliable estimates for the parameters. In segmentation, the parameterized function can

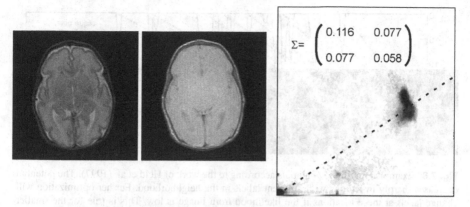

$$\Sigma = \begin{pmatrix} 0.116 & 0.077 \\ 0.077 & 0.058 \end{pmatrix}$$

Fig. 7.7 The covariance matrix Σ in 2d feature space is a 2×2 matrix. The high value of off–diagonal entries compared to the variances in the diagonal show that there is a lot of covariance between the two features. The redundancy, which is causing the co-variance, is indicated by the *dashed line* in the 2d histogram

often be used directly. A posteriori probabilities of class membership (foreground and background) are computed from features of a scene element $\mathbf{v}$, and $\mathbf{v}$ is then assigned to the class with highest probability.

7.1.3 Computing the A Priori Probability

A priori probabilities represent knowledge about the objects irrespective of the data. The simplest kind of a priori knowledge for a segmentation between the foreground and background is an estimate of the ratio of foreground to background pixels. This can be computed from the training data that were used to compute the likelihood functions. It is important that this reflects the correct ratio. If, for instance, segmentation based on the classification of scene elements is carried out as part of a process chain where first an approximate region of interest (ROI) is computed, ratios have to be computed from the ROIs.

A priori knowledge may also include neighbor information because segment membership is spatially correlated. The necessary model would predict that it is more likely that neighboring scene elements belong to the same class. This can be represented by a Markov Random Field (MRF). The model is similar to the one used in image enhancement (Chap. 4). If we assume a normal distribution for the likelihood function this is done by replacing the likelihood function of (4.47) by the term derived in (7.5) resulting in

$$P(\mathbf{f}|\mathbf{g}) \propto P(\mathbf{g}|\mathbf{f}) \cdot P(\mathbf{f}) = \frac{1}{Z_1} \exp\left(-\frac{(f(\mathbf{v}) - \mu)}{2\sigma^2}\right) \cdot \frac{1}{Z_2} \exp\left(-U(\omega)\right). \quad (7.15)$$

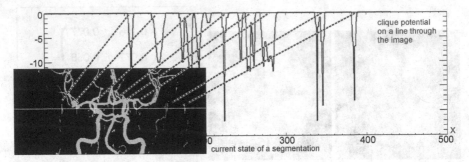

Fig. 7.8 Examples for clique potentials according to the work of Held et al. (1997). The potential decreases sharply in regions with different labels in the neighborhood. Further optimization will change labels at these locations if the likelihood from image is low. This is true for the smaller structures cut by the *line*

For segmentation, Geman and Geman (1984) suggested the generalized Ising model to model clique potentials V_c that make up $U(\omega)$

$$V_c = \begin{cases} \xi_c, & \text{if all sites of the clique have the same label,} \\ -\xi_c, & \text{otherwise.} \end{cases} \quad (7.16)$$

The potential ξ_c is specific to the clique type.

Instead of explicitly computing clique potentials U from all cliques in a given neighborhood, an approximation of U can be defined that describes the desired segmentation properties. Since segmentation should produce as few segments as possible, the a priori probability can simply decrease with the number of different labels in the neighborhood of **v**. This has been used for MRF-based MRI brain segmentation by Held et al. (1997) (see Fig. 7.8)

$$P(\mathbf{f}) = \frac{1}{Z_2} \exp\left(- \sum_{\mathbf{w} \in Nb(\mathbf{v})} \delta\big(f(\mathbf{v}) \neq f(\mathbf{w})\big)\right), \quad (7.17)$$

where δ is the delta function

$$\delta(x) = \begin{cases} 1, & \text{if } x = 0, \\ 0, & \text{otherwise.} \end{cases} \quad (7.18)$$

Iterative optimization of the MRF is then done using simulated annealing or other means [e.g., ICM (Besag 1986), mean-field optimization (Zhang 1992; Celeux et al. 2003), graph cuts (Boykov et al. 2001)] or by introducing a hidden measure model (Marroquin et al. 2003), see also Sect. 14.1 on MRFs and their optimization). A good initialization (e.g., by optimizing the function without considering the a priori knowledge using an EM algorithm) helps to arrive at acceptable computation times.

Another option for fast MRF computation is to use multiresolution MRFs. In Bouman and Shapiro (1994) and Cheng and Bouman (2001) a system of Markov Random Fields is developed and parameterized, which defines neighbor systems on a multiscale representation of the image. Results at each scale are included as a priori knowledge in the segmentation of the next scale. The segmentation is initialized by computing a labeling at the coarsest scale and then proceeding through the scales. It allows to define a small neighborhood system since dependencies across larger ranges are captured at coarser scales. It also speeds up computation since the initialization from the previous scale is a good predictor for the optimal result at the current scale.

7.1.4 Extension to More than Two Classes

Likelihood functions and a priori probabilities can be computed for more than two classes if the scene shall be segmented into several different objects. Segmentation is then given by classification to the most probable class.

7.2 Clustering in Feature Space

So far, segmentation required the classes to be known to which scene elements should be assigned. This type of segmentation is actually a combination of segmentation and object detection since scene elements are assigned a meaning. Segmentation in feature space, however, is possible without having to make this assumption. This is particularly useful if it is not known a priori into how many and which classes scene elements should be grouped.

The process is called *clustering*. The underlying assumption is that scene elements from the same object have more similar features than those that belong to different objects. Similar to classification, clustering is a generic methodology that is able to group features of any kind. It makes sense to differentiate between clustering techniques for low-dimensional densely populated features spaces and those for high-dimensional sparsely populated features spaces. Hence, we will discuss the topic twice (here and in Chap. 12).

Clustering for segmentation works in low-dimensional feature space. In 2D feature space (and with some difficulty in 3D as well), the simplest way of clustering is to do it interactively. The 2D distribution is displayed and the user points out or delineates clusters. The resulting segmentation is then displayed and clustering may then be corrected (see Fig. 7.9). However, since this process is highly subjective, it may be more appropriate for a quick first look at the data and should be replaced by some automatic clustering if a series of data sets is to be analyzed.

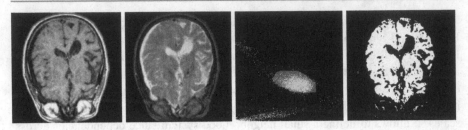

Fig. 7.9 If feature space is low-dimensional (in this case $d = 2$), clustering may be done interactively in the histogram and results are immediately displayed

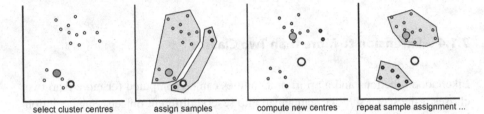

| select cluster centres | assign samples | compute new centres | repeat sample assignment ... |

Fig. 7.10 Partitional clustering starts with initial cluster centers to which samples are assigned according to distance. New cluster centers are computed after the assignment phase. The process is repeated until there are no changes in cluster membership

7.2.1 Partitional Clustering and k-Means Clustering

The objective of a *partitional clustering* method is to find cluster centers $CC = \{c_1, \ldots, c_K\}$ in feature space such that the distance of all samples to their center is minimal:

$$CC_{\min} = \arg\min_{CC} d_{CC}(\mathbf{f}) = \arg\min_{CC} \sum_{i=1}^{M} \left\| \mathbf{f}_i - \mathbf{c}(\mathbf{f}_i) \right\|, \qquad (7.19)$$

where $\mathbf{c}(\mathbf{f}_i)$ delivers the cluster center $\mathbf{c}_k$ that is closest to $\mathbf{f}_i$.

A heuristic strategy is employed for finding optimal cluster centers. First, cluster centers are fixed and samples are assigned to clusters that minimize d_{CC} given the cluster centers. Then, a new center $\mathbf{c}_c$ is defined for each cluster c that minimizes $\sum_{f_i \in c_c} \|\mathbf{f}_i - \mathbf{c}_k\|$. The process is repeated until no further change of cluster assignment takes place (see Fig. 7.10).

Partitional clustering is initialized by assigning the K cluster centers to K arbitrary samples in the data set and by minimizing $\sum_{f_i \in c_c} \|\mathbf{f}_i - \mathbf{c}_k\|$ for the initial centers. The process is heuristic since the assignment to clusters (the first step) and determination of new cluster centers (the second step) are optimized separately although they depend on each other. The procedure may not produce the optimal result and is not guaranteed to converge. Providing a good initial guess for the cluster centers is advisable.

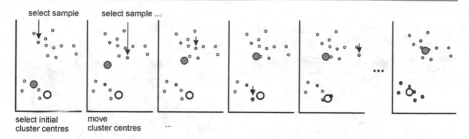

select sample   select sample ...

select initial   move
cluster centres   cluster centres   ...

Fig. 7.11 First pass of the k-means clustering algorithm. Samples are selected at random and assigned to the nearest cluster center. After each assignment, cluster center locations are updated

Fig. 7.12 Second phase in k-means clustering. Given the estimates for cluster centers from the first step, all samples are analyzed according to their distance to the nearest cluster center and potentially re-assigned

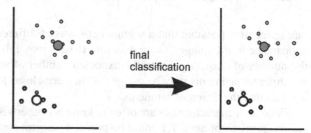

final classification

As opposed to partitional clustering *k-means clustering* (Duda et al. 2000) always terminates, as it requires just two iterations. The objective remains the same. However, instead of assigning all samples to the current estimate for cluster centers before computing a new cluster center, the two objectives are interleaved by computing new cluster centers after each assignment of a feature to a cluster.

The method is initialized similarly to partitional clustering by selecting K samples to act as initial cluster centers. Again, the results will improve when the initial guess is close to the true location of the cluster centers. The process iterates once through the complete data set (including the samples that were chosen to represent the initial cluster centers) by randomly removing samples from it. The selected sample is assigned to its closest cluster center. This cluster now has a new member so that its center has to be moved to the centroid of all samples (see Fig. 7.11).

The process is repeated until all samples have been chosen once. After that, the final cluster center locations are assumed to have been found. Initial uncertainties stemming from a small number of samples determining a cluster center have been compensated by the later addition of samples from the data base. Uncertainty about cluster center locations at an early stage may have led to unreliable early cluster assignments. Hence, in a second iteration, cluster centers are kept constant and samples are assigned according to their distance to these centers (see Fig. 7.12).

Knowing the number of clusters and a good initialization for cluster center positions are necessary to employ k-means clustering successfully for segmentation. The number of clusters is often assumed to be larger than the number of different segment classes expected in the image. The main reason for this lies in the nature of clustering algorithms. Clusters are groups of samples that are close together in fea-

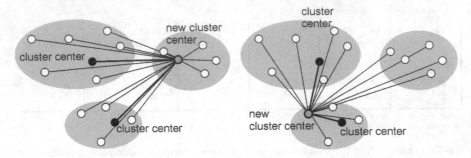

Fig. 7.13 The diversity measure D rates the closest distance $d_{\min}^c$ of the new center to all other centers with respect to the furthest distance of the new center to any of the unassigned samples

ture space. It is possible that a segment consists of different tissues with a different appearance in the image. These different tissues may fall into different clusters. If the number of clusters is set to the expected number of segments, clusters separating different segments may be merged if they are closer to each other than clusters representing the different segments.

Since such characteristics are often unknown—otherwise the more direct classification approach of Sect. 7.1 could be pursued—segmentation by k-mean clustering is often a trial-and-error procedure. The user starts with a first guess about the number of clusters, visualizes the members of the computed clusters, and then varies (increases or decreases) k until an acceptable solution is reached.

The results of k-means clustering depend on a good initialization for cluster centers. Since distribution in feature space is usually unknown, random selection is used to start the procedure. The simplest way is to separate the feature space into K compartments at random and compute the centers of gravity from the samples in each compartment. Peña et al. (1999) compared four methods and found that this simple random selection had a similar performance as a nonrandom procedure suggested by Kaufman and Rousseeuw (2005) that took the distribution characteristics into account. The latter did, however, terminate less likely in a bad partitioning.

The method of Kaufman and Rousseeuw (2005) started with sample locations, but they selected the samples according to a heuristic diversity criterion. Iteratively, a sample is selected as new cluster center that maximizes this diversity measure until K clusters have been selected. The diversity measure D rates the distance of the newly selected cluster center $\mathbf{C}_{\text{new}}$ to all already selected centers $\mathbf{C}_1, \dots, \mathbf{C}_k, k < K$ with respect to distances of $\mathbf{C}_{\text{new}}$ to all nonselected samples $\mathbf{s}_i$ in the following way (see also Fig. 7.13):

$$d_{\min}^c = \min_k \left(\| \mathbf{C}_{\text{new}} - \mathbf{C}_k \| \right), \tag{7.20}$$

$$D = \max_i \left(0, d_{\min}^c - \| \mathbf{C}_{\text{new}} - \mathbf{s}_i \| \right). \tag{7.21}$$

A different strategy was presented by Bradley and Fayyad (1998) who used modes of an estimated density function for improving a given set of initial cluster centers. The samples in feature space are assumed to approximate a mixture of probability density functions (similar to the Gaussian mixture used in Sect. 7.1.1 to represent a likelihood function). The modes of this mixture are then the local maxima of the density and are assumed to be potential cluster centers. Searching for the modes is the subject of mean shift clustering described in the next section. The approach of Bradley and Fayyad (1998) does not require all modes to be detected, but moves the initially selected cluster centers closer to the likely locations of the modes.

K-means clustering can be used as a preprocessing step to segmentation. The number of possible cluster centers is then set high to segment the scene into many regions (which may be thought of as a kind of superpixel). These are then postprocessed for the final segmentation. The method is less sensitive to the selection of cluster centers compared to a direct attempt of doing classification via clustering. It has been used, for instance, by Ng et al. (2006) for providing a watershed transform with large enough regions so that noise removal can be done by intensity averaging in the superpixels.

7.2.2 Mean-Shift Clustering

K-means clustering requires the number of clusters to be known. Misjudging the number of different clusters may lead to unwanted results. *Mean-shift clustering* is an alternative that does not require this kind of information (Fukunagu and Hostetler 1975; Comaniciu and Meer 2002). Instead, mean-shift clustering attempts to find all possible cluster centers in feature space. The samples are assumed to stem from a density function, which is a mixture of an unknown number of probability density functions. Each of the probability functions describes the probability of a sample to belong to one cluster. Ideal clustering would identify the probability functions of the mixture model and then assign cluster membership based on this probability.

Determining parameters of an unknown number of probability functions of an unknown type will be difficult or even impossible. In mean-shift clustering, heuristics are employed to arrive at a feasible solution. The following conditions are assumed.

- The probability density functions of the mixture model have only one maximum and that this maximum represents the mean of the function.
- Combining the probability functions in the mixture model preserves the maxima, so that the local maxima of the mixture function represent the means of the underlying probability functions. The local maxima are the modes of the density function.
- The local minima of the mixture model segment the feature space so that each segment contains only one of the local maxima.

Finding the local maxima of the mixture model under these assumptions produces the clusters in feature space. The mean shift algorithm proceeds as follows.

- For each location in feature space a marker is shifted toward the next local maximum by applying a gradient ascent algorithm.
- If a local maximum has been found and it has no cluster label, it is labeled.

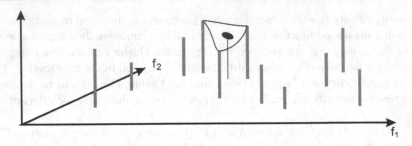

Fig. 7.14 The gradient at some location in feature space is approximated by interpolation over a predefined neighborhood using a suitable kernel function

- Irrespective of whether the local maximum has been labeled at this step or previously, the location from which it has been found receives the label as cluster label.

Gradient ascent requires computing a gradient of the density function. Since the density function is only approximated by a distribution of samples, the gradient can only be approximated as well (see Fig. 7.14). This is done by a kernel window estimator. If the feature space is isotropic, the kernel is rotationally symmetric (Comaniciu and Meer 2002):

$$k(\mathbf{x}) = k(\|\mathbf{x}\|^2), \tag{7.22}$$

where k is a one-dimensional function on distance such as the Gaussian $k(x) = \exp(-x^2/2)$. The kernel density estimation for some location $\mathbf{x}$ in d-dimensional feature space with samples $\mathbf{x}_1, \ldots, \mathbf{x}_N$ is then

$$f_{h,K}(\mathbf{x}) = \frac{c_{K,d}}{Nh^d} \sum_{i=1}^{N} k\left(\frac{\|\mathbf{x} - \mathbf{x}_i\|^2}{h}\right). \tag{7.23}$$

The value of h determines the width of the kernel and $c_{K,d}$ is a normalizing constant. If k is differentiable and g is the derivative of $-k$, the gradient is

$$\nabla f_{h,K}(\mathbf{x}) = \frac{c_{K,d}}{Nh^{d+2}} \sum_{i=1}^{N} g\left(\frac{\|\mathbf{x} - \mathbf{x}_i\|^2}{h}\right)\left[\frac{\sum_{i=1}^{N} g(\frac{\|\mathbf{x} - \mathbf{x}_i\|^2}{h})}{\sum_{i=1}^{N} x_i g(\frac{\|\mathbf{x} - \mathbf{x}_i\|^2}{h})} - \mathbf{x}\right]. \tag{7.24}$$

The gradient consists of two parts with different meanings. The first part is a kernel estimator using the derivative g instead of the original function k, and the second represents the error between the actual position $\mathbf{x}$ and its estimate by the kernel estimator. The latter is called the mean shift $m_{h,G(\mathbf{x})}$ of $\mathbf{x}$.

The parts can be separated if a new normalizing constant $c_{G,d}$ for g is introduced and the parts are rearranged:

$$\nabla f_{h,K}(\mathbf{x}) = \frac{c_{G,d}}{Nh^d} \sum_{i=1}^{N} g\left(\frac{\|\mathbf{x} - \mathbf{x}_i\|^2}{h}\right) \frac{c_{K,d}}{c_{G,d}h^2}\left[\frac{\sum_{i=1}^{N} g(\frac{\|\mathbf{x} - \mathbf{x}_i\|^2}{h})}{\sum_{i=1}^{N} x_i g(\frac{\|\mathbf{x} - \mathbf{x}_i\|^2}{h})} - x\right]. \tag{7.25}$$

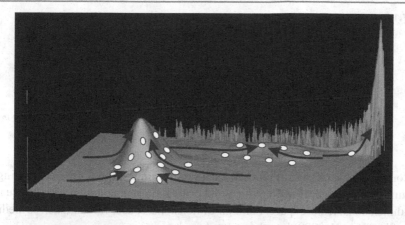

Fig. 7.15 The mean-shift algorithm starts moving from every position in feature space towards the local maxima in the function

The kernel estimator is then

$$\nabla f_{h,G}(\mathbf{x}) = \frac{c_{G,d}}{Nh^d} \sum_{i=1}^{N} g\left(\frac{\|\mathbf{x} - \mathbf{x}_i\|^2}{h}\right) \qquad (7.26)$$

and the mean shift is

$$m_{h,G}(\mathbf{x}) = \frac{c_{K,d}}{c_{G,d}h^2}\left[\frac{\sum_{i=1}^{N} g\left(\frac{\|\mathbf{x} - \mathbf{x}_i\|^2}{h}\right)}{\sum_{i=1}^{N} x_i g\left(\frac{\|\mathbf{x} - \mathbf{x}_i\|^2}{h}\right)} - \mathbf{x}\right]. \qquad (7.27)$$

Starting with some initial position $\mathbf{x}$ the algorithm proceeds by repeatedly changing the position by the mean shift until the gradient length is zero and a local maximum is reached. If this is done for all sample points and cluster labels are created and assigned as described above, it results in finding all modes in feature space and assigning each location in feature space to its corresponding mode (see Fig. 7.15).

In Comaniciu and Meer (2002), 2D images were segmented using color information and the pixel coordinates as features. Since the mean-shift algorithm is a very general method, it has found many applications. Its biggest advantage is that it is parameter-free. The determination of the number of clusters and of the clustering itself does not depend on user input.

Such a data-driven decision has disadvantages, however. Segmentation by mean-shift often results in oversegmented images since every local maximum in feature space forms its own cluster (Tuzel et al. 2008). In Tuzel et al. (2009) additional constraints in feature space were used to override the decision of the mean-shift procedure (the so-called must-link constraints that forced cluster elements to stay bound together).

Fig. 7.16 Topology of a
Kohonen network

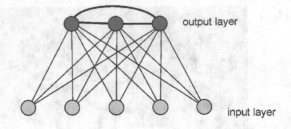

Computing the mean shift for each location in feature space is time-consuming if the dimension is high. However, this is not critical for segmentation with its usually low-dimensional feature space. For high-dimensional space, variants such as median shift (Shapira et al. 2009) have been developed.

7.2.3   Kohonen's Self-organizing Maps

Neural networks may be used for unsupervised clustering as well. Clustering is done by the association of a feature vector to a model cluster vector using a similarity measure.

A well-known network of this kind is Kohonen's *self-organizing map* (*SOM* or Kohonen network; Kohonen 1995). The network shares some similarities with mean-shift clustering discussed in the previous section in that it attempts to cluster data based on some inherent attributes. In an SOM this attribute is the similarity between feature vectors. Furthermore, an SOM also assumes some underlying structure between different clusters and attempts to find this structure as well. The structure information can be used to steer the clustering procedure.

The network consists of a single output layer that is fully connected to all nodes in the input layer (see Fig. 7.16). Each node in the input layer represents a feature in feature space. Each node in the output layer corresponds to a potential cluster.

The network is called self-organizing as it learns feature patterns and the organization of the feature distribution without supervision. Feature patterns are represented by weight vectors $\mathbf{w}_j = (w_{1j} w_{2j}, \ldots, w_{Nj})^{\mathrm{T}}$ leading to output nodes j. The organization of the feature distribution is represented by connecting output nodes to a one- or two-dimensional map and letting output at a node j influence the adjacent nodes in some neighborhood $N_\delta(j)$. In its simplest form, the neighborhood between output nodes is $N_\delta(j) = 0$ (i.e., there is no influence between output nodes). In this case, the network is a simple *association network*.

Given that the feature vector has components $i = 1, \ldots, N$ to be assigned to $j = 1, \ldots, C$ clusters, $N \cdot C$ edges connect the input nodes with the output layer with weights w_{ij}. The activation signal $f_j(\mathbf{f})$ at an output node j is the norm of the difference between the feature vector and the vector of nodes $\mathbf{w}j = (w_{1j} w_{2j}, \ldots, w_{Nj})^{\mathrm{T}}$

connecting input nodes with the output node

$$f_j(\mathbf{f}) = \|\mathbf{f} - \mathbf{w}_j\| = \sqrt{\sum_{i=1}^{N}(f_i - w_{ij})^2}. \tag{7.28}$$

The output of an association network is not f_j but the index of the node which has the highest value. If weights w_{ij} are set properly so that $\mathbf{w}_j$ is the center of a cluster $\mathbf{c}_j$, the result will be the index of that cluster.

Training the network seeks to move cluster centers $\mathbf{w}_j$ closer to the feature vectors. As training is unsupervised, the true cluster centers and the true clusters are not known. It is called *reinforcement learning* or *competitive learning*. The weights are initially set to random values. Feature vectors from samples are then fed to the network. The winning neuron in the output layer is determined. Weights leading to the winning neuron are adapted so that it becomes more similar to the feature vector:

$$\mathbf{w}_j^{(n+1)} = \mathbf{w}_j^{(n)} + \alpha(\mathbf{f} - \mathbf{w}_j), \tag{7.29}$$

where α is the learning rate. The value of α must be less than 1 to let the network memorize previous activations ($\alpha = 1$ would cause a perfect adaptation of the weight vector $\mathbf{w}_j$ to the pattern presented by $\mathbf{f}$, and the network "forgets" enforcements due to other vectors presented earlier). Initial values for α between 0.25 and 0.5 are quite common.

Another variant of it (the one that was originally introduced by Kohonen) requires normalization of the weights and gradually reduces the angle between $\mathbf{w}_j$ and $\mathbf{f}$:

$$\mathbf{w}_j^{(n+1)} = \frac{\mathbf{w}_j^{(n)} + \alpha\mathbf{f}}{\|\mathbf{w}_j^{(n)} + \alpha\mathbf{f}\|}. \tag{7.30}$$

Training is done for all samples. Since the neuron j wins for which $\mathbf{f}$ is most similar to $\mathbf{w}_j$, correction is done only for those weights that need the minimum amount of change. If samples are clustered in feature space, different output neurons will win for different samples causing a gradual separation of the weights of the weight vectors leading to the different output neurons. Hence, the weight vectors learn feature patterns that are present in the data.

The process is repeated several times (called epochs) until a stable state is reached (i.e., weight change falls below some threshold). The learning rate decreases with time so as to enable major corrections in the beginning of the process and increasing the influence of "memory" with time.

Several influences may affect the convergence of the system.

- The selection of the first samples has a much stronger influence on weight changes and cluster assignment than later training. If several artificial cluster centers for a single cluster are generated that are similar to each other, it leads to weak reinforcement of these clusters, as later samples will change only one of these centers.

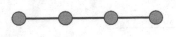 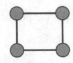 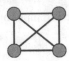

Fig. 7.17 Different neighborhood activation schemes for the same number of nodes in the output layer make different assumptions about relations between the clusters

- If the number of cluster centers does not match the true number of centers some of the weight vectors $\mathbf{w}_j$ will only receive weak enforcement either because superfluous centers divert reinforcement or because some cluster centers actually represent two or more true clusters.
- The initial random distribution of weights may inadvertently have produced patterns that misguide the pattern search, as this represents inappropriate a priori knowledge introduced into the system.

The remedy for slow convergence, convergence to a false optimum, or no convergence is to stop the training if the improvement of clustering indicates problems and to repeat it with a new set of randomly selected weights and a new random order of selecting samples.

The success of clustering using an association network depends very much on a good initialization and a correctly selected number of clusters. By Kohonen's introduction of the *neighborhood activation* a different representation of patterns in the data is achieved (see Fig. 7.17 for examples of neighborhood systems). It acknowledges possible relations between patterns of different clusters. A Kohonen network arranges output neurons in a line or in a regular grid so that every neuron is connected to two or four other neurons.

Reinforcement learning with the consideration of neighboring neurons does not vary much from the strategy stated above. The difference is that—besides updating the weights of the winning neuron j—also those of neurons in the neighborhood $N_\delta(j)$ of j are updated. If, e.g., $\delta = 5$, $N_\delta(j)$ contains all neurons that are less than five neurons away from j (using the maximum norm).

Training a Kohonen network produces a feature map that does not associate samples to cluster centers, but maps out regions in the grid of output neurons. Hence, the number of output neurons in a Kohonen network must be larger than the number of clusters expected. Essentially, the Kohonen network detects clusters in high-dimensional feature space by mapping it to the low-dimensional space of node connectivity in the network.

Separation into clusters is a separate step after training the network. It requires some supervision. Representative samples from different clusters are mapped to the network. The response points out representative regions for the clusters. They are either found interactively by displaying the network response (which is much easier than displaying a potential high-dimensional feature distribution) or segmented automatically by observing the activation difference for samples from different clusters.

Training is not guaranteed to converge to an optimal clustering. Techniques to recognize and remedy convergence problems that were suggested for association networks apply here as well. However, introducing the concept of possible interdependency between clusters by connecting output neurons and being able to represent clusters by more than a single neuron simplifies the choice of the number of output nodes.

The number of nodes depends on the complexity of the cluster boundaries to be represented. The reduction of dimensionality from feature space to a self-organizing map requires that all attributes that characterize a certain class in feature space must be representable by the map. Hence, if the map is too small, different patterns in feature space may not be separable in the map. On the other hand, the map also generalizes cluster attributes. A large map does not only require too much time to train, but it may also learn how to represent the noise in the sample data.

The neighborhood distance usually decreases with time. Initially, δ is set to a large value. It may comprise half the size of the output grid since—in the beginning—the optimal dimensionality reduction for clusters in feature space to the Kohonen network is unknown. Neighborhood size is decreased with time because a large neighborhood inhibits the separation of regions in different clusters.

Kohonen networks have been used for similar applications as clustering approaches (e.g., for segmenting MR brain images using intensity with Jiang et al. 2003 and without spatial features Reddick et al. 1997).

7.3   Concluding Remarks

Segmentation as the classification of scene elements solves two problems at the same time. It detects an object and it delineates its boundary. It requires discriminating features of the scene elements such as intensity or a vector of intensities from different imaging channels (e.g., color channels or T_1- and T_2-weighted images in MRI). If discriminating features exist, classification is simple and leads to an automatic segmentation method. All necessary parameters can be learned from the training data.

Compared to classification in general, the dimension of feature space is low and the sample density of training data is high. This allows estimation of the likelihood functions from training data and consequently classification by computing conditional a posteriori probabilities. Clustering techniques may even relieve the user from the tedious manual delineation of objects in the training data.

Problems arise when the contrast between different structures (e.g., different organs) is low or if the noise level is too high. Training data should be selected carefully to assure their representativeness for the classification problem.

7.4   Exercises

- Why is it not always appropriate to assume a Gaussian distribution for the likelihood function? Give examples for cases where this is unjustified.

- What is the goal when using a kernel density estimator? What criteria influence the selection of the kernel? Why is it reasonable to consider different kernels for different classes?
- Consider the CT image in Fig. 7.1. How can training data be generated to separate the bone structures from the background for these kinds of images?
- What are the requirements for computing the parameters of a Gaussian mixture model? Sketch a situation or give an example where a Gaussian mixture model is the appropriate means.
- What are the parameters that have to be computed for a multidimensional Gaussian distribution?
- What kind of information can be represented by the a priori probability term? How is it parameterized for the different kinds of information?
- What kind of knowledge is encoded when the segmentation is defined as the probability of a Markov Random Field?
- How does clustering differ from classification? What roles can clustering play as part of image segmentation? Please give examples.
- What kind of criterion is attempted to be optimized by partional clustering? Why is the result not necessarily optimal?
- How does k-means clustering differ from partitional clustering? What are the advantages of this difference?
- What needs to be initialized for k-means clustering? How can this initialization be carried out so that knowledge about the distributions of samples in feature space is included?
- What is the major difference between mean-shift clustering and k-means clustering?
- What is meant by "mean shift" and how is this used in the clustering method?
- Explain why mean shift clustering is slow when feature space is high.
- What is the purpose of an association network and how can it be used for clustering?
- How is an association network trained?
- How does a Kohonen network differ from an association network? What are the consequences when the two network types are used for clustering?

References

Besag J (1986) On the statistical analysis of dirty pictures. J R Stat Soc B (Methodol) 48(3):259–302

Bouman CA, Shapiro M (1994) A multiscale random field model for Bayesian image segmentation. IEEE Trans Image Process 3(2):162–177

Boykov Y, Veksler O, Zabih R (2001) Fast approximate energy minimization via graph cuts. IEEE Trans Pattern Anal Mach Intell 23(11):1222–1239

Bradley PS, Fayyad UM (1998) Refining initial points for k-means clustering. In: Proc 15th intl conf machine learning, pp 91–99

Celeux G, Forbes F, Peyrard N (2003) Procedures using mean field-like approximations for Markov model-based image segmentation. Pattern Recognit 36(1):131–144

Cheng H, Bouman CA (2001) Multiscale Bayesian segmentation using a trainable context model. IEEE Trans Image Process 10(4):511–525

Comaniciu D, Meer P (2002) Mean shift: a robust approach toward feature space analysis. IEEE Trans Pattern Anal Mach Intell 24(5):603–619

Duda RO, Hart PE, Stork DG (2000) Pattern classification: pattern classification. Pt 1, 2nd edn. Wiley, New York

Fukunagu K, Hostetler LD (1975) The estimation of the gradient of a density function with applications in pattern recognition. IEEE Trans Inf Theory 21:32–40

Geman S, Geman D (1984) Stochastic relaxation, Gibbs distributions, and the Bayesian restoration of images. IEEE Trans Pattern Anal Mach Intell 6(6):721–741

Held K, Kops ER, Krause BJ, Wells WW III, Kikinis R, Muller-Gartner HW (1997) Markov random field segmentation of brain MR images. IEEE Trans Med Imaging 16(6):878–886

Jiang Y, Chen KJ, Zhou ZH (2003) SOM based image segmentation. In: Lecture notes in computer science. LNCS, vol 2639, pp 640–643

Kaufman L, Rousseeuw PJ (2005) Finding groups in data: an introduction to cluster analysis. Wiley, New York

Kohonen T (1995) Self-organizing maps. Springer, Berlin

McLachlan GJ, Krishnan T (1996) The EM algorithm and extensions. Wiley-Interscience, New York

Marroquin JL, Santana EA, Botello S (2003) Hidden Markov measure field models for image segmentation. IEEE Trans Pattern Anal Mach Intell 25(11):1380–1387

Ng HP, Ong SH, Foong KWC, Goh PS, Nowinski WL (2006) Medical image segmentation using k-means clustering and improved watershed algorithm. In: IEEE Southwest Symposium on Image Analysis and Interpretation, pp 61–65

Peña JM, Lozano JA, Larrañaga P (1999) An empirical comparison of four initialization methods for the k-means algorithm. Pattern Recognit Lett 20(10):1027–1040

Reddick WE, Glass JO, Cook EN, Elkin TD, Deaton RJ (1997) Automated segmentation and classification of multispectral magnetic resonance images of brain using artificial neural networks. IEEE Trans Med Imaging 16(6):911–918

Shapira L, Avidan S, Shamir A (2009) Mode-detection via median-shift. In: Intl conf computer vision (ICCV), pp 1909–1916

Tuzel O, Porikli F, Meer P (2008) Pedestrian detection via classification on Riemannian manifolds. IEEE Trans Pattern Anal Mach Intell 30(10):1713–1727

Tuzel O, Porikli F, Meer P (2009) Kernel methods for weakly supervised mean shift clustering. In: Intl conf computer vision (ICCV 2009), pp 59–68

Zhang J (1992) The mean field theory in EM procedures for Markov random fields. IEEE Trans Signal Process 40(10):2570–2583

Segmentation as a Graph Problem

8

Abstract

2D and 3D images can be mapped on a graph where scene elements are nodes and neighborhood is expressed by edges connecting the nodes. Assigning weights to edges that represent local properties of a good segmentation allows finding a segmentation using optimization methods on graphs.

Two such techniques that have been used for segmentation are minimum cost graph cuts and minimum cost paths. Methodology, parameterization, advantages, and problems for algorithms that are based on either of the two techniques are discussed in this chapter.

Concepts, notions and definitions introduced in this chapter

> Interactive graph cuts
> Graph cuts to optimize a Markov Random Field
> Normalized graph cuts
> Fuzzy connectedness and its mapping to a minimum cost path problem
> The image foresting transform
> Random walks

A number of segmentation techniques that were discussed in Chap. 6 treat the image as a graph. Examples are region merging techniques, region growing, or live wire segmentation. While the former two use a graph as convenient way to represent the segmentation process, live wire employs a simple graph theoretic concept to compute a result that is guaranteed to be optimal with respect to some criterion. Representing segmentation as an optimization task on a graph taps into the multitude of efficient methods for computing the desired result. Two types of strategies from this field have been specialized to compute a segmentation.

- Graph cuts are a way for automatic or semi-automatic segmentations based on region, boundary, and external attributes.

K.D. Toennies, *Guide to Medical Image Analysis*,
Advances in Computer Vision and Pattern Recognition,
DOI 10.1007/978-1-4471-2751-2_8, © Springer-Verlag London Limited 2012

- Optimal paths on graphs can be used to associate scene elements to seeds representing different segments.

For the two strategies, various methods will be presented and discussed in the following sections. All solutions apply to images of an arbitrary dimension. However, for increased readability, we will discuss the methods at the example of 2D images with pixels as scene elements.

8.1   Graph Cuts

A *graph cut* creates two or more disconnected subgraphs by removing edges from a connected graph. Graph cuts can be applied to many areas in image processing and image understanding of which segmentation is just one. Representing a segmentation of an image by a graph cut is straightforward (Boykov and Jolly 2001; Boykov et al. 2001). Pixels are represented by nodes, and pairs of nodes representing neighboring pixels are connected by edges. The graph cut consists of a set of edges that specify the segments. The concept is powerful because of its versatility and generality. Graph cuts can be computed for scenes of any dimension and—at least in principle—for any neighborhood system between scene elements.

While cutting a graph into more than two subgraphs is difficult, expensive, and not yet fully understood, simple and fast algorithms exist for producing the cut of a graph into two subgraphs. Each of these two subgraphs may consist of several disconnected components, but each of the components of a subgraph will be associated to the same label. Hence, graph cuts are well suited to solve a foreground segmentation problem. Nodes of the graph then represent pixels and edges represent the adjacencies between pixels. If a scene shall be separated into subgraphs with more than two labels, graph cuts are either employed hierarchically by cutting a subgraph again or they are used to correct an existing multilabel segmentation that has been created by some other means.

8.1.1   Graph Cuts for Computing a Segmentation

A *minimum cost graph cut* consists of a set of edges so that the sum of edge weights in the cut is minimal for all possible cuts. In the case of segmentation, edge costs will be defined in a way so as to let the minimum cost cut represent a good foreground segmentation. The criterion for an interactive graph cut will combine user knowledge ("this node belongs to the foreground") and local image attributes.

Finding the minimum cut is solved as a maximum flow problem (see Fig. 8.1). Each edge is assigned a flow capacity. All nodes $\mathbf{p} \in P$ representing pixels are connected to two special nodes, the *source S* and the *sink T*, via *terminal links* (t-links). Edges connecting neighboring pixels are called *neighbor links* (n-links). The set of all n-links is N. Let us now presume that water is flowing from the source through the graph to the sink.

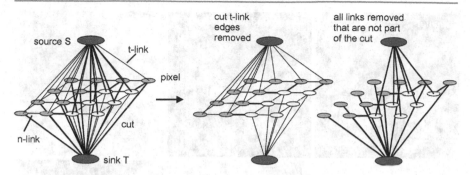

Fig. 8.1 Graph cuts for image segmentation: All pixels are connected to their neighbors via *n*-links and to a source and a sink via *t*-links. The cut separates the source from the sink. All *t*-links that are part of the cut indicate association of a pixel either to foreground (*t*-link to the source) or to the background

If the segmentation would be known, the weights for all links can be preset to describe the desired segmentation. Terminal links from the source to foreground pixels and from the sink to background pixels are attributed a "0," the remaining *t*-links are attributed a "1." Neighbor links connecting foreground or background pixels are attributed a "1" and *n*-links connecting a foreground pixel with a background pixel receive a "0" as an attribute.

The optimal cut consists of all *t*-links and *n*-links that have a value of "0" since the total cost of all edges in this case is 0. The set of edges of the cut consists of all edges connecting the foreground pixels with the source, all edges connecting the background pixels with the sink, and all edges at region boundaries between the foreground and background pixels. Hence, edges to one of the terminal nodes in the cut define the segment label of the segmentation. Edges of the cut that are *n*-links represent the boundary between segments. Note that neither foreground nor background pixels need to be a single connected component.

Computing a segmentation that is already known is not particularly useful, but the strategy outlined above can be employed as well if the assignment of a pixel to the foreground or background is less clear. Instead of attributing pixels with the certainty of belonging to the foreground, $R_p(\text{"frg"}) = 0$, $R_p(\text{"bkg"}) = 1$, or background, $R_p(\text{"frg"}) = 1$ and $R_p(\text{"bkg"}) = 0$, the probabilities of a pixel of belonging to the foreground or background are used to assign weights to the *t*-links. If these probabilities P for some pixel **p** with coordinates $(p_1, p_2, \ldots,)$ are $P(\mathbf{p} \in \text{"frg"})$ and $P(\mathbf{p} \in \text{"bkg"})$, then a possible measure suggested by the inventors of foreground graph cuts for segmentation (Boykov and Jolly 2001) is

$$R_p(\text{"frg"}) = -\ln P(\mathbf{p} \in \text{"frg"}) \quad \text{and} \quad R_p(\text{"bkg"}) = -\ln P(\mathbf{p} \in \text{"bkg"}). \quad (8.1)$$

The probabilities P are specified based on domain knowledge (such as "bone" in CT has a range of $60, \ldots, 3000$ HU) or they can be estimated from histogram analysis from training data. The value of this measure is close to zero if the prob-

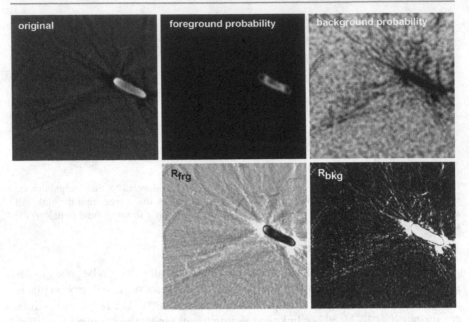

Fig. 8.2 Flow values from source to pixels (foreground) and from pixels to sink (background) are inversely proportional to the probability of these pixels belonging to the foreground or background

ability of a pixel belonging to the foreground or background is high and increases with decreasing probability (see Fig. 8.2).

If nothing else about the segment membership is known, all n-links would receive a constant weight, and the application of a graph cut algorithm would be similar to histogram-based thresholding. The power of graph cut algorithms, however, stems from combining this local region attribute with boundary attributes.

Generally, segment boundaries are indicated by the change of intensity, texture, or color. Given that a function $f(\mathbf{p})$ exists for each pixel $\mathbf{p}$ that combines these three attributes in a proper manner for the segmentation, the difference $\| f(\mathrm{p}) - f(\mathrm{q}) \|$ for two pixels $\mathbf{p}$ and $\mathbf{q}$ being connected by an n-link may serve as a weight for this link. Boykov and Jolly (2001) suggested the following measure (see Fig. 8.3):

$$B_{p,q} = \exp\left[-\frac{\| f(\mathbf{p}) - f(\mathbf{q}) \|^2}{2\sigma^2} \right] \cdot \frac{1}{\|\mathbf{p} - \mathbf{q}\|}. \tag{8.2}$$

The function resembles a nonnormalized Gaussian distribution. The value of σ is set so that it separates the high frequency and high amplitude noise from true edge variation. The latter is assumed to have a lower amplitude in the high frequency range than the noise.

If the n-link weights are used with all t-links having the same weights, the method produces results similar to the watershed transform (which finds all boundaries at zero crossings). However, combining the two measures compensates the

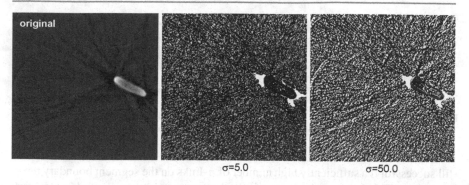

Fig. 8.3 The boundary term depends on the local intensity difference and a smoothing parameter σ. A large value for σ means that small intensity differences are counted as noise and do not receive a low flow value

Table 8.1 Weights for t-links and n-links for computing a segmentation by graph cuts

Edge type	Weights	Edges
n-link	$B_{p,q} = \exp\left[-\frac{\|f(\mathbf{p})-f(\mathbf{q})\|^2}{2\sigma^2}\right] \cdot \frac{1}{\|\mathbf{p}-\mathbf{q}\|}$	all $(p,q) \in N$
t-link	$R(\mathbf{p}, S) = \lambda \cdot (-\ln P(\mathbf{p} \in \text{"frg"}))$	all $(S, p), p \in P$
t-link	$R(\mathbf{p}, T) = \lambda \cdot (-\ln P(\mathbf{p} \in \text{"bkg"}))$	all $(T, p), p \in P$

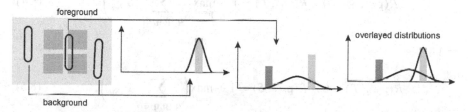

Fig. 8.4 Interactive input for foreground and background produces two distributions that overlap to such a large extent that a segmentation based on intensity alone will not produce the desired grouping into a single foreground object surrounded from background

deficiencies of one of the measures by the other measure. The weights for all the links are summarized in Table 8.1.

Finding a cut C separating S and T that minimizes the cost of all edges in C minimizes

$$E(C) = \lambda \cdot \left(\sum_{p \in S_c} R(\mathbf{p}, S) + \sum_{p \in T_{c_c}} R(\mathbf{p}, T) \right) + \sum_{(p,q) \in N_C} B_{p,q}. \qquad (8.3)$$

Here, N_C is the subset of all edges in N that are part of the cut C, and S_C and T_C are subsets of edges $(\mathbf{p}, S)$ and $(\mathbf{p}, T)$, respectively, that are part of C. The value of λ governs the relative influence of the boundary term with respect to the region term. A small value for λ would be selected if the probability distributions of the region attribute overlap or if they are very flat (see Fig. 8.4). The segmentation could be

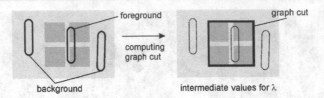

Fig. 8.5 An intermediate range of values for λ results in the desired segmentation (sketch of results that can be achieved using the method presented in Boykov and Jolly 2001)

still successful if a sufficiently high number of n-links on the segment boundary have low values. This behavior has been nicely demonstrated by an example presented in Boykov and Jolly (2001) (Fig. 8.5 shows a sketch of the behavior for different values of λ).

Graph cuts have been extended further to include a priori knowledge about region membership. If the foreground or background membership of some pixels is known, their t-link weights can be set accordingly so as to ensure that the minimum cost cut does cut the corresponding link. The t-link weight for the known foreground pixels $\mathbf{p}_{\text{frg}}$ and background pixels $\mathbf{p}_{\text{bkg}}$ are

$$R(\mathbf{p}_{\text{frg}}, S) = 0 \wedge R(\mathbf{p}_{\text{frg}}, T) = 1 + \max_{\mathbf{p} \in P} \left(\sum_{\mathbf{q}:(\mathbf{p},\mathbf{q}) \in N} B_{p,q} \right) \tag{8.4}$$

and

$$R(\mathbf{p}_{\text{bkg}}, T) = 0 \wedge R(\mathbf{p}_{\text{bkg}}, S) = 1 + \max_{\mathbf{p} \in P} \left(\sum_{\mathbf{q}:(\mathbf{p},\mathbf{q}) \in N} B_{p,q} \right). \tag{8.5}$$

It will always be costlier to cut the t-link from T to a $\mathbf{p}_{\text{frg}}$ or from S to a $\mathbf{p}_{\text{bkg}}$ than to cut any n-link leading to pixel $\mathbf{p}_{\text{frg}}$ or $\mathbf{p}_{\text{bkg}}$, respectively.

Introducing the known foreground and background pixels enables user interaction at runtime. Histograms of interactively specified $f(\mathbf{p}_{\text{frg}})$ and $f(\mathbf{p}_{\text{bkg}})$ may be used to estimate region membership probabilities.

The computation of the minimum cut is done by computing the maximum flow between the source and sink. The flow from source to sink will be limited by a set of edges that are saturated with flow. This set of edges forms a closed boundary separating the source from the sink[1] irrespective of the dimension of the scene that is represented by the graph.

The iterative Floyd–Fulkerson algorithm computes the maximum flow. It augments flow until saturation (see Fig. 8.6). The algorithm keeps a copy G_{residual} of the graph $G = \{V, E\}$ with nodes $V = \{v_i\}$ and edges $E = \{e_j\}$. The weights $w_{\text{res}}(e_i)$

---

[1] If the boundary is not closed, at least one non-saturated edge between source and sink would exist. Flow could be increased until this edge is saturated as well.

Fig. 8.6 The Ford–Fulkerson algorithm finds a sequence of edges with maximal flow capacity at each step. Total flow is increased accordingly and remaining capacity is reduced

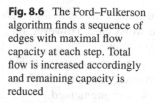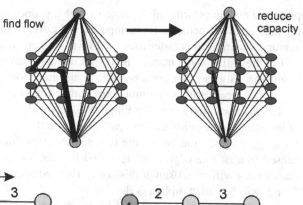

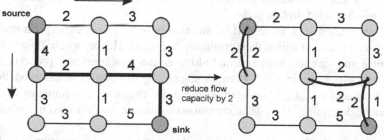

Fig. 8.7 Computation of the path with maximal remaining capacity is done by computing a minimum cost path on the capacity

of edges in $G_{residual}$ are the residual flow capacity, which, at initialization, is equal to the capacity $w(e_i)$ of edges in G.

At each iteration, the minimum cost path from S to T is determined in $G_{residual}$ (see Fig. 8.7). The flow from S to T is augmented by the capacity of the edge with smallest weight w_{min} along this path. Residual capacity along the edges of the path is reduced by w_{min}. Edges E with $w_{res}(e) = 0$ are removed and are part of the graph cut.[2] The process continues until T becomes unreachable from S. The set of edges removed from the residual capacity graph constitute the minimum cost graph cut.

The algorithm above is efficient in worst-case analysis for arbitrary graphs. The average performance for computing graph cuts for segmentation can be improved, however, if the specific structure of graphs from images is taken into account (i.e., that all pixels are connected by t-links to S and T and that all n-links are local) (Boykov and Kolmogorov 2004).

The essence of Boykov's algorithm is the reuse of information from a path search between the source and sink instead of starting the path search at each iteration after a flow augmentation from scratch. The disadvantage of this approach is that

---

[2]It is possible that edges between two neighboring pixels are removed by this procedure which may make a pixel unreachable from S and T. This corresponds to segmentation boundaries that are broader than a pixel in methods such as the watershed transform. If this is undesirable, similar strategies as in WST have to be followed for assigning these pixels either to foreground or background.

paths are not necessarily minimum cost paths. It does not change the optimality of the solution, but increases the computational costs in the worst case. However, on average, the method is faster than the Floyd–Fulkerson algorithm.

For the initial augmentation, Boykov's method searches a minimum cost path by simultaneously carrying out a breadth-first search from source S and sink T. If the two search trees meet, a minimum cost path is found and flow is augmented.

The method differs from the Floyd–Fulkerson algorithm in the next step. Instead of initiating a new minimum cost path search on the updated residual capacity graph $G_{residual}$, it reuses the net of the two search trees. Since augmentation will have caused at least one edge to be removed because of saturation, at least one of the search trees will be broken at this edge. The nodes that are no longer connected to S or T will be called orphan nodes.

In a restoration step, there will be an attempt to be reconnect orphan nodes to the one search tree to which they originally belonged. Hence, a new flow between the source and sink has been restored although the minimum cost property is not necessarily given. Again, the bottleneck edge along this path is determined, flow is augmented, and $G_{residual}$ is updated accordingly. The process terminates when no path can be determined (i.e., when orphan nodes remain unconnected in the restoration step).

The algorithms above assume that weights along edges are positive, which can be easily assured and which is true for the weighting scheme given by (8.2) to (8.5).

For a given image, the computation of a graph cut needs to be repeated from scratch when the weights are changed. This may happen, for instance, if the user adds foreground or background pixels because the current segmentation result is unsatisfactory.

The complete recomputation of maximum flow can be avoided using a simple trick. This will be demonstrated by the example of adding new foreground nodes $\mathbf{p}_{frg,1}, \ldots, \mathbf{p}_{frg,N}$. It changes the flow capacity at edges $(S, \mathbf{p}_{frg,i})$ by the positive value $(K - \lambda) \cdot R_{bkg}(\mathbf{p}_{frg,i})$. It also changes the flow capacity at edges $(T, \mathbf{p}_{frg,i})$ by the negative value $-\lambda \cdot R_{frg}(\mathbf{p}_{frg,i})$. Computing maximum flow can be continued using the previous result in the residual capacity graph $G_{residual}$ instead of starting with G if the residual capacities of edges $(S, \mathbf{p}_{frg,i})$ and $(T, \mathbf{p}_{frg,i})$ are changed accordingly. If one of these edges no longer exists in $G_{residual}$ because it was saturated, it has to be included again.

Updating the residual capacity graph as explained above may assign negative weights to some edges. This is remedied by computing $w_{min} = \min_{e \in G_{res}} w(e)$ and subtracting it from all edge weights. It changes the maximum flow by a constant but does not change the the set of edges in C (see Fig. 8.8).

8.1.2 Graph Cuts to Approximate a Bayesian Segmentation

The graph cut technique outlined above can also be used as part of a segmentation procedure that optimizes label classification based on a Markov random field model presented in Sect. 7.1.3. In Boykov et al. (2001) the problem is defined as an energy

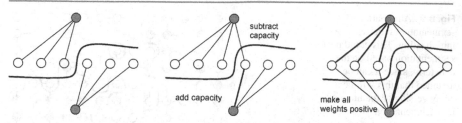

Fig. 8.8 Adding a foreground node after a cut requires updating the capacities to this node from source and sink accordingly. Since this may result in edges with negative weight, a constant factor is added to all edges (including those removed because they are saturated)

minimization task, which makes it conceptually similar to some of the active contour segmentation schemes presented in the next chapter.

- *Interaction costs* $V(f(\mathbf{p}), f(\mathbf{q}))$ represent what is the a priori probability term of the MRF formulation and what is called internal energy in active contours. Interaction costs are a smoothing term that is assumed to be minimal if labels $f(\mathbf{p})$ of a pixel $\mathbf{p}$ and those of its neighbors $\mathbf{q}$ are equal. The neighborhood for the set of neighbor pairs N can be defined in an arbitrary manner.
- *Data costs* $D(f(\mathbf{p}))$ represent what the likelihood function is in the MRF formulation and what is the external energy in active contours. The value of $D(f(\mathbf{p}))$ is assumed to be minimal if the features of pixels $\mathbf{p} \in G$ having some label are similar to the feature values expected for this kind of segment.

The goal of segmentation is to find a labeling S_{opt} that minimizes a weighted combination of internal and external energies:

$$S_{\mathrm{opt}} = \arg\min_{S} E(S) = \sum_{(\mathbf{p},\mathbf{q}) \in N} V\big(f(\mathbf{p}), f(\mathbf{q})\big) + \gamma \sum_{\mathbf{p} \in G} D\big(f(\mathbf{p})\big). \tag{8.6}$$

The weight γ depends on the kind of image and has to be specified by the user. Data costs are weighted high if data are reliable (high contrast, low noise), while otherwise interaction costs are weighted higher. Data costs $D(f(\mathbf{p}))$ can be any nonnegative function of $f(\mathbf{p})$. It could be, for instance, the difference of the actual value of $\mathbf{p}$ compared to an expected value $E_f(\mathbf{p})$ for pixels belonging to a segment labeled with f. Interaction costs need to be a metric or a semimetric on the labels l. It is a reasonable constraint that requires nonnegativity, symmetry, and $V(f(\mathbf{p}), f(\mathbf{p})) = 0$. If it is a metric, the triangle inequality must hold as well.

Automatic segmentation by graph cut requires some initial labeling that assigns a segment label to each pixel. In principle, this labeling can be arbitrary. There are two reasons why segmentation should be initiated with a good guess nonetheless.

- Most optimization schemes are iterative local relabeling procedures that are not guaranteed to terminate in the global minimum.
- It is not guaranteed that the global minimum really is the desired segmentation.

Hence, the initial labeling should be as close as possible to the desired final result. Such an initial segmentation can be created by first omitting the interaction term V. The initial label $f(\mathbf{p})$ for a scene element $\mathbf{p}$ is then the label of which the expected

Fig. 8.9 Automatic
segmentation requires an
initialization. This could be a
segmentation based on the
data term, since it can be
assumed that this will be a
noisy version of the unknown
true segmentation

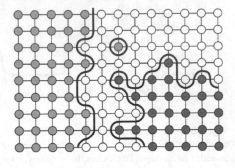

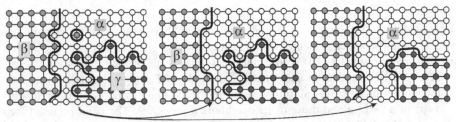

Fig. 8.10 An $\alpha-\beta$ swap finds an optimal label swap between all sites labeled with α and β. Other regions are not changed. An α-expansion expands the region labeled with a into all other regions

feature vector is closest to the feature vector observed at **p**. It is a reasonable strategy since the interaction costs serve as a smoothness constraint to reduce the effects of noise on the segmentation (see Fig. 8.9 for a schematic view). If the omission of the smoothness constraint does not produce a good initial segmentation, the noise level is so high that the final segmentation is mainly influenced by the a priori knowledge. In such a case, using such a simple model of a priori knowledge is inappropriate altogether and a different segmentation strategy should be employed.

Given the initialization, graph cut optimizes the labeling according to the interaction term enforcing equal labels between neighboring scene elements and to the data term given by the likelihood function. Two different methods have been presented to achieve this goal (Boykov et al. 2001, see also Fig. 8.10).

- $\alpha-\beta$ *swap moves* find an optimal swap of labels between all scene elements having the labels α and β.
- α-*expansion moves* expand regions labeled with α into all regions with other labels.

If the scene is separated into two different regions (e.g., foreground and background) both methods produce optimal results. If the scene has more than two different segment types, it has been shown by Boykov et al. (2001) that the α-expansion moves produces a result of which the total energy is at most twice the minimum energy that is searched. No such assertion can be made for $\alpha-\beta$ swap moves.

A segmentation can be achieved by either iterating several times through all possible $\alpha-\beta$ swap moves for all label combinations (α, β) or by repeatedly carrying out α-expansion moves. A set of moves through all possible (α, β) combinations for $\alpha-\beta$ swaps or through all possible labels α for α-expansions is called a *cycle*. The

Fig. 8.11 Graph of all nodes currently labeled α or β for an α–β-swap move

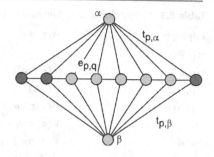

Table 8.2 Weights for an α–β swap

Edge type	Weight	Edges
$e(\mathbf{p}, \mathbf{q})$	$V(f(\mathbf{p}), f(\mathbf{q}))$	All $(\mathbf{p}, \mathbf{q}) \in P_{\alpha,\beta}$, $(\mathbf{p}, \mathbf{q}) \in N$
$t(\mathbf{p}, \alpha)$	$\sum_{q \in N_p, q \notin P_{\alpha,\beta}} V(f(\mathbf{p}), f(\mathbf{q})) + \gamma D(f(\mathbf{p}))$	All $\mathbf{p} \in P_{\alpha,\beta}$
$t(\mathbf{p}, \beta)$	$\sum_{q \in N_p, q \notin P_{\alpha,\beta}} V(f(\mathbf{p}), f(\mathbf{q})) + \gamma D(f(\mathbf{p}))$	All $\mathbf{p} \in P_{\alpha,\beta}$

iterative procedure stops when iterating through a cycle does not reduce the total energy $E(S)$. Termination after a fixed number of cycles is guaranteed since D is nonnegative and V is at least a semimetric.

Although it sounds as if α-expansion moves should be preferred to swap moves this should be taken with a grain of salt. Assuring that the energy of the final labeling is at most twice as high as the minimal energy tells little about the actual labeling error (i.e., the number and location of mislabeled scene elements).

For computing each move (swap move or expansion move) a graph has to be created from the scene. The nodes in this graph represent a subset of the scene elements. Two nodes are connected by an edge if the corresponding scene elements are neighbors by some neighborhood definition. The neighborhood could be the usual four- or eight-neighborhood for pixels (6- or 26-neighborhood for voxels), but in general, every kind of neighborhood is admissible.

The graphs for α–β swap moves and for α-expansion moves are different from each other. The graph for an α–β swap move consists of the subset of all nodes $\{\mathbf{p}_\alpha\} \cup \{\mathbf{p}_\beta\}$ representing scene elements labeled with $f(\mathbf{p}) = \alpha$ or $f(\mathbf{p}) = \beta$ and two terminal nodes $\boldsymbol{\alpha}$ and $\boldsymbol{\beta}$. Nodes $\mathbf{p}, \mathbf{q} \in \{\mathbf{p}_\alpha\} \cup \{\mathbf{p}_\beta\}$ are connected by an edge $e(\mathbf{p}, \mathbf{q})$ if they are neighbors. All nodes $\mathbf{p}$ are connected with the two terminal links by edges $t(\mathbf{p}, \alpha)$ and $t(\mathbf{p}, \beta)$, respectively (see Fig. 8.11). Table 8.2 lists the weights given to the edges.

This table has some similarities to the table for interactive graph cuts. Again, for all edges in the graph, interaction costs V are computed. The main difference is in the definition of the cost for the edges to the two terminals. Additionally to the data cost D of scene element $\mathbf{p}$, interaction costs are added from neighboring nodes that are labeled neither α nor β. This is necessary because a cut that results in a relabeling also changes potential relabeling costs to other nodes (the interaction cost between label α and another label γ may be different to the cost between labels β and γ). The set of edges in the graph cut contains edges connecting pixel nodes with terminal

Table 8.3 Weights for an α-expansion move

Edge type	Weight	Edge
$t(\mathbf{p}, \bar{\alpha})$	∞	All $\mathbf{p} \in P_\alpha$
$t(\mathbf{p}, \bar{\alpha})$	$\gamma D(f(\mathbf{p}))$	All $\mathbf{p} \notin P_\alpha$
$t(\mathbf{p}, \alpha)$	$\gamma D(\alpha)$	All $\mathbf{p} \in P$
$e(\mathbf{p}, \mathbf{a})$	$V(f(\mathbf{p}), \alpha)$	All $(\mathbf{p}, \mathbf{q}) \in N, f(\mathbf{p}) \neq f(\mathbf{q})$
$e(\mathbf{a}, \mathbf{q})$	$V(\alpha, f(\mathbf{q}))$	
$t(\mathbf{a}, \bar{\alpha})$	$V(f(\mathbf{p}), f(\mathbf{q}))$	
$e(\mathbf{p}, \mathbf{q})$	$V(f(\mathbf{p}), \alpha)$	All $(\mathbf{p}, \mathbf{q}) \in N, f(\mathbf{p}) \neq f(\mathbf{q})$

Fig. 8.12 The graph for an α-expansion consists of all nodes whether being labeled α or not, plus auxiliary nodes between neighboring nodes with label α and some other label

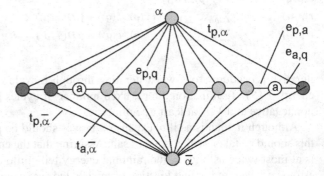

label nodes. Pixels are assigned the label of these terminal nodes. It has been shown in Boykov et al. (2001) that relabeling nodes according to the minimum cut on this graph using the edge costs from Table 8.2 maximally decreases the total energy with respect to the two labels. It is not the global optimum, however, since the swap does not consider the costs from pixels with other labels γ.

The graph for an α-expansion consists of all nodes representing pixels in the scene and two terminal nodes α and $\bar{\alpha}$. Auxiliary nodes $\mathbf{a}$ are introduced between each pair of nodes $\mathbf{p}$ and $\mathbf{q}$ that have different labels $f(\mathbf{p}) \neq f(\mathbf{q})$ (see Fig. 8.12). These auxiliary nodes are connected by edges to nodes $\mathbf{p}$ and $\mathbf{q}$ via edges $e(\mathbf{p}, \mathbf{a})$ and $e(\mathbf{a}, \mathbf{q})$ and to the terminal node $\bar{\alpha}$ via $t(\mathbf{a}, \bar{\alpha})$. The introduction of auxiliary nodes is necessary to represent the costs that incur when a label change takes place. Edge costs for all edges are listed in Table 8.3.

Similar to the $\alpha-\beta$ swap, it can be shown that computing a minimum cut using the graph with edge weights as given above and relabeling nodes according to the links to either α or $\bar{\alpha}$ produces the maximum decrease in total energy that can be achieved by expanding the α-labels into all other pixels. The graph changes after every step since the number, placement, and weights of the auxiliary nodes change.

Fig. 8.13 The blob
constraint penalizes cutting
through edges between pixels
the more the orientation
varies from the orientation of
a line between the blob center
and the pixel. In this example,
cutting the edge depicted in
(**a**) is cheaper than cutting the
edge depicted in (**b**)

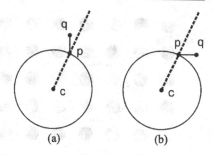

8.1.3 Adding Constraints

Basic graph cut segmentation produces segments based on homogeneity in the segments and boundary length. Its performance can be enhanced if additional domain knowledge is integrated into the cost function.

A blob component has been used (Funka-Lea et al. 2006) to separate the heart from the background in CT images. The blob component is realized by adding a term to (8.6) that penalizes the direction deviations of a line segment **pq** of a cut to a line from a prespecified blob center **c** to the location of **p** (see Fig. 8.13). This is a way to promote convex structures around a prespecified blob center (which in this case is a location in the center of the heart specified by the user). The approach has been generalized by Veksler (2008) who extended the approach to use arbitrary star-convex shapes around a selected center. It allows to include a variety of generic shape constraints into the graph cut formulation.

The segmentation of line-like extrusions of a structure has been made possible by a method presented by Vicente et al. (2008). Such extrusions are cut by regular graph cut segmentation, as it requires too many edges to be part of the cut. In Vicente et al. (2008) an additional user-specified constraint augments an existing segmentation (e.g., from graph cut segmentation) to add missing extrusions to the result. The required user input consists of placing seed points into extremal points of the missing extrusion. The constraint then requires these points to be connected to the existing segmentation. Different kinds of conditions are given for this connection. A heuristic solution is presented that combines the graph cut with a Dijkstra-like path searching algorithm to connect the seeds with the original segmentation.

Priors can be more specific than the ones here if a model predicts a specific shape. This will be discussed in Chap. 11 on the use of shape models.

8.1.4 Normalized Graph Cuts

Graph cuts sometimes produce undesired results because the minimum-cut-maximum-flow tends to cut as few edges as possible (see Fig. 8.14). In interactive graph cuts it may produce segments with boundaries very close to the foreground or background seed points. This is particularly so if the data terms for the foreground and background have very different characteristics (e.g., when one of them has to allow

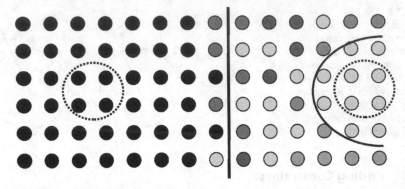

Fig. 8.14 A graph cut segmentation may stop too early because the inhomogeneous foreground *on the right* results in a weak data constraint. Hence, smoothness overtakes, which causes a short boundary close to the initialization

for a much higher variation of feature values than the other). In such a case, it can be helpful to add a size constraint into the equation that requires segments to have a similar size. It makes sense if the goal of segmentation is not to extract a specific object—of which the size may be very different from that of the background—but to produce agglomerations of pixels that shall be further processed for analysis. Normalizing the segmentation by segment size is comparable with similar segmentation methods such as the watershed transform or region merging, however, with the difference that it optimizes a criterion that includes both region and boundary terms.

In Shi and Malik (2000) a method is suggested that incorporates such a normalization criterion into the graph cut procedure. The *normalized graph cut* segments an image into regions with one of two labels, **a** or **b**, with minimal costs. The costs consist of the original graph cut costs *cut*(**a**,**b**) weighted by association costs *assoc*(**a**,**v**) and *assoc*(**b**,**v**) between nodes of a segment to all nodes **v** in the scene. The total cost of a normalized cut is then

$$NCut(\mathbf{a}, \mathbf{b}) = \frac{cut(\mathbf{a}, \mathbf{b})}{assoc(\mathbf{a}, \mathbf{v})} + \frac{cut(\mathbf{a}, \mathbf{b})}{assoc(\mathbf{b}, \mathbf{v})}. \tag{8.7}$$

Unfortunately, computing the optimal cut is NP-complete. Hence, Shi and Malik (2000) presented an approximation of the result. The problem is mapped on a linear equation system representing the graph as a matrix and the unknown labeling by an indicator vector. The indicator vector **x** for nodes $\mathbf{N} = \{\mathbf{n}_1, \ldots, \mathbf{n}_M\}$ in the graph has elements x_i as follows:

$$x_i = \begin{cases} 1, & \text{if } \mathbf{n}_i \in A, \\ -1, & \text{if } \mathbf{n}_i \in B. \end{cases} \tag{8.8}$$

An $M \times M$ weight matrix $\mathbf{W}$ denotes the costs of the edge between nodes n_i and n_j. The value of an element w_{ij} is

$$w_{ij} = \begin{cases} e(i, j), & \text{if } \mathbf{n}_i \text{ and } \mathbf{n}_j \text{ are connected by an edge,} \\ 0, & \text{otherwise.} \end{cases} \quad (8.9)$$

Furthermore, a diagonal matrix $\mathbf{D}$ is created with entries d_{ii} representing the association costs of a node $\mathbf{n}_i$ to all other nodes:

$$d_{ii} = \sum_{j=1,M} w_{ij}. \quad (8.10)$$

The cost function can then be rewritten as

$$NCut(A, B) = NCut(\mathbf{x}) = \frac{\sum_{\{(i,j)\}, x_i > 0, x_j < 0} -w_{ij} x_i x_j}{\sum_{\{i\}, x_i > 0} d_{ii}}$$

$$+ \frac{\sum_{\{(i,j)\}, x_i < 0, x_j > 0} -w_{ij} x_i x_j}{\sum_{\{i\}, x_i < 0} d_{ii}}. \quad (8.11)$$

Introducing a cost ratio k for the association costs of scene elements with label $\mathbf{a}$ to the total association cost

$$k = \frac{\sum_{\{i\}, x_i > 0} d_{ii}}{\sum_i d_{ii}} \quad (8.12)$$

and setting

$$\mathbf{y} = (1 + \mathbf{x}) - \frac{k}{1 - k} (1 - \mathbf{x}) \quad (8.13)$$

it can be shown (Shi and Malik 2000) that the cost of a cut specified by an indicator vector $\mathbf{x}$ is given by

$$NCut(\mathbf{x}) = \frac{\mathbf{y}^T (\mathbf{D} - \mathbf{W}) \mathbf{y}}{\mathbf{y}^T \mathbf{D} \mathbf{y}}. \quad (8.14)$$

Finding an optimal cut requires finding a vector $\mathbf{y}$ that minimizes $NCut(\mathbf{x})$. Solving the associated eigenproblem can generate solutions for

$$(\mathbf{D} - \mathbf{W})\mathbf{y} = \lambda \mathbf{D} \mathbf{y}. \quad (8.15)$$

The solution for the second largest eigenvalue (i.e., the associated eigenvector) produces the vector $\mathbf{y}$ and consequently the vector $\mathbf{x}$ to create the labeling. The result only approximates the optimal solution since $\mathbf{x}$ may contain values that are neither 1 nor -1. In a final step, the real-valued vector is mapped onto an indicator vector.

Fig. 8.15 Fuzzy
connectedness between two
pixels is defined by the
maximal local affinity of all
paths between the two pixels

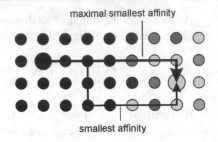

The NCut algorithm can be extended to separate an image into more than two labels in two ways. Further separations can be generated by repeated subdivision if the NCut algorithm is applied again on a labeled scene. This is the most stable, but a rather slow solution for multilabel segmentation. Another option is to use eigenvectors associated to smaller eigenvalues. Due to the way to approximate eigenvalues and due to the fact that the result is only an approximation of the true optimal decomposition, this is much less stable, however. Alternative ways to solve the multilabel segmentation problem were proposed (e.g., by Ng et al. 2002 and Tolliver and Miller 2006).

8.2   Segmentation as a Path Problem

Instead of using graph cuts, segmentation can also be modeled as a minimum cost path problem. This is the underlying principle of the live wire method of Sect. 6.9, where part of a segment boundary has been modeled as a path in a graph representing a 2D scene. It has been extended to segmentations based on regional attributes in several ways, which will be presented below. Common to all approaches is that there is no restriction on the number of dimensions of the scene to be segmented. Another common aspect is that all approaches require seed elements similar to seeded region growing. Segmentation is then solved as a minimum cost path problem between each pixel and the seed elements. A pixel receives the label of a seed pixel, which can be reached with the lowest cost.

8.2.1   Fuzzy Connectedness

Fuzzy connectedness is an old concept to describe the connectivity between sets that have a spatial component so that the neighborhood between elements of the set can be defined. The concept has been exploited for image segmentation by relating connectedness to segmentation goals (Udupa and Samarasekera 1996). An exact, but rather mathematical description can be found in Udupa and Saha (2003).

Fuzzy connectedness between two scene elements is given by *local affinity* values a of a path between the two elements. The affinity of a path is given by the smallest local affinity between neighboring elements along the path. Fuzzy connectedness μ

between two elements $\mathbf{p}_j$ and $\mathbf{p}_k$ is then the minimum affinity of the strongest path between the elements (see Fig. 8.15):

$$\mu(\mathbf{p}_j, \mathbf{p}_k) = \max_{p(\mathbf{p}_j,\mathbf{p}_k) \in P(\mathbf{p}_j,\mathbf{p}_k)} \left[\min_{(\mathbf{p}_{s1},\mathbf{p}_{s2}) \in p(\mathbf{p}_j,\mathbf{p}_k)} a(\mathbf{p}_{s1}, \mathbf{p}_{s2}) \right], \tag{8.16}$$

where $P()$ is the set of all paths between two pixels, $p()$ is a path, and $(\mathbf{p}_{s1}, \mathbf{p}_{s2})$ are adjacent pixels under some adjacency relationship.

The affinity value a between two pixels is a local property that depends on the distance between the two pixels, on the homogeneity of the feature values of the two pixels, and on the deviation of the feature values from the expected values. Affinity decreases with increasing distance, inhomogeneity, and dissimilarity of the features to the expected features.

In principle, any reasonable measure for distance, homogeneity, and dissimilarity to some expected value can be used to measure affinity. In Udupa and Saha (2003), however, an elegant way was presented to relate homogeneity and dissimilarity to the expected semantics. Details can be found in Udupa and Saha (2003), but the essence of the argumentation is that inhomogeneity can be caused by two effects: random fluctuation and the fact that the two pixels $\mathbf{p}_j$ and $\mathbf{p}_k$ belong to different objects. Since only the latter is relevant in terms of the affinity measure, the authors

- estimated homogeneous regions of interest around the two scene elements,
- computed measures of deviation under two different hypotheses ($\mathbf{p}_j$ is brighter than $\mathbf{p}_k$ or $\mathbf{p}_k$ is brighter than $\mathbf{p}_j$),
- made the assumption that the higher of the two deviation measures ($d_{\max}, d_{\min}$) depends on random variation plus any variation caused by $\mathbf{p}_j$ and $\mathbf{p}_k$ belonging to different objects, while the other represent just variation by random noise (which simply means that the SNR should be better than 1),
- and finally used the difference $d_{\max} - d_{\min}$ for computing a homogeneity measure.

A similar approach is used for computing the dissimilarity from the expected feature values. The main difference is that the weighting does not depend on the relative difference in appearance at $\mathbf{p}_j$ and $\mathbf{p}_k$, but on a probability given some expected intensity distribution functions.

Given the affinity measure, fuzzy connectedness can be used to associate pixels to user-specified seed elements. In Herman and Carvalho (2001) it was shown that computing fuzzy connectedness for every pixel with respect to given seed pixels can be done efficiently by applying Dijkstra's algorithm to compute a minimum cost path.

Fuzzy connectivity for segmentation can be applied in an absolute and a relative manner (see Fig. 8.16). Absolute connectivity is specified if a threshold on fuzzy connectivity can be given that is required for all pixels of a segment. Given a seed pixel, all pixels are detected that fulfill this criterion with respect to the seed. This bears some similarity to region growing methods such as those presented in Chap. 6. However, different to those, fuzzy connectivity is not heuristic and guarantees to optimize a (fuzzy) membership function. Furthermore, region growing

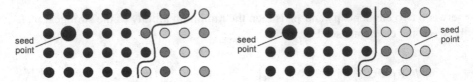

Fig. 8.16 Segmentation using absolute fuzzy connectedness puts the segment boundary between pixels of which fuzzy connectedness falls below some pre-specified threshold. In relative fuzzy connectedness, connectedness for each pixel to a set of seed pixels is computed. Pixels receive the label of the seed to which the connectedness is maximal

works only with a simple neighborhood relationship and homogeneity features cannot be defined. The latter leads to serious problems when the implicit homogeneity assumption of region growing (the region has a constant intensity value) is not true.

As a relative method, segmentation using fuzzy connectedness is even more versatile. In this case, fuzzy connectivity of a pixel to each of K different seed pixels is computed. The pixel receives the label of the one seed to which it has the highest fuzzy connectedness. The segmentation produces as many connected segments as there are seed pixels and does not require a predefined threshold on fuzzy connectedness.

8.2.2 The Image Foresting Transform

Using the *image foresting transform* (IFT) (Falcao et al. 2004) for segmentation bears some similarity to segmentation by interactive graph cut segmentation. The IFT creates a segmented image by finding minimum cost paths in a graph with nodes representing pixels and edges representing the neighborhood between pixels. The IFT allows separation of a scene into an arbitrary number of differently labeled segments. Minimum cost paths to each pixel may originate at arbitrary pixels, but specific seed locations may be selected by proper definition of the initial path costs at every pixel. The result is a forest of trees. Pixels being roots of a tree connect to all nodes of the graph that can be reached from this root by a minimum cost path (see Fig. 8.17).

The graph $G = \{V, E\}$, for which the IFT is computed, consists of nodes $V = \{\mathbf{p}_1, \mathbf{p}_2, \ldots\}$ representing pixels and edges $E = \{e_1, e_2, \ldots\}$ connecting adjacent pixels. Adjacency may be defined such that two pixels are adjacent if they share a common corner, edge, or surface. Other adjacency relationships are possible as well (similar to graph cuts). An edge e_j connecting $\mathbf{p}_{j,1}$ with $\mathbf{p}_{j,2}$ carries a cost $c(e_j) = c(\mathbf{p}_{j,1}, \mathbf{p}_{j,2})$. If region-based segmentation is the objective, this cost is related to the likelihood of $\mathbf{p}_{j,1}$ and $\mathbf{p}_{j,2}$ belonging to the same region. Furthermore, nodes $\mathbf{p}$ carry a cost $h(\mathbf{p})$, which is called the *node load*. In region-based segmentation, the node load reflects the likelihood of this node being a potential seed of a segment. Given a scene represented by a graph, the IFT will compute the shortest path from one of the seeds to every node in the graph. The method for computing the IFT is a modified and optimized version of Dijkstra's method for computing minimum cost paths.

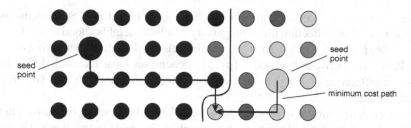

Fig. 8.17 The image foresting transform computes minimum cost path from seed pixels to all other pixels. Segmentation is then given by assigning labels from the seed which can be reached with lowest costs. The method bears similarity to segmentation using fuzzy connectedness, however, the length of the path influences computed costs

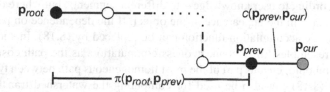

Fig. 8.18 Sketch of path cost computation according to (8.17)

Path costs $\pi(\mathbf{p}_{root}, \mathbf{p}_{cur})$ between a root node $\mathbf{p}_{root}$ and the current node $\mathbf{p}_{cur}$ are defined by an accumulation function $\pi_{acc}[\pi(\mathbf{p}_{root}, \mathbf{p}_{prev}), c(\mathbf{p}_{prev}, \mathbf{p}_{cur})]$ of the path cost $\pi(\mathbf{p}_{root}, \mathbf{p}_{prev})$ to the parent node $\mathbf{p}_{prev}$ of node $\mathbf{p}_{cur}$ and the edge cost $c(e) = c(\mathbf{p}_{prev}, \mathbf{p}_{cur})$ of an edge connecting $\mathbf{p}_{prev}$ with $\mathbf{p}_{cur}$ (see Fig. 8.18). Various definitions of the path cost function π_{acc} are possible such as

$$\pi_{acc}\big[\pi(\mathbf{p}_{root}, \mathbf{p}_{prev}), c(\mathbf{p}_{prev}, \mathbf{p}_{cur})\big] = \pi(\mathbf{p}_{root}, \mathbf{p}_{prev}) + c(\mathbf{p}_{prev}, \mathbf{p}_{cur}), \qquad (8.17)$$

which adds the edge cost to the cost of the path from $\mathbf{p}_{root}$ to $\mathbf{p}_{prev}$, or

$$\pi_{acc}\big[\pi(\mathbf{p}_{root}, \mathbf{p}_{prev}), c(\mathbf{p}_{prev}, \mathbf{p}_{cur})\big] = \max\big[\pi(\mathbf{p}_{root}, \mathbf{p}_{prev}), c(\mathbf{p}_{prev}, \mathbf{p}_{cur})\big], \quad (8.18)$$

which computes the maximum edge cost along the path. Any accumulation function that fulfills

$$\pi(\mathbf{p}_{root}, \mathbf{p}_{cur}) \geq \pi(\mathbf{p}_{root}, \mathbf{p}_{prev}) \qquad (8.19)$$

is acceptable. If (8.19) is violated, a minimum cost path of finite length does not always exist.

Using the concept for segmentation is straightforward. Each node is assigned a label and labels are propagated from the root of each tree in the forest to all children. After computing the IFT, labels are interpreted as segment membership.

Selecting appropriate node loads and path cost accumulation functions produces a variety of different segmentation methods. Additive path costs defined by (8.17) are useful for representing a seeded region growing by a minimum cost path search.

In this case, a set of seeds s with labels l_s have to be predefined. Seed elements $\mathbf{s}$ receive a load $h(\mathbf{s})$ reflecting the homogeneity in a local neighborhood around $\mathbf{s}$. All other nodes $\mathbf{p}$ receive loads $h(\mathbf{p}) = \infty$, which excludes them from being roots of the IFT. Path costs between two nodes $(\mathbf{p}_1, \mathbf{p}_2)$ depend on local intensity differences or on the difference of $f(\mathbf{p}_2)$ to the function value at the root to which $(\mathbf{p}_1, \mathbf{p}_2)$ is added as path.

After carrying out the IFT, pixels have been labeled according to the root label of the minimum cost path leading to the corresponding node in the graph. The segmentation depends on the homogeneity along paths from the seed pixels to all pixels of a segment and on the length of the path.

The latter is often a desired behavior in interactive segmentation, as it allows the user to place seeds of different labels close to each other at subregions that belong—according to user knowledge—to different segments, but where there is no visible difference in the appearance of the object. If the dependence on path length is unwanted, the accumulation function can be replaced by (8.18). In such a case, the method resembles fuzzy connectedness computation, as the path cost depends on the most inhomogeneous part of the most homogeneous path between two pixels.

Equation (8.18) can also be used for computing the watershed transform. For a watershed transform with markers, the above-mentioned seeds play the role of markers. The cost function is the intensity at the seeds. The IFT will find a path to the marker with lowest intensity. For a WST without markers, loads for each pixel are set to infinity so that pixels become a source of a water basin if they are local minima.

The IFT can be thought of as a generalization of the concepts that underlie the live wire and the fuzzy connectedness approaches presented earlier, as the authors have shown that many of the graph-oriented methods can be seen as special cases of the IFT. It is different from the graph cut strategy, as the assignment of seeds (whether explicitly or implicitly by being roots in the IFT forest) predetermines the topology of segments, whereas in graph cut segmentation pixels with the same label may belong to several different components. Whether graph cut or IFT is the appropriate strategy when representing a segmentation problem as path search in a graph depends on the domain knowledge about the desired kind of segmentation.

8.2.3 Random Walks

An effective and almost parameter-free variant to apply seeded segmentation on a graph are *random walks* (Grady 2006). Given seed pixels with labels $l_1, \ldots, l_K$, the algorithm computes for each unseeded pixel $\mathbf{p}$ the probability $P_k(\mathbf{p})$ that a random walk reaches the seed with label l_k first. Random walks define the desired segmentation similar to segmentation based on fuzzy connectedness or the image foresting transform (see Fig. 8.19). However, the search strategy goes from unlabeled pixels to the seeds instead of starting from the seeds. At first sight, this appears to be less efficient since the walk to the seed is governed by probabilities to walk along edges of the path between pixel and seed. Indeed, sampling random walks starting from

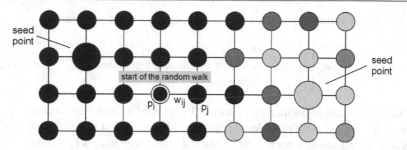

Fig. 8.19 Random walk segmentation computes for each start pixel the probability of reaching each of the seeds given the probability w_{ij} of walking from pixel $\mathbf{p}_i$ to pixel $\mathbf{p}_j$

every pixel would be unfeasible. Fortunately, the probability of reaching a seed from an unlabeled pixel can be directly computed without having to carry out the walk.

The walk is governed by probabilities to reach a pixel $\mathbf{p}_i$ from a neighboring pixel $\mathbf{p}_j$. This constitutes the data term. The probability is higher the more likely the two pixels belong to the same segment. A probability function suggested by Grady (2006) for the data term is

$$w_{ij} = \exp\left(-\beta\left(f\left(\mathbf{p}_i\right) - f\left(\mathbf{p}_j\right)\right)^2\right), \tag{8.20}$$

where f is the intensity of the pixel. The parameter β influences how quickly the probability decreases with increasing intensity differences. The function is similar to Boykov's term for interactive graph cuts (8.2), except for the fact that the spatial distance between neighbors is not accounted for.

Segmentation by random walks first computes the probabilities for each pixel and each seed. Pixels are assigned a label that corresponds to the seed in which the random walk most likely ends. It is guaranteed that all pixels of a segment with label l_k are connected to the seed pixel with label l_k.

Computing the probabilities is associated to other equilibrium problems that can be calculated directly by solving a system of linear equations, as was shown by Grady (2006). The strategy to solve the problem is similar to that used in the computation of normalized cuts by expressing the optimization task on the graph as an optimization task on matrices. However, the optimized entity is completely different. As opposed to the Normalized Graph Cut algorithm, the result is not an approximation since its domain is the solution space.

In Grady (2006) it was shown that finding the probabilities for a walk starting at some pixel to arrive at some seed pixel is related to minimizing

$$D\left(\mathbf{x}\right) = \frac{1}{2} \sum_{e_{ij} \in E} w_{ij}(x_i - x_j) = \frac{1}{2}\mathbf{x}^T \mathbf{L} \mathbf{x}, \tag{8.21}$$

where $\mathbf{L}$ is a symmetric, positive semidefinite, sparse matrix with entries

$$L_{ij} = \begin{cases} d_i, & \text{if } i = j \\ -w_{ij}, & \text{if } v_i \text{ and } v_j \text{ are adjacent nodes} \\ 0, & \text{otherwise.} \end{cases} \qquad (8.22)$$

The nodes V are regrouped into a subset V_M of marked nodes and a subset V_U of unmarked nodes. The list of nodes is reordered so that the first nodes are the marked ones and the remaining ones are the unmarked nodes. The matrix $\mathbf{L}$ is reordered accordingly consisting now of two submatrices $\mathbf{L}_M$ and $\mathbf{L}_U$, which represent edge weights among the marked and unmarked nodes, and a submatrix $\mathbf{B}$ containing weights between the marked and unmarked nodes. The equation to minimize reads now (see Grady 2006 for details):

$$\begin{aligned} D(\mathbf{x}) &= \frac{1}{2} \begin{pmatrix} \mathbf{x}_M^T & \mathbf{x}_U^T \end{pmatrix} \begin{pmatrix} \mathbf{L}_M & \mathbf{B} \\ \mathbf{B}^T & \mathbf{L}_U \end{pmatrix} \begin{pmatrix} \mathbf{x}_M \\ \mathbf{x}_U \end{pmatrix} \\ &= \frac{1}{2} (\mathbf{x}_M^T \mathbf{L}_M \mathbf{x}_M + 2\mathbf{x}_U^T \mathbf{B}^T \mathbf{x}_M + \mathbf{x}_U^T \mathbf{L}_U \mathbf{x}_U). \end{aligned} \qquad (8.23)$$

Since this needs to be minimized with respect to the unknown $\mathbf{x}_U$, the equation is differentiated with respect to $\mathbf{x}_U$, yielding

$$\partial \left[\frac{1}{2} (\mathbf{x}_M^T \mathbf{L}_M \mathbf{x}_M + 2\mathbf{x}_U^T \mathbf{B}^T \mathbf{x}_M + \mathbf{x}_U^T \mathbf{L}_U \mathbf{x}_U) \right] \Big/ \partial \mathbf{x}_U = \frac{1}{2} (2\mathbf{B}^T \mathbf{x}_M + 2\mathbf{L}_U \mathbf{x}_U). \quad (8.24)$$

This is set to zero for finding the minimum of D, which results in a system of linear equations

$$\mathbf{B}^T \mathbf{x}_M + \mathbf{L}_U \mathbf{x} = 0 \quad \Leftrightarrow \quad \mathbf{L}_U \mathbf{x} = -\mathbf{B}^T \mathbf{x}_M. \qquad (8.25)$$

For determining probabilities to reach some seed location $\mathbf{x}_s$, the potential for the marked nodes $\mathbf{x}_M$ is set to 1 for the location $\mathbf{x}_s$ and 0 for all other locations, resulting in a vector $\mathbf{m}^s$ with elements m_j^s

$$m_j^s = \begin{cases} 1, & \text{if node } j \text{ has the label } s, \\ 0, & \text{otherwise.} \end{cases} \qquad (8.26)$$

The equation system to be solved for this label is then

$$\mathbf{L}_U \mathbf{x} = -\mathbf{B}^T \mathbf{m}^s. \qquad (8.27)$$

Instead of solving for a single seed, the solution can be found for all seeds when a matrix $\mathbf{M}$ is created from all possible vectors $\mathbf{m}^s$ and a matrix $\mathbf{X}$ is created by duplicating $\mathbf{x}$ for every seed. Now, the equation system reads

$$\mathbf{L}_U \mathbf{X} = -\mathbf{B}^T \mathbf{M}. \qquad (8.28)$$

The complete algorithm then consists of the following four steps.
1. Create a graph from the image and compute the edge weights based on the image intensities.
2. Generate a list of k seed nodes (interactively or by some automatic analysis).
3. Solve the equation system for the first $k - 1$ seeds (since probabilities are computed, the probability $p(k)$ for the kth seed is $1 - \sum_{i=1...k-1} p(i)$).
4. Assign a label to each pixel that belongs to the seed that is most likely reached from this pixel.

The code for this algorithm can be obtained from the web page of the author (www.cns.bu.edu/~lgrady/random_walker.matlab_code.zip).

Random walks have been applied to medical image segmentation for brain and cardiac MRI (Grady and Funka-Lea 2004) and have been shown to have a good performance on natural images (Duchenne et al. 2008). Similar to all other methods presented in this chapter, random walks are independent of the dimension of the data. A fast GPU implementation has been presented in Grady et al. (2005).

8.3 Concluding Remarks

Mapping an image on a graph is straightforward as are the definitions of global and local criteria for a good segmentation as node costs. The methods presented in this chapter show different ways to compute an optimal segmentation based on cost functions using (sometimes adapted) standard algorithms on graphs. The beauty of using graphs as a representation lies in the independence from dimensionality and in the versatility to define different cost functions that represent different segmentation goals. The behavior of all segmentation methods presented here can be changed by parameterization. The basic algorithm always remains the same.

The selection of cost functions requires some insight into the underlying problem that is solved by the optimization procedure. A good example for this is the use of graph cuts to solve an MRF minimization problem. It shows the common features between two segmentation strategies that, at first sight, appear to be very different. However, coming up with this solution will be difficult for a domain expert (e.g., a radiologist), unless he or she also possesses expert knowledge about the underlying principles of these two approaches. Hence, the potential versatility will be of more interest to the developer, who may generate a toolbox of different segmentation methods by reusing the representational power of a graph for characterizing the various attributes of different segmentation strategies. The paper of Kolmogorov and Zabih (2004) is a helpful resource as far as graph cut segmentation is concerned as it addresses energy functions and the graphs to construct for their minimization for binary problems such as foreground segmentation.

8.4 Exercises

• What kind of information is introduced by defining source and sink nodes in graph cut segmentation? How is it introduced?

- How is the influence of noise implicitly reduced in interactive graph cut segmentation?
- Explain the strategy that is used to avoid the complete recomputation of the maximum flow when additional foreground or background nodes are specified in interactive graph cuts.
- How is an initial labeling created for graph-cut-based automatic segmentation? Why is it important that this labeling is a good approximation of the final result?
- What are the differences in using swap moves and expansion moves? Given a three-label-segmentation, which of the two moves would be faster? Explain why.
- Why is it impossible to estimate the quality of a swap move optimization with respect to the unknown optimal solution?
- What would be the characteristics of a segmentation problem where regular graph cuts would be preferred to normalized graph cuts?
- What is meant by normalization in normalized graph cuts?
- At what step and how does it become apparent that the solution for finding an optimal normalized graph cut is approximate?
- Why is fuzzy connectedness an appropriate criterion to characterize a good segmentation? How is it used for this characterization?
- What is the difference between relative and absolute fuzzy connectedness? How is this reflected in segmentation methods based on fuzzy connectedness?
- Explain how the concept of fuzzy connectedness is related to the image foresting transform.
- What are the similarities and what are the differences between image foresting transform and interactive graph cuts? Characterize a segmentation problem where the IFT would be preferred over interactive graph cuts.
- Explain how the foresting transform can be used to produce a watershed transform.
- How does a random walker differ from the image foresting transform?
- How is information about the smoothness of segment boundaries represented in a segmentation by a random walker?

References

Boykov Y, Jolly MP (2001) Interactive graph cuts for optimal boundary and region segmentation of objects in n-d images. In: 8th intl conf computer vision (ICCV'01), vol 1, pp 105–112

Boykov Y, Veksler O, Zabih R (2001) Fast approximate energy minimization via graph cuts. IEEE Trans Pattern Anal Mach Intell 23(11):1222–1239

Boykov Y, Kolmogorov V (2004) An experimental comparison of min-cut/max-flow algorithms for energy minimization in vision. IEEE Trans Pattern Anal Mach Intell 26(9):1124–1137

Duchenne O, Audibert JY, Keriven R, Ponce J, Segonne F (2008) Segmentation by transduction. In: IEEE conf computer vision and pattern recognition, CVPR2008, pp 1–8

Falcao AX, Stolfi J, de Alencar Lotufo R (2004) The image foresting transform: theory, algorithms, and applications. IEEE Trans Pattern Anal Mach Intell 26(1):19–29

Funka-Lea G, Boykov Y, Florin C, Jolly MP, Moreau-Gobard R, Ramaraj R, Rinck D (2006) Automatic heart isolation for CT coronary visualization using graph-cuts. In: 3rd IEEE intl symp biomedical imaging: nano to macro, pp 614–617

Grady L, Funka-Lea G (2004) Multi-label image segmentation for medical applications based on graph-theoretic electrical potentials. In: Computer vision and mathematical methods in medical and biomedical image analysis. LNCS, vol 3117, pp 230–245

Grady L, Schiwietz T, Aharon S, Westermann R (2005) Random walks for interactive organ segmentation in two and three dimensions: implementation and validation. In: Medical image computing and computer-assisted intervention—MICCAI 2005. LNCS, vol 3750, pp 773–780

Grady L (2006) Random walks for image segmentation. IEEE Trans Pattern Anal Mach Intell 28(11):1768–1783

Herman GT, Carvalho BM (2001) Multiseeded segmentation using fuzzy connectedness. IEEE Trans Pattern Anal Mach Intell 23(5):460–474

Kolmogorov V, Zabih R (2004) What energy functions can be minimized via graph cuts? IEEE Trans Pattern Anal Mach Intell 26(2):147–159

Ng A, Jordan M, Weiss Y (2002) On spectral clustering: analysis and an algorithm. In: Proc 14th ann conf advances in neural information processing systems, pp 849–856

Shi J, Malik J (2000) Normalized cuts and image segmentation. IEEE Trans Pattern Anal Mach Intell 22(8):888–905

Tolliver DA, Miller GL (2006) Graph partitioning by spectral rounding: applications in image segmentation and clustering. Proc - IEEE Comput Soc Conf Comput Vis Pattern Recognit 1:1053–1060

Udupa JK, Samarasekera S (1996) Fuzzy connectedness and object definition: theory, algorithms, and applications in image segmentation. Graph Models Image Process 58(3):246–261

Udupa JK, Saha PK (2003) Fuzzy connectedness and image segmentation. Proc IEEE 91(10):1649–1669

Veksler O (2008) Star shape prior for graph-cut image segmentation. In: Computer vision—ECCV 2008. LNCS, vol 5304, pp 454–467

Vicente S, Kolmogorov V, Rother C (2008) Graph cut based image segmentation with connectivity priors. In: IEEE conf comp vision and pattern recognition, CVPR 2008: 1–8.

Active Contours and Active Surfaces

9

Abstract

Active contours and active surfaces are means of model-driven segmentation. Their use enforces closed and smooth boundaries for each segmentation irrespective of the image content. They are particularly useful if such properties cannot be derived everywhere from the data.

In this chapter, we will discuss explicit and implicit active contours, their definition, parameterization, and properties. Different fitting methods for active contours will be presented in detail since their understanding is necessary to understand parameterization and stability issues.

Concepts, notions and definitions introduced in this chapter

> Explicit active contours and surfaces
> Snakes
> Intrinsic and extrinsic attributes of active contours
> Optimization of explicit active contours
> Constraints for the evolution of explicit active contours
> Implicit active contours in the level set framework
> Stationary and dynamic level sets
> Level set evolution by front propagation
> Geodesic active contours, variational level sets

The Bayesian formulation of the segmentation problem and its solution as a graph problem are examples for a data-driven segmentation. The underlying model for most of these methods is that objects in an image appear homogeneous. The use of active contours and active surfaces (i.e., active boundaries) is *model-driven*. The model predicts properties of an ideal segment, which are imposed on the data. In the case of active contours or surfaces, the attributes of the outline of an ideal object boundary are predicted. The boundary is assumed to be smooth and closed. This kind of domain knowledge allows a successful segmentation of objects even if they

K.D. Toennies, *Guide to Medical Image Analysis*,
Advances in Computer Vision and Pattern Recognition,
DOI 10.1007/978-1-4471-2751-2_9, © Springer-Verlag London Limited 2012

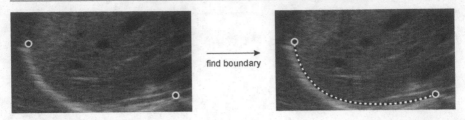

Fig. 9.1 Finding the segment boundary between the two points will be very difficult if additional information about the smoothness and closedness of the course of the boundary cannot be included in the procedure

are only partially contrasted against the background (see Fig. 9.1). Since the model does not predict the shape or appearance of an object, it may be applied to a wide variety of different objects (and not just, e.g., to livers in ultrasound images).

Using such a model of an ideal segment is best suited for foreground segmentation. It requires the representation of a deformable ideal segment that balances model attributes against data information. The importance of the model with respect to the data is usually parameterizable so that it can be set according to assumptions about the reliability of data and model. Since model-driven segmentation is a fitting process, the quality of a given estimate for the true segment boundary needs to be computable. Furthermore, a process is required to determine the best fit.

The model can either be represented explicitly or implicitly. An *explicit representation* describes the boundary as a parameterizable curve or surface in space. Locations in space that are not on the boundary are not defined by this representation. An *implicit representation* describes the boundary as a function of the space in which it is embedded. Hence, locations that are not part of the boundary are defined as well as the inner or outer points.

An explicit representation is often more intuitive than an implicit representation because the searched boundary is explicitly described. It has the disadvantage that the behavior of an evolving instance of such representation, when being fitted to the data, is difficult to control. A location to which a boundary may move is defined in terms of the representation only when the boundary is placed on this location. This is different for an implicit representation. Each location in space is part of the representation at any time. Evolving boundaries may change their topology if necessary.

In the next section, explicit representations of active contours will be discussed. They are based on the snake model presented by Kass et al. (1988). This is followed by a discussion on implicit active contours presented by Osher and Sethian (1988).

9.1 Explicit Active Contours and Surfaces

Active contours were first presented by Kass et al. (1988) who called their model a *snake*. The snake is a curve that is fitted to the data while retaining certain smoothness properties. The goal is to find a contour that separates (part of) an object from

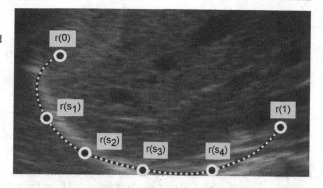

Fig. 9.2 A snake is a deformable curve $\mathbf{r}(s)$ with points $0 \leq s \leq 1$ that is placed into an image

the background. The course of the snake smoothly follows high intensity gradients if the gradients reliably reflect the object boundary. Otherwise, a smooth boundary is generated bridging regions of noisy data or missing gradients. Such an active contour is particularly well suited to segment an object instance in an image where the data are distorted by noise or artefacts.

The extent of regions with missing or distorted gradient information should be relatively small because otherwise the smooth boundary completion by the active contour may not reflect the true course of the object boundary.

9.1.1 Deriving the Model

An active contour is a deformable curve $\mathbf{r}(s)$, $0 \leq s \leq 1$ that is placed into a 2D image (see Fig. 9.2). The vector $\mathbf{r}(s)$ contains the (x, y) coordinates of points s on the curve. The model enforces smoothness by minimizing the first and second derivatives along the curve:

$$E_{\text{internal}}\big(\mathbf{r}(s)\big) = w_1 \frac{\partial \mathbf{r}(s)}{\partial s} + w_2 \frac{\partial^2 \mathbf{r}(s)}{\partial s^2} = \min, \quad w_1, w_2 > 0. \quad (9.1)$$

The term E_{internal} models the *internal energy* of a linear-elastic band. It behaves similarly to a rubber band, except in extreme situations (a rubber band close to rupture no longer stretches linearly with the exerted force).

The first derivative in E_{internal} is the *elasticity* and the second derivative is the *stiffness* of the rubber band. The weights w_1 and w_2 rate stiffness against elasticity and balance this term against an external energy E_{external} from the image. *External energy* is often related to the image gradient for causing the active contour to follow high gradients in the image. An example is

$$E_{\text{external}}\big(\mathbf{r}(s)\big) = -\big\|\nabla f\big(\mathbf{r}(s)\big)\big\| = \min, \quad (9.2)$$

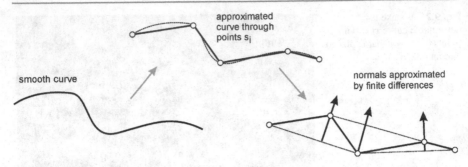

Fig. 9.3 The smooth snake curve defined everywhere on the curve is approximated by a finite sequence of curve points s_i with derivatives estimated from finite differences

where $f(\mathbf{r}(s))$ is the image intensity at position $\mathbf{r}(s)$. Finding the optimal curve now requires minimization of the two energies along s:

$$\int_0^1 E_{\text{internal}}(\mathbf{r}(s)) + E_{\text{external}}(\mathbf{r}(s)) \, ds = \min. \tag{9.3}$$

Using variational calculus (see Sect. 14.2) to find a function $\mathbf{r}(s)$ that minimizes the functional in (9.3) leads to the following Euler–Lagrange equation:

$$-w_1 \frac{1}{\partial s}\left(\frac{\partial \mathbf{r}(s)}{\partial s}\right) + w_2 \frac{1}{\partial s^2}\left(\frac{\partial^2 \mathbf{r}(s)}{\partial s^2}\right) + \nabla E_{\text{external}}(\mathbf{r}(s)) = 0. \tag{9.4}$$

The derivative of the external force (e.g., the gradient length as in (9.2)) will be zero at the maxima of E_{external}. Hence, it is an influence vector field that points to the closest feature in the data. Minimizing (9.4) simulates placing an elastic band in this vector field. The band then moves to the closest features while trying to achieve an energy-minimal state.

In the absence of an external energy, this state is either a straight line or a point to which the curve shrinks. It is a straight line when the boundary conditions of (9.4) are given by two separate end points of the curve. It shrinks to a point when the boundary conditions are given by a closed curve (i.e., a periodic function $\mathbf{r}(s)$).

In practice, the curve $\mathbf{r}(s)$ is defined only at a finite number of locations $0 \leq s_1 < s_2 < \cdots < s_n \leq 1$ (see Fig. 9.3). Derivatives through the curve are approximated by finite differences:

$$\frac{\partial \mathbf{r}(s_i)}{\partial s} \approx \frac{\mathbf{r}(s_i) - \mathbf{r}(s_{i-1})}{h}, \tag{9.5}$$

$$\frac{\partial^2 \mathbf{r}(s_i)}{\partial s^2} \approx \frac{\mathbf{r}(s_{i+1}) - 2\mathbf{r}(s_i) + \mathbf{r}(s_{i-1})}{h^2}, \quad h = \|\mathbf{r}(s_i) - \mathbf{r}(s_{i-1})\|. \tag{9.6}$$

Differentiating this according to (9.4) we arrive at the following expressions for the terms of the Euler–Lagrange equation:

$$-\left(w_1\frac{\partial \mathbf{r}(s_i)}{\partial s}\right)' \approx \frac{w_1}{h}\left((\mathbf{r}(s_i)-\mathbf{r}(s_{i-1}))-(\mathbf{r}(s_{i+1})-\mathbf{r}(s_i))\right)$$

$$= \frac{w_1}{h}\left(-\mathbf{r}(s_{i-1})+2\mathbf{r}(s_i)-\mathbf{r}(s_{i+1})\right), \qquad (9.7)$$

$$\left(\frac{\partial^2 \mathbf{r}(s_i)}{\partial s^2}\right)'' \approx \frac{w_2}{h^2}\Big[\left(\mathbf{r}(s_{i-2})-2\mathbf{r}(s_{i-1})+\mathbf{r}(s_i)\right)-2\left(\mathbf{r}(s_{i-1})-2\mathbf{r}(s_i)+\mathbf{r}(s_{i+1})\right)$$

$$+ \left(\mathbf{r}(s_i)-2\mathbf{r}(s_{i+1})+\mathbf{r}(s_{i+2})\right)\Big]. \qquad (9.8)$$

The derivative of the external energy $\nabla E = [\partial E/\partial x \ \partial E/\partial y]^{\mathrm{T}}$ is approximated by differences as well.

The results are two linear equation systems, one for each coordinate

$$\mathbf{Ax}+\frac{\partial E(s)}{\partial x}=\mathbf{0}, \quad \mathbf{x}=\left(x_1 \ \ldots \ x_N\right), \quad \frac{\partial E(s)}{\partial x}=\left(\frac{\partial E(s_1)}{\partial x} \ \ldots \ \frac{\partial E(s_N)}{\partial x}\right)$$

$$(9.9)$$

$$\mathbf{Ay}+\frac{\partial E(s)}{\partial x}=\mathbf{0}, \quad \mathbf{y}=\left(y_1 \ \ldots \ y_N\right), \quad \frac{\partial E(s)}{\partial y}=\left(\frac{\partial E(s_1)}{\partial y} \ \ldots \ \frac{\partial E(s_N)}{\partial y}\right)$$

$$(9.10)$$

where $\mathbf{0}$ is the zero vector. The matrix $\mathbf{A}$ is a band matrix. It contains the weights from (9.7) and (9.8):

$$\mathbf{A}=\begin{pmatrix} -2w_1+6w_2 & w_1-4w_2 & w_2 & \ldots & 0 \\ w_1-4w_2 & -2w_1+6w_2 & w_1-4w_2 & \ldots & \\ w_2 & w_1-4w_2 & -2w_1+6w_2 & & w_2 \\ \ldots & \ldots & \ldots & \ldots & w_1-4w_2 \\ 0 & 0 & 0 & \ldots & -2w_1+6w_2 \end{pmatrix}.$$

$$(9.11)$$

Equations (9.9) and (9.10) can be solved analytically by inverting $\mathbf{A}$. It can be done in $O(N)$ time since $\mathbf{A}$ is pentadiagonal. If weights w_1 and w_2 are kept constant, the matrix does not change and the inversion does not need to be repeated.

Given $\mathbf{A}$, an iterative scheme for the displacement of the active contour over time can be developed. If node positions $\mathbf{r}(s)$ vary with time, their location at time t is $\mathbf{r}^{(t)}(s)$ with $\mathbf{r}^{(t)}(s) = (\mathbf{x}^{(t)} \ \mathbf{y}^{(t)})$. The active contour will stop moving if a local minimum of the energy function has been found. In the local minimum, $\mathbf{x}^{(t+1)} - \mathbf{x}^{(t)} = \mathbf{0}$ and $\mathbf{y}^{(t+1)} - \mathbf{y}^{(t)} = \mathbf{0}$ must hold. This can be plugged in into (9.9) and (9.10), yielding

$$\mathbf{Ax}^{(t)}+\frac{\partial E(s^{(t)})}{\partial x}=\gamma\left(\mathbf{x}^{(t+1)}-\mathbf{x}^{(t)}\right) \qquad (9.12)$$

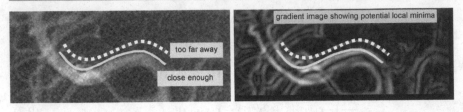

Fig. 9.4 The energy function has many local minima. Hence, the snake will find the contour only if placed close enough to the boundary

and

$$\mathbf{A}\mathbf{y}^{(t)} + \frac{\partial E(\mathbf{s}^{(t)})}{\partial y} = \gamma \left(\mathbf{y}^{(t+1)} - \mathbf{y}^{(t)}\right). \tag{9.13}$$

Resolving this for the node locations at time $t + 1$ results in the following iteration step

$$\mathbf{x}^{(t+1)} = (\mathbf{A} - \gamma \mathbf{I})^{-1} \left(\mathbf{x}^{(t)} - \frac{\partial E(\mathbf{s}^{(t)})}{\partial x}\right) \tag{9.14}$$

and

$$\mathbf{y}^{(t+1)} = (\mathbf{A} - \gamma \mathbf{I})^{-1} \left(\mathbf{y}^{(t)} - \frac{\partial E(\mathbf{s}^{(t)})}{\partial y}\right), \tag{9.15}$$

where $\mathbf{I}$ is the identity matrix and γ is a parameter that controls the step size. The matrix $(\mathbf{A} + \gamma \mathbf{I})$ is still pentadiagonal and does not change for given values of w_1, w_2, and γ. Hence, it can be inverted with an $O(N)$ computational cost and does not need to be inverted again as long as the parameters do not change.

Unfortunately, the energy function has many local minima. It is not guaranteed that the iterative procedure fits the active contour to the desired object boundary. Hence, most active contour methods require the user to place the model contour sufficiently close to the object to be segmented (see Fig. 9.4).

9.1.2 The Use of Additional Constraints

Several variants of the active contour for boundary representation in 2D and 3D exist. The *balloon model* presented as an active contour in 2D (Cohen 1991) and in 3D (Cohen and Cohen 1993) adds an additional inflating force that causes a closed active contour or surface to move away from its initial position (see Fig. 9.5). The inflation force is included as additional external force

$$\mathbf{f}_{\text{external}}\left(\mathbf{r}(s)\right) = k_1 \mathbf{n}(s) - k_2 \frac{\nabla E_{\text{external}}(\mathbf{r}(s))}{\|\nabla E_{\text{external}}(\mathbf{r}(s))\|}. \tag{9.16}$$

The vector $\mathbf{n}(s)$ is normal to the curve $\mathbf{r}(s)$ at a point s. The two external influences are weighted with respect to each other by k_1 and k_2 using application-specific weights. The inflation force causes the curve to move beyond spurious

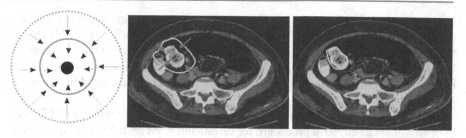

Fig. 9.5 A balloon force is an additional force for a closed active contour that drives the contour outward or inward. In this example, an inward driving force was chosen that lets the contour move towards the boundary when placed around the structure of interest

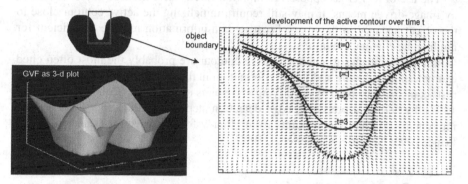

Fig. 9.6 Gradient vector flow (Xu and Prince 1998) drives a contour from everywhere in the image to the segment boundary

gradients caused by noise. Balloon forces have been used in many applications in medical image analysis (McInerney and Terzopoulos 1995a; Honea et al. 1999; Ladak et al. 2000) since their behavior is intuitive and often effective.

Another strategy to influence the behavior of an active contour is the introduction of *gradient vector flow*, as presented by Kichenassamy et al. (1995) and Xu and Prince (1998). An introduction and examples can be found at the authors' webpage at http://www.iacl.ece.jhu.edu/static/gvf/. The method is available as Matlab code.

The authors observed that displacement, as defined by the gradient of external forces, vanishes if the active contour is too far away from image features (such as high gradients). They defined a static, smooth attraction field that is defined everywhere in the image. This field is called gradient vector flow (GVF) and it replaces the gradient of external energy $\nabla E_{\text{external}}$ in (9.4).

A gradient vector field $\mathbf{v}(\mathbf{x}) = \mathbf{v}(x_1, x_2) = [u(x_1, x_2)v(x_1, x_2)]$ in a 2D image with locations $\mathbf{x} = (x_1 x_2)$ is computed by minimizing (see Fig. 9.6 for an example)

$$\varepsilon = \iint \lambda \left[\left(\frac{\partial u}{\partial x_1} \right)^2 + \left(\frac{\partial u}{\partial x_2} \right)^2 + \left(\frac{\partial v}{\partial x_1} \right)^2 + \left(\frac{\partial v}{\partial x_2} \right)^2 \right] + \|\nabla f\|^2 \|\mathbf{v} - \nabla f\|^2 \, dx_1 \, dx_2,$$

$$(9.17)$$

where f is the image function and $\nabla f(\mathbf{x})$ the desired image feature. A GVF function that minimizes ε produces values $\mathbf{v}(\mathbf{x})$ that are close to $\nabla f(\mathbf{x})$ if $\nabla f(\mathbf{x})$ is large. Otherwise, the first term of (9.17) enforces a smooth variation of $\mathbf{v}$ in space. The weight λ is application-specific. If the data contain noise, high values for λ will result in a smoothly varying gradient vector field that is not influenced by spurious gradients in the data.

The GVF needs to be computed only once. It is done by discretizing (9.17) and then arriving at an iterative procedure for estimating $\mathbf{v}$. At each location $\mathbf{x}$, the current estimate for $\mathbf{v}$ is adapted as to minimize the difference of $\mathbf{v}(\mathbf{x})$ to $\mathbf{v}(\mathbf{x}_{nb})$ in neighboring locations $\mathbf{x}_{nb}$. Simultaneously, the difference between the current estimate of $\mathbf{v}(\mathbf{x})$ to the image gradient $\nabla f(\mathbf{x})$ is minimized.[1]

The use of a GVF as opposed to inflation forces finds the true object boundary by image-driven means. It may still require initializing the active contour close to the object instance in the image because data information may be insufficient for guiding the contour evolution.

The two strategies to guide an active contour are probably the most often cited examples for including additional information in the process. Other methods are to restrict the search space by specifying end points of the curve (Cohen and Kimmel 1997), by adding a preceding edge detection step (Park and Keller 2001), or by introducing continuity constraints from already found structures (Davatzikos and Prince 1995; Neuenschwander et al. 1997).

9.1.3 T-snakes and T-surfaces

A constraint that sometimes inhibits a good segmentation is the preservation of topology. Although it is most welcome when the topology is known, it makes segmentation by active contours cumbersome when the segment consists of an unknown number of regions with smooth boundaries. In such a case, topology-adaptive snakes (*T-snakes*) presented by McInerney and Terzopoulos (1995b) and McInerney and Terzopoulos (2000) can be applied.

T-snakes receive their ability of topological adaptation by a combination of an explicit active curve representation with an implicit representation of the curve. Hence, they behave somewhat similarly to the implicit active contours to be described in the next section.

A T-snake is a closed active contour together with an implicit representation, by which space is separated into interior and exterior scene elements. The T-snake develops in a sequence of deformation steps. Within a deformation step the contour behaves like a regular snake but additionally updates the implicit representation (see Fig. 9.7). The update step between two deformation steps uses the implicit representation for splitting the enclosed regions into two or more regions or for merging regions.

---

[1]The procedure is similar to optical flow computation by simultaneous minimization of the error for the Horn–Schunck constraint and the difference between neighboring displacement vectors.

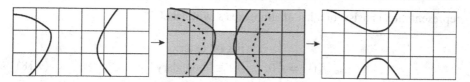

Fig. 9.7 A T-snake moves as an explicit representation but it includes an update step where an additional implicit representation is used to decide whether the explicit topology needs to be changed

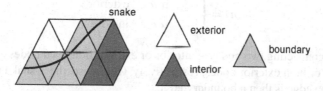

Fig. 9.8 For ease of computation the griding is a simple grid. Grid elements are either interior, exterior or boundary elements depending on the location of simplex node inside or outside of the object

The snake evolution is governed by an inflation or deflation force. During a deformation step, the contour either shrinks or grows, but may alternate between growing and shrinking from step to step.

The T-snake differs from a regular snake in the existence of the implicit representation and reparameterization after each deformation step. These two aspects are now described in more detail.

The implicit representation for a T-snake is a list of element features of a cell enumeration representation. A cell enumeration representation decomposes a finite space into a finite number of elements. Every point in space belongs to exactly one of the elements. Pixel and voxel representations are examples for 2D and 3D cell enumeration representations.

Although the T-snakes can be defined on a pixel or a voxel representation, it is easier to work with simplexes.[2] In 2D this is a representation by triangles, in 3D it is a representation by tetrahedrons (the representation is then called a *T-surface*).

To make things not overly complicated, simplex cells are usually similar to each other and arranged in a simple grid (such as the one shown in Fig. 9.8). A simplex is fully inside or outside of an active contour if all its boundary nodes are interior or exterior nodes. The active contour is passing through the simplex if some of the simplex nodes are interior and some of them are exterior. Hence, the implicit

---

[2]The advantage over using a pixel or voxel grid is that unique surface representations for a surface passing the cell exist. This is important for an active contour because it is a surface in 2D or 3D. Using a pixel or voxel grid requires an additional mechanism to resolve ambiguities, which are known, for instance, from the Marching Cube algorithm on a voxel grid.

representation consists of a list of simplexes s with labels f_s

$$f_s(s) = \begin{cases} -1 & \text{if } s \in \text{``exterior''} \\ 0 & \text{if } s \in \text{``boundary''} \\ 1 & \text{if } s \in \text{``interior''.} \end{cases} \tag{9.18}$$

A similar function exists for all nodes n of the simplex

$$f_n(n) = \begin{cases} -1 & \text{if } n \in \text{``exterior''} \\ 1 & \text{if } n \in \text{``interior''.} \end{cases} \tag{9.19}$$

An edge connecting two nodes is interior or exterior if the two nodes are both interior nodes or both exterior nodes, respectively. Otherwise, the T-snake must cross the edge: The edge is then a boundary edge.

The T-snake is initially defined by a vertex sequence with all vertices lying on the boundary edges. The evolution of the T-snake will cause snake vertices no longer to lie on boundary nodes. Hence, the intersection points of the evolved T-snake with grid edges are computed during reparameterization and denoted potential snake vertices. Given the T-snake, nodes of the cell representation are tested as to whether their label (interior or exterior) should change.

The update may be ambiguous if a T-snake intersects itself or is intersected by other T-snakes. In such a case, a cell node may be exterior with respect to one part of the T-snake and interior with respect to another part. The ambiguity is resolved by assuming that a T-snake either shrinks or grows. If it grows, then a node once being interior can never be declared exterior. The opposite is true for a shrinking T-snake.

After updating cell nodes, labels of cells and cell edges are updated accordingly.

In the next step it is tested whether all vertices of the updated T-snake are still on boundary edges. If a part of the T-snake intersects interior edges because the T-snake intersected itself or touched other T-snakes, the respective vertices are removed and the T-snakes are merged. A T-snake vertex may also lie on an exterior edge. In this case, the vertices are removed resulting in two separate T-snakes.

If T-snakes are extended to T-surfaces on a 3D grid, the algorithm does not change except for the fact that the grid now consists of nodes, edges, faces, and cells and the computation time increases with the amount of data.

9.2   The Level Set Model

T-snakes already show the advantage of an implicit boundary representation. However, T-snakes use different representations for different tasks. The implicit representation of a T-snake consists of an enumeration of function values in discrete space. Derivatives, curvatures, and other smoothness properties cannot be represented in this space. It requires changing between a discrete, implicit representation

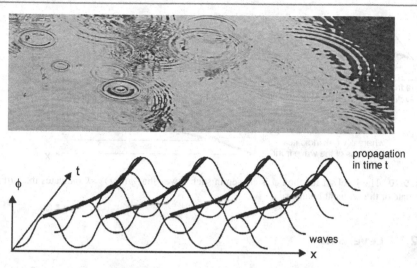

Fig. 9.9 The level set model can be thought of a function representing waves moving over time. A specific wave front represents the current estimate of the segment boundary

and a continuous, explicit representation during the evolution of the active contour.

The *level set model* integrates smoothness properties, correspondence to the data, and evolution of a representation of interior and exterior points in a common, continuous implicit representation (Sethian 1998; Osher and Paragios 2003). The level set model is an implicit function of image space $\mathbf{x} = (x_1, x_2, \ldots, x_N)$. Every location in space can be uniquely assigned a label "interior," "exterior," or "boundary." Self-intersections, which may happen in an explicit representation, are impossible. Topological changes during the adaptation of a level set representation to the data may happen. The goal of a level set representation in segmentation is to define a continuous, smooth representation of a segment boundary and let it evolve so that it adapts to boundary locations in the image in some optimal fashion. Just what is optimal is defined similarly to the criteria used for explicit active contours and surfaces.

The level set function can be thought of as a wave (see Fig. 9.9). Wave propagation guides a specific wave front to the segment boundary. To represent this propagation in time, the level set model embeds an implicit N-dimensional active contour in $(N + 1)$-dimensional space. The first N dimensions represent locations $\mathbf{x} = (x_1, x_2, \ldots, x_N)$ in the image. The additional dimension is the time t.

An initial level set function $\phi(\mathbf{x}, t_0)$ at time t_0 is given by the user. Its level $\phi(\mathbf{x}, t_0) = k(t_0)$ describes the initial guess of the segment boundary. It usually does not coincide with the true object boundary. The level set function is then evolved toward the object while maintaining the smoothness of the wave front.

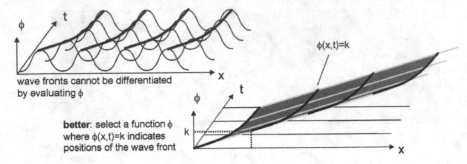

Fig. 9.10 The level set function ϕ is chosen in such a way that $\phi(\mathbf{x}, t) = k$ indicates the current estimate of the segment boundary

9.2.1 Level Sets

Wave propagation in the level set framework does not rely on the specific shape of a wave. Hence, a wave function ϕ is selected so that the position of a wave front is given by all points having a specific value (see Fig. 9.10). A k-level set of a function $\phi(\mathbf{x})$ consists of all points $\mathbf{x}$ for which $\phi(\mathbf{x}) = k$. For differentiable functions ϕ, which are defined on a real number domain, the level set consists of closed boundaries separating $\phi(\mathbf{x}) > k$ from $\phi(\mathbf{x}) < k$.

A level set is said to be the *interface* between two sets of points. If used to represent a segmentation, discretized values of $\mathbf{x}$ denote coordinates of scene elements (e.g., pixels, voxels) and $\phi(\mathbf{x}) = k$ is the segment boundary. Since the level k is arbitrary, it is usually the 0-level set that is evolved.

The level set method evolves the interface based on its intrinsic properties, extrinsic image properties, and domain knowledge. An intrinsic property could, for instance, enforce a smooth segment boundary. Extrinsic properties (e.g., related to the intensity gradient) cause the 0-level set to terminate on segment boundaries. An example for domain knowledge is the placement of the initial level set.

Level sets are in many respects similar to the snakes introduced in the previous section. Hence, the terms active contour and active surface apply to level sets as well. A number of differences should be noted, however.

- Snakes represent curves explicitly. Changing the topology during snake evolution is impossible unless the representation is transferred to an implicit representation (such as in T-snakes). The level set definition is an implicit representation by some function $\phi(\mathbf{x})$ without having this restriction (see Fig. 9.11).
- Snake-like representations can be defined for arbitrary dimensions only if the explicit representation is adapted accordingly (and possibly also the optimization scheme). The level set formulation is independent of the dimension.
- Snakes are discretized in terms of the explicit representation which may require reparameterization if adjacent nodes become too far apart in image space. This is not necessary for level sets, as they are defined—and will be evolved—in continuous space.

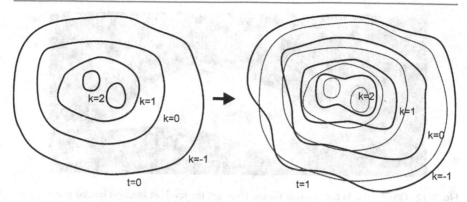

Fig. 9.11 Level sets are implicitly defined on f. Hence, topology of the explicit boundary may change (in the example above, this happens for $\phi(\mathbf{x}, t) = 2$)

These are good reasons to consider an implicit active contour for segmentation. It does not mean, however, that explicit active contours should be disregarded in any case. If, for instance, the topology of a segmentation is known, this is already represented in an explicit formulation.

The great advantage of the level set representation is its generality. It enables solutions for many different applications under the same concept.

Before applying level sets to segmentation, several questions need to be answered.

- What is an appropriate function ϕ for representing the interface?
- How can interface motion be represented in a parameterizable fashion so that different evolving interfaces can be generated by changing parameters?
- Which parameters are useful to let the interface evolve toward the segment boundaries?

The level set function and the evolution methods will be discussed in the next section. This is then followed by a treatment of techniques to speed up the computation. Finally, we will explain strategies to parameterize the level set method.

9.2.2 Level Sets and Wave Propagation

The evolution of a level set is the propagation of a wave ϕ. The current estimate of segment boundaries at some time t consists of all locations $\mathbf{x}$ for which $\phi(\mathbf{x}, t) = 0$. The wave ϕ can be defined as the level set function:

$$\phi(\mathbf{x}, t) = \begin{cases} d(\mathbf{x}, C(t)), & \text{if } \mathbf{x} \text{ is inside the segment,} \\ -d(\mathbf{x}, C(t)), & \text{otherwise.} \end{cases} \tag{9.20}$$

The function $C(t)$ is the set of points in the 0-level set at time t, and $d(\mathbf{x}, C(t))$ is the shortest distance of $\mathbf{x}$ to this curve. In other words, the level set function is a signed distance function (see Fig. 9.12).

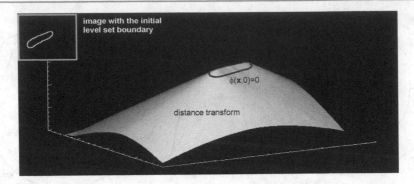

Fig. 9.12 Given some initial position for the level set, the level set function can be generated as distance transform for the distance from this initial boundary

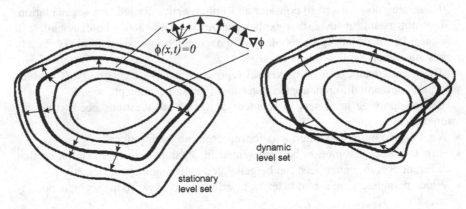

Fig. 9.13 Level sets propagate orthogonal to the wave front. Stationary level sets either move outward or inward. Dynamic level sets may change the propagation direction

The wave is propagated orthogonal to the wave front. Domain knowledge about expected segment properties and a data term influence the propagation speed at each point. Ideally, the interface stops (at least it slows down) at the segment boundary. Interface motion can be of two kinds (see Fig. 9.13).

- A *stationary level set* is a function of arrival times for a level set for each location **x**. Being a function, a point **x** in image space never gets reached twice. Hence, the interface is either moving to the inside or the outside starting from the initial level set. A segmentation is then a set of points which are reached at the same time.
- A *dynamic level set* defines the level set as function of **x** and time t. The interface may change direction during its evolution and may cross a point **x** several times. A segmentation is the location of the interface at some point in time.

Fig. 9.14 Level set evolution of a dynamic level set over time

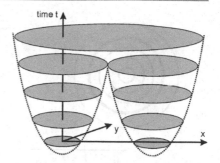

Computing the propagation of stationary level sets is simple. Given a speed F the arrival time $T(\mathbf{x})$ at some location $\mathbf{x}$ uses the fact that traveled distance dx during time interval dT equals speed multiplied by dT. In one dimension this gives

$$F \cdot dT = dx \quad \Leftrightarrow \quad F \cdot \frac{dT}{dx} = 1, \tag{9.21}$$

and for spaces of arbitrary dimensions it is

$$F \cdot |\nabla T| = 1, \quad \text{with } T = 0 \text{ on the initial segment boundary } \Gamma. \tag{9.22}$$

The gradient ∇T is inverse to the velocity vector. Computing the level set evolution requires finding arrival times T for every scene element such that the condition in (9.21) is fulfilled. The speed F is a function of locations $\mathbf{x}$. $F(\mathbf{x})$ will be based on internal and external properties. Internal properties guarantee, for instance, the smoothness of the interface. External properties cause the interface to slow down at potential segment boundaries. Examples for different speed functions will be given in Sect. 9.2.6. If the speed function is defined properly, the segment boundary is found if progression per time interval falls below some threshold.

However, using stationary level sets for segmentation severely restricts their applicability. They behave similarly to region growing. Dynamic level sets are required if the active contours should be able to reverse the propagation direction when, for instance, stretching modeled by internal energies causes a currently expanding front to shrink.

The wave front of a dynamic level set is represented by embedding the level set function for an N-dimensional image into an $(N + 1)$-dimensional space, with time being the additional dimension. The 0-level set $\phi(\mathbf{x}, t) = 0$ represents the current segment boundary at time t. Level set evolution traces changes $d\phi/dt$ of ϕ over time (see Fig. 9.14).

The equation governing dynamic level set evolution bears some similarity to (9.21) for stationary level sets. It is

$$\phi_t = -F |\nabla \phi|, \tag{9.23}$$

where ϕ_t is the derivative of ϕ at any point $\mathbf{x}$ over time.

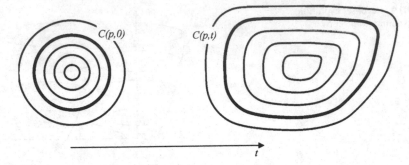

Fig. 9.15 Definitions for the level set curve C and its evolution over time

The evolution of an initial level set function ϕ consists of repeatedly solving an initial value problem using the current level set function $\phi(\mathbf{x}, t)$ as initial value and solving for $\phi(\mathbf{x}, t + \Delta t)$ using the derivative in (9.23). It requires some care in the selection of appropriate differences to approximate the differential and in the selection of the step size. This will be detailed in the next section. First, however, we will need to derive (9.23) to understand the meaning of its components.

For arriving at (9.23), an abstract formulation of all points on the level set is defined, plugged into the level set term, and then differentiated with respect to time t (see Fig. 9.15):

- The level set function at time t is $\phi(\mathbf{x}, t)$;
- The set of points $\mathbf{p}$ on the level set interface C at time $t = 0$ is $C(\mathbf{p}, 0) = \{\mathbf{x}|\phi(x, 0) = 0\}$;
- The set of points $\mathbf{p}$ on the level set interface C at time t is $C(\mathbf{p}, t) = \{\mathbf{x}| \phi(\mathbf{x}, t) = t\}$;
- All points on the interface at time t are $C(t) = \phi^{-1}(t)$.

The definitions are used to differentiate the level set equation $\phi(\mathbf{x}, t) = 0 \Leftrightarrow \phi(C(t), t) = 0$:

$$\frac{d\phi(C(t), t)}{dt} = 0. \tag{9.24}$$

Applying the chain rule[3] results in

$$\frac{\partial \phi(C(t), t)}{\partial t} = \frac{\partial \phi(C(t), t)}{\partial C(t)} \frac{\partial C(t)}{\partial t} + \frac{\partial \phi(\mathbf{x}, t)}{\partial t}. \tag{9.25}$$

The different terms on the left-hand side describe the propagation of the interface. Since $C(t)$ are the points on the interface at time t, the expression $\partial \phi(C(t), t)/\partial C(t)$ is the partial derivative of the level set function with respect to

---

[3]The chain rule for a function g of several functions $f_1, f_2, \ldots, f_n$ is

$$\frac{d[g(f_1(t), f_2(t), \ldots, f_n(t))]}{dt} = \frac{dg}{df_1}\frac{df_1}{dt} + \frac{dg}{df_2}\frac{df_2}{dt} + \cdots + \frac{dg}{df_n}\frac{df_n}{dt}.$$

the interface. This is just the gradient of the level set function. It is abbreviated by

$$\nabla\phi(\mathbf{x}, t) = \frac{\partial\phi(C(t), t)}{\partial C(t)}. \tag{9.26}$$

The reference to the domain is often omitted. The term is referred to as $\nabla\phi$.

The term $\partial C(t)/\partial t$ is the derivative of the interface with respect to time. It describes the (intended) propagation speed of the evolving interface. This term will be the container of curve- and image-dependent information that governs interface evolution.

Finally, the term $\partial\phi(\mathbf{x}, t)/\partial t$ describes the change of the level set function over time. Since this entity needs to be computed to evolve the level set, the equation is rearranged accordingly. With setting $\phi_t = \partial\phi(\mathbf{x}, t)/\partial t$ (again omitting the domain variable), the evolution equation is compactly written as

$$\phi_t = -\nabla\phi \frac{\partial C(t)}{\partial t}. \tag{9.27}$$

Level set evolution is orthogonal to the interface. With unit vector $\nabla\phi/|\nabla\phi|$, which is orthogonal to C, the speed F of the curve evolution $\partial C(t)/\partial t$ in this direction is

$$F = \frac{\partial C(t)}{\partial t} \frac{\nabla\phi}{|\nabla\phi|} \quad \Leftrightarrow \quad \frac{\partial C(t)}{\partial t} = F \frac{|\nabla\phi|}{\nabla\phi}. \tag{9.28}$$

Hence, speed F can be included in (9.27) arriving at the formulation $\phi_t = -F|\nabla\phi|$ of (9.23).

Given an appropriate speed function F, (9.23) is the base for computing a level set segmentation. Internal and external properties will be defined for F so that the interface slows down at the segment boundaries. The decrease in speed can be used for terminating the evolution.

The formulation of the level set evolution in (9.21) and (9.23) is attractive because it separates considerations for stable computation (how to set Δt for approximating the update of the level set function, how to approximate $\nabla\phi$) from definitions of segmentation constraints in F. Hence, given an appropriate implementation of the approximation scheme, a user can change segmentation characteristics without having to worry about stability issues. It is worthwhile to understand the approximation nonetheless since the selection of a speed function F may influence the speed of interface progression.

9.2.3 Schemes for Computing Level Set Evolution

Level set evolution can be computed explicitly or implicitly. Although implicit computation is by far the most often applied solution, we will begin with a short characterization of an explicit level set evolution. It is very similar to the evolution of explicit active contours and shares its advantages and disadvantages. The method is called a *Lagrangian solution* or *marker particle solution*. The latter describes the

Fig. 9.16 In the marker particle solution, markers on the 0-level set are tracked over time

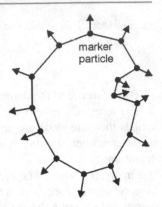

approach pretty well (see Fig. 9.16). The current location of the interface is discretized by uniform sampling. Each sample point is a marker particle that is tracked over time. Since evolution is orthogonal to the interface, normals are estimated and evolved according to the speed function. The solution is easy to implement but has some problems.

- Changes of topology are difficult to deal with. The Lagrangian solution defines topology explicitly by initial adjacencies between marker particles. An extra rule is needed that produces a change of topology.
- Particle tracking requires regular resampling since the evolution of the interface will change the density of the distribution of marker particles along the level set.

Hence, the marker particle solution is only appropriate when the initial level set placement is already close to the expected final result, so that neither of the two problems arises.

The implicit solution (called the *Eulerian solution*) computes the value of the level set function ϕ at each point in time at each location $\mathbf{x}$ in the scene. Hence, the level set function is represented instead of the interface. Sampling depends on image resolution and not on marker locations on the interface. The topology of the interface is a result of evaluating $\phi(\mathbf{x}, t) = 0$.

A detailed derivation of the Eulerian solution is given in Sethian (1998). We will highlight aspects that relate to the robustness of the evolution process.

Given the level set equation $\phi_t = -F|\nabla\phi|$, the evolution process for $\phi(t)$ is

$$\phi(t + \Delta t) = \phi(t) + \Delta t \cdot \phi_t = \phi(t) - \Delta t \cdot F|\nabla\phi|. \tag{9.29}$$

An appropriate step size for the time step Δt needs to be found and an appropriate approximation for the gradient $\nabla\phi$ has to be computed. It will turn out that the gradient approximation depends on the local propagation of the interface resulting in a so-called *upwind scheme*. The step size will depend on the fastest propagation speed in the domain.

To illustrate this, we will follow the explanation in Sethian (1998) and discuss the solution in a 1D domain. We will begin with a simple 1D wave $u(x, t)$ that travels with constant unity speed in direction of the positive x-axis (see Fig. 9.17). Given

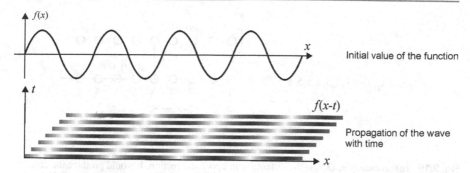

Fig. 9.17 Example of a simple wave $f(x)$ propagating with constant speed *from left to right*

Fig. 9.18 For computing the level set propagation, differentials need to be approximated by differences in x- and t-direction

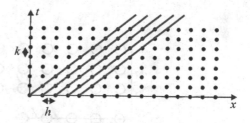

an initialization $u(x, 0) = f(x)$, the solution for this propagation is

$$u(x, t) = f(x - t) \qquad (9.30)$$

and the representation by a differential equation is

$$u_x = -u_t \quad \Leftrightarrow \quad u_x + u_t = 0, \qquad (9.31)$$

where the subscripts denote differentiation with respect to x and t, respectively.

If $u(x, 0) = f(x)$ is the initial placement of a level set, the speed function for this process would be $F = 1$. For computing the evolution, the two differentials have to be approximated (see Fig. 9.18). There is one possible solution for u_t:

$$u_t \approx D^{+t}u \equiv u_t(x, t) = \frac{u(x, t + k) - u(x, t)}{k}, \qquad (9.32)$$

where k is the step size along the time axis.

Since the function is evolved along t, the approximation of the differential in x can be in arbitrary direction, resulting in the following three possible solutions:

$$u_x \approx D^{+x}u \equiv u_x(x, t) = \frac{u(x + h, t) - u(x, t)}{h}, \qquad (9.33)$$

$$u_x \approx D^{-x}u \equiv u_x(x, t) = \frac{u(x, t) - u(x - h, t)}{h}, \qquad (9.34)$$

$$u_x \approx D^{0x}u \equiv u_x(x, t) = \frac{u(x + h, t) - u(x - h, t)}{2h}, \qquad (9.35)$$

where h is the step size along the x axis.

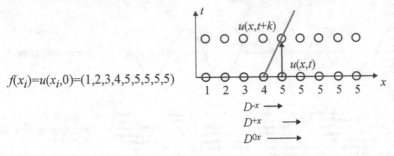

$$f(x_i)=u(x_i,0)=(1,2,3,4,5,5,5,5,5)$$

Fig. 9.19 In this example, D^{-x} is the difference in upwind direction. It would produce the correct estimate $u(5, t+k) = 4$. Choosing D^{+x} would produce $u(5, t+k) = 5$ and choosing D^{0x} would result in $u(5, t+k) = 4.5$

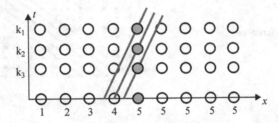

Fig. 9.20 The step size for the time steps has to be chosen so that estimates of derivatives in upwind direction result in an interpolation. In the example, step k_1 would be unstable, while k_2 and k_3 would result in a stable estimate

It depends on the wave propagation which of the three differences should be taken. The wave in this example does not change its shape. Hence, the differential at time t travels along the propagation direction to another position at time $t + k$. Estimating the differential by a difference should therefore interpolate at time t over an interval that contains the location of the differential $u_x(x, t + k)$. D^{+x} must be chosen, if the wave propagates from right to left, and D^{-x} otherwise (see Fig. 9.19 for an example).

If the waves were real ocean waves, this direction would be against the direction of the wind that drives the waves. Hence, it is called an *upwind scheme*. Taking the downwind difference instead would always extrapolate the differential, which would make the solution unstable.

Choosing the upwind scheme does not automatically guarantee that the approximation is always interpolating. Extrapolation is avoided only if a step size k is chosen such that the wave propagation does not exceed the propagation h of the wave everywhere on the line x (see Fig. 9.20).

In the example of (9.31), the direction toward the origin is upwind since the wave moves to the right. Thus, D^{-x} is the difference to select. Since the wave is moving with constant speed everywhere, the appropriate step size must ensure that $k \leq h$.

Fig. 9.21 If the direction of propagation depends on location, the upwind direction has to be selected accordingly

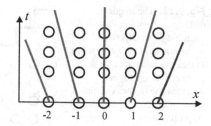

The evolution of the wave $u_x + u_t = 0$ is then approximated by

$$\frac{u(x, t+k) - u(x, t)}{k} + \frac{u(x, t) - u(x-h, t)}{h} = 0, \qquad (9.36)$$

leading to the following iteration step

$$u(x, t+k) = u(x, t) - kD^{-x}u(x, t) = u(x, t) - \frac{k}{h}[u(x, t) - u(x-h, t)]. \quad (9.37)$$

There is not much change if propagation is a function of x or $u(x)$ that may be positive at some locations x and negative at others (see Fig. 9.21). For an arbitrary propagation $a(x)$, selecting a switch function

$$\nabla u = \max(0, a(x))D^{-x}u - \min(0, a(x))D^{+x}u \qquad (9.38)$$

always chooses the upwind direction.

9.2.4 Computing Stationary Level Set Evolution

Stationary level set evolution uses the upwind scheme for stable estimates of arrival times. It will be explained for 2D level sets but easily extends to 3D. Arrival times $T(x, y)$ need to be computed at every location (x, y) given an initial level set based on (9.21). Resolving (9.21) with respect to arrival times results in

$$|\nabla T(x, y)| = \frac{1}{F(x, y)} \quad \Rightarrow \quad \sqrt{(\nabla T(x, y))^2} = \frac{1}{F(x, y)} \qquad (9.39)$$

for a given speed function F. The approximation $|\nabla T|$ by upwind differences is then

$$[\max(D^{-x}T(x, y), 0)^2 + \min(D^{+x}T(x, y), 0)^2 + \max(D^{-y}T(x, y), 0)^2$$

$$+ \min(D^{+y}T(x, y), 0)^2]^{\frac{1}{2}} = \frac{1}{F(x, y)}. \qquad (9.40)$$

This is a set of nonlinear equations where $T(x, y)$ are the unknowns. It is solved by the following iterative algorithm.

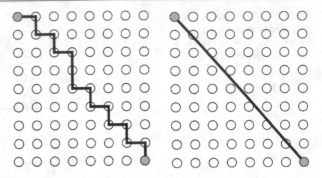

Fig. 9.22 The major difference between Fast Marching and Dijkstra's minimum cost path algorithm is that the latter always proceeds along edges, whereas the former estimates costs in the correct direction of propagation

- Initialize T with $T(x, y) = 0$ for all locations on the initial boundary Γ and $T(x, y) = \infty$ for all other locations.
- Correct all equations of the equation system iteratively.
- Terminate the process when the change of all T's falls below some threshold.

The method requires several runs since the equations are dependent on each other via the difference operators D (hence, correcting one equation will change T-values in other equations).

Computing arrival times in this fashion is stable but very slow. In the first runs, only pixels in the immediate vicinity of the boundary Γ will converge quickly to their true values. Far away pixels correct T-values based on equally wrong T-values in their vicinity.

It is more efficient to restrict updates to those pixels that are neighbored by pixels of which the correct arrival time is known. This is done by the *fast marching method* of Sethian (1996). The initial level set Γ can be an infinitesimal circle indicating the location of the structure to be segmented or it may already roughly approximate the true object boundary.

Since the level set function is stationary, the speed can be computed in advance for each location $\mathbf{x}$. The shortest arrival times are then computed by turning the problem into a shortest path computation. Local costs at a location $\mathbf{x}$ depend on the speed with which the moving front passes $\mathbf{x}$.

This is similar to Dijkstra's minimum cost path algorithm used (e.g., for the image foresting transform). However, Dijkstra's algorithm computes the shortest connections along edges between two locations $\mathbf{x}_1$ and $\mathbf{x}_2$. This is not necessarily the shortest connection in the underlying continuous Euclidean space of the level set function (see Fig. 9.22). Thus, the fast marching algorithm computes arrival times by propagating the front in Euclidean space.

The fast marching algorithm for computing arrival times from a set of start pixels $\mathbf{X}_0 = \{\mathbf{x}_{0,i}\}$ keeps (see Fig. 9.23)

- a list of *known* nodes for which arrival times have already been computed and which are completely surrounded by other known nodes,
- a list of *far* nodes to which arrival times have not yet been computed,
- a list of *trial* nodes to which arrival times have been computed and which are adjacent to at least one far node.

Fig. 9.23 The Fast Marching Method proceeds by extending the wave front from nodes with known arrival times into trial nodes that are adjacent to known nodes

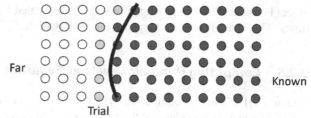

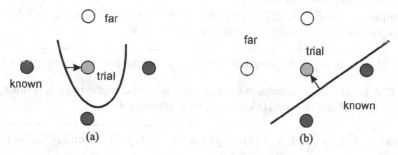

Fig. 9.24 The two different cases for computing arrival time: (**a**) the two closest nodes are opposite from each other. (**b**) The two closest nodes are at a 90° angle

Initially, all nodes except those in X_0 are far nodes. The nodes in X_0 are known nodes if they are completely surrounded by other nodes in X_0. Otherwise, they are trial nodes. The algorithm iteratively selects the a trial node x_{min} with the shortest arrival time, removes it from the trial set, puts it into the known-node set, and computes the propagation into the adjacent nodes of x_{min}.

Computing arrival times for a node x neighboring x_{min} requires the estimation of the front passing known nodes in the vicinity of x_{min}. Two cases have to be differentiated (see Fig. 9.24).

1. The two nodes x_{n1} and x_{n2} with the lowest arrival time $u(x_{n1})$ and $u(x_{n2})$ of all four neighbors of x are opposite to each other. In this case, the front is moving from $x_{closest} = \mathrm{argmin}(u(x_{n1}), u(x_{n2}))$. The arrival time at x is $u(x) = u(x_{closest}) + c(x)$.

2. The two nodes x_{n1} and x_{n2} are at a 90° angle with respect to x. The front has passed through these nodes. The propagation direction is computed under the assumptions that
   - the front moves orthogonal to its boundary,
   - that this boundary can be approximated by a straight line between x_{n1} and x_{n2}, and
   - that the speed does not accelerate between x_{min} and x.

Iterative propagation is stopped when the current level set best approximates the object boundary. The stopping criterion depends on the evolution of the front. Since local propagation speed (the speed term) is usually defined in a way so that the speed is low when the gradient is high, the front should move slowly when reaching the object boundary. A slow propagation speed is indicated by a fast increase of arrival times. This is a criterion for stopping the propagation.

9.2.5 Computing Dynamic Level Set Evolution

The upwind scheme for computing dynamic level set evolution represented by $\phi_t = -F|\nabla\phi|$ needs to consider that the sign of ϕ is unknown. Hence, the switch has to be applied first to select the correct upwind direction depending on the sign of ϕ. For the simple case of $F = 1$, (9.23) simplifies to $\phi_t + |\nabla\phi| = 0 \Rightarrow \phi_t + \sqrt{(\nabla\phi)^2} = 0$ resulting in the following iteration step for a 1D level set

$$\phi^{t+1}(x) = \phi^t(x) + \Delta t\sqrt{\max\left(D^{-x}\phi^t(x),0\right)^2 + \min\left(D^{+x}\phi^t(x),0\right)^2}. \quad (9.41)$$

If $F \neq 1$ and its sign is unknown, the switch has to be applied again, resulting in the final upwind scheme for 1D level sets with arbitrary F

$$\phi^{t+1}(x) = \phi^t(x) + \Delta t\Big[\max\left(F(x),0\right)\sqrt{\max\left(D^{-x}\phi^t(x),0\right)^2 + \min\left(D^{+x}\phi^t(x),0\right)^2}$$

$$+ \min\left(F(x),0\right)\sqrt{\max\left(D^{+x}\phi^t(x),0\right)^2 + \min\left(D^{-x}\phi^t(x),0\right)^2}\Big]. \quad (9.42)$$

Changing the dimension does not change much in this scheme, except that the upwind direction has to be selected based on the gradient direction $\nabla\phi$ in multi-dimensional space. For a 3D space, for instance, the upwind scheme is

$$\phi^{t+1}(x,y,z) = \phi^t(x,y,z) + \Delta t\Big[\max\left(F(x,y,z),0\right)\sqrt{\nabla^+}$$

$$+ \min\left(F(x,y,z),0\right)\sqrt{\nabla^-}\Big] \quad (9.43)$$

with

$$\nabla^+ = \Big[\max\left(D^{-x}\phi^t(x,y,z),0\right)^2 + \min\left(D^{+x}\phi^t(x,y,z),0\right)^2$$

$$+ \max\left(D^{-y}\phi^t(x,y,z),0\right)^2 + \min\left(D^{+y}\phi^t(x,y,z),0\right)^2$$

$$+ \max\left(D^{-z}\phi^t(x,y,z),0\right)^2 + \min\left(D^{+z}\phi^t(x,y,z),0\right)^2\Big] \quad (9.44)$$

and

$$\nabla^- = \Big[\max\left(D^{+x}\phi^t(x,y,z),0\right)^2 + \min\left(D^{-x}\phi^t(x,y,z),0\right)^2$$

$$+ \max\left(D^{+y}\phi^t(x,y,z),0\right)^2 + \min\left(D^{-y}\phi^t(x,y,z),0\right)^2$$

$$+ \max\left(D^{+z}\phi^t(x,y,z),0\right)^2 + \min\left(D^{-z}\phi^t(x,y,z),0\right)^2\Big]. \quad (9.45)$$

Given appropriate time differences Δt, this scheme can be repeatedly applied to update the level set function. However, the computation would be very slow since the equation has to be evaluated for every time step and every location. Furthermore, since the step size is restricted by the fastest progress anywhere in the scene,

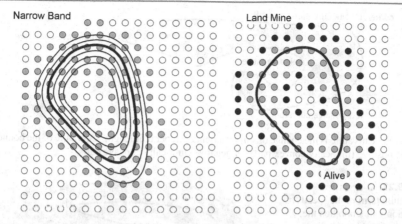

Fig. 9.25 The narrow band method computes the level set function only in a narrow band around the 0-level set. The boundary locations of the narrow band are labeled "land mines." Hitting a land mine with the 0-level set requires re-computing the level set function in the narrow band around the current 0-level set

progress can be slow when the interface slowly reaches the segment boundary but ϕ is changing very fast somewhere else in the image.

The *narrow band method* (Adalsteinsson and Sethian 1995) makes use of the fact that the state of ϕ is only of interest close to the 0-level set. The time-consuming computation of the level set everywhere is replaced by a method where ϕ is computed only for positions $\mathbf{x}$ that are close to the current level set (i.e., where $\phi(\mathbf{x}, t) = 0$, see Fig. 9.25). The computation is still slower than fast marching because ϕ has to be updated in a band $|\phi(\mathbf{x}, t_0)| < k_{max}$ around the initial level set $\phi(\mathbf{x}, t_0) = 0$ instead of just propagating a front $\phi(\mathbf{x})$. It surpasses fast marching capabilities in that it computes a dynamic level set in the band, hence enabling a front that shrinks and grows according to the data information as long as the level set $\phi(\mathbf{x}, t) = 0$ does not exceed the initial band $|\phi(\mathbf{x}, t_0)| < k_{max}$.

Pixel sites in the narrow band are labeled *alive* since their correct level set value is known and can be used for level set propagation. Sites at the border of the narrow band are called *land mines*. If the level set hits a land mine at some time t_e, the level set function $\phi(\mathbf{x}, t_e) = k(t_e)$ has to be computed for all values $k(t_e)$ since the function ϕ has not been evolved outside the band and derivatives there are not valid. The time t_e is constant for $\phi(\mathbf{x}, t_e) = k(t_e)$ and may be rewritten as $\phi_{te}(\mathbf{x}) = k_{te}$. Since $\phi_{te}(\mathbf{x})$ does not depend on t, it can be computed using the fast marching method. Then, a new band $|\phi(\mathbf{x}, t_e)| < k(t_e)$ is defined and the algorithm proceeds.

9.2.6   Segmentation and Speed Functions

The initial placement of the level set at time t_0 introduces position information into the segmentation. A boundary described by a level set is placed somewhere close to an object in an image. The object may consist of several segments. If forces

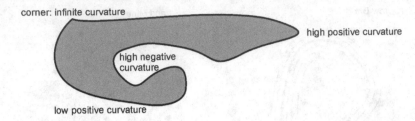

Fig. 9.26 Curvature is the change of surface orientation per unit length. Curvature of the boundary can be positive (in locally convex parts) or negative (in locally concave parts)

Fig. 9.27 A negative curvature term in the speed function will smoothen the boundary and keep it from developing sharp corners

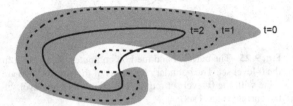

attract the level set towards an object boundary and pushes it away from interior or exterior points (e.g., by using intensity gradient information), the level set will evolve into several closed boundaries following the gradients in the vicinity of the initial placement. Using the curvature term lets the level set disregard small regions with high gradients caused by noise.

The level set approach can also be used for a nonlocalized search. The initial level set (possibly representing boundaries of several disconnected objects) is then placed in such a way that it encloses the whole image. The level set will still evolve in a set of smooth boundaries close to high gradient regions.

The *speed function* is the only parameterizable entity, which influences the result of a level set segmentation. It encodes interface properties and data-driven properties. A simple speed function is

$$F = F_{\text{img}}(v - \varepsilon \kappa). \tag{9.46}$$

The term v is an advection force. It drives the interface either to the outside (positive advection, $v > 0$) or to the inside (negative advection, $v < 0$). It is a necessary component if segmentation shall be started from some seed element, which is so far away from the segment that the data term cannot guide the evolution of the interface.

The second term relates level set evolution to curvature κ weighted by ε (see Fig. 9.26). It keeps the interface from developing local high curvature details if the curvature term increases with negative curvature. High curvature details may eventually develop into sharp corners (see Fig. 9.27). Since this is unwanted in most applications in the medical field (there are few structures in the human body with sharp corners), the curvature term is used almost always in this fashion.

Curvature in 2D is the second derivative of the curve. The solution is more difficult in higher dimensions since infinitely many curves pass a point on a surface. An average curvature for interfaces in arbitrary dimensions can be defined using the

Fig. 9.28 Divergence characterizes the flow of a vector field

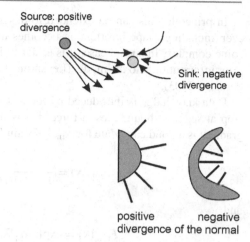

Source: positive divergence

Sink: negative divergence

Fig. 9.29 The divergence of the normal of the 0-level set is the curvature of this level set

positive   negative
divergence of the normal

divergence of surface normals. The divergence $\nabla \bullet \mathbf{f}$ of a vector field $\mathbf{f}$ describes the degree of dispersion of the field at source (positive divergence) and the degree of concentration at sinks (negative divergence) (see Fig. 9.28). Divergence is

$$\nabla \bullet f = \sum_{i=1}^{n} \frac{\partial}{\partial x} f_i. \tag{9.47}$$

The divergence of the normal of a 0-level set is positive at convex locations and negative at concave locations (see Fig. 9.29). Using the definition above, the divergence for a 2D level set is

$$\kappa_{2d} = \nabla \bullet \mathbf{n} = \nabla \frac{\nabla \phi}{|\nabla \phi|} = \frac{\partial [\frac{\phi_x}{(\phi_x^2 + \phi_y^2)}]}{\partial x} + \frac{\partial [\frac{\phi_y}{(\phi_x^2 + \phi_y^2)}]}{\partial y} = -\frac{\phi_{xx} - 2\phi_x \phi_y \phi_{xy} + \phi_{yy}}{(\phi_x^2 + \phi_y^2)^{\frac{3}{2}}}.$$

$$\tag{9.48}$$

Computing curvature in higher dimensions follows the same structure adding derivatives of the derivative of the level set function with respect to all directions.

To some extent, the curvature term may even be used to fill in missing information. If salient image features are missing in some parts of the image but the shape of objects is known and simple, curvature can represent this shape. An example would be the segmentation of circles or spheres of unknown size. The curvature of a sphere is constant and the reciprocal of its radius. Penalizing deviation from this expectation will cause a level set to evolve into circles or spheres if no image information is present. Hence, if such a circle is partially visible by having high gradients only at parts of its boundary, the level set will evolve into a boundary following these high gradient regions as long as the curvature is close to the expected curvature. If this is not true because the gradients do not represent the circle boundary, the level set will follow the circular shape instead.

In principle, this can be extended to describe arbitrary expected shapes. However, including shape information becomes increasingly difficult when shapes become complex. In such a case, it is easier to integrate explicit shape knowledge as prior information into the model (Leventon et al. 2000; Rousson and Paragios 2002; Paragios 2003).

Data knowledge is introduced by the last term F_{img}. Since the interface should stop at segment boundaries, a force that is inversely proportional to the intensity gradient is a good candidate for F_{img}. Examples suggested in the literature are

$$F_{img}(\mathbf{x}) = \frac{1}{1 + \alpha |\nabla(G_\sigma * I(x))|}, \tag{9.49}$$

and

$$F_{img}(\mathbf{x}) = \exp\big(-\alpha \big|\nabla\big(G_\sigma * I(x)\big)\big|\big). \tag{9.50}$$

In both cases, α controls the strength with which the speed is influenced by this term and G_σ denotes a convolution of the intensity function I with a Gaussian with standard deviation σ.

On inspection, it becomes obvious that the image term will never be 0 and consequently the propagation according to (9.46) will never be 0 as well. Keeping the image term from stopping the propagation is intentional as it is usually not known beforehand what the exact gradient strength is at a boundary and whether this is a unique feature for the segment boundary (otherwise segmentation would be trivial).

Since the level set evolution will not stop automatically, a termination criterion has to be given. Commonly used criteria are to stop evolution if the average or maximum evolution speed falls below some threshold or if an evolution step does not change the current pixel labeling (i.e., no foreground pixels become background or vice versa).

9.2.7 Geodesic Active Contours

The minimization problem for computing a snake can be formulated in the level set framework. It is not dependent on the dimension of the active contours and allows topology changes during evolution of the active contour.

The approach received its name because the problem is formulated as finding a locally shortest contour in a non-Euclidean space. For doing this, the original snake is altered by removing the second derivative from the minimization equation. Caselles et al. (1997) showed that this does not substantially influence the smoothness constraint of the curve.

The condition for an ideal curve $C(p)$ is then to minimize

$$E(C) = \int_0^1 |C'(p)|^2 \, dp + \lambda \int_0^1 g\big(|\nabla I(C(p))|^2\big) \, dp = E_{internal}(C) + \lambda E_{external}(C), \tag{9.51}$$

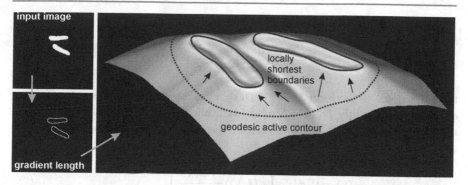

Fig. 9.30 If the strength of the gradient is used as 3rd dimension for the embedding of a 2d object in 3d space, locally shortest curves on this surface (the geodesics) are the segment boundaries that are found by geodesic active contours (which may change topology if needed)

where $p = p(\mathbf{x})$ are locations on the curve, I is the image function, ∇I its gradient, g an arbitrary function that strictly decreases with the gradient, and λ is a parameter that controls the influence of the internal energy versus the external energy of C.

Caselles et al. showed that this corresponds to a search for a minimum length curve in a Riemannian space that is induced by the image information (see Fig. 9.30). Riemannian space is a curved space that may be thought as being embedded in a higher-dimensional Euclidean space. Distances are computed on the curved manifold. Hence, they depend on the distance traveled along the manifold and on the local curvature. This may sound a bit complicated but representing the energy minimization problem of active contours as a shortest path problem in well-defined non-Euclidean space provides a simple solution to the optimization problem. It enables us to make use of theorems about shortest distances in this space. It can be shown that the solution to (9.51) is to evolve the curve in time t in the following manner[4]

$$\frac{\partial C(t)}{\partial t}(p) = \big[g\big(I(p)\big)\kappa - \big(\nabla g(p) \bullet \mathbf{n}\big)\big]\mathbf{n}, \qquad (9.52)$$

where κ is the curvature of the curve and $\mathbf{n}$ is normal to the curve pointing inward. Hence, the curve will move toward high gradient areas, where g is small, while attempting to smooth out its course by minimizing the curvature.

The explicit evolution of C, however, may pose a problem when optimization requires a change of topology. Hence, the optimization is formulated using the level set approach. The curve $C(t)$ is taken as the 0-level set of a level set function $f(x, t)$. Optimization is not by wave propagation, but by using variational calculus (see Sect. 14.2) to minimize (9.51). Hence, level sets of this kind are referred to as *variational level sets*.

---

[4]It is a solution under some specializing assumptions that are necessary to define a unique optimum because the formulation contains a free parameter. Details are described in Caselles et al. (1997). It does not restrict the use of this formalism to find an optimal active contour.

The Euler–Lagrange equation

$$\frac{dE}{df} = \frac{d}{dx}\frac{\partial F}{\partial f'} - \frac{\partial F}{\partial f} = 0 \tag{9.53}$$

for a functional of the form $F(f(x), f'(x), x)$ is created if we substitute $f(x)$ by $\phi(\mathbf{x})$ and consequently $f'(x)$ by $\nabla\phi(\mathbf{x})$. In Caselles et al. (1997) the authors showed in Appendixes B and C that this derivative results in the following evolution of $\phi(\mathbf{x}(t), t)$ with respect to time

$$\frac{\partial\phi}{\partial t}(\mathbf{x}) = |\nabla\phi| \operatorname{div}\left(g(I(\mathbf{x}))\frac{\nabla\phi(\mathbf{x})}{|\nabla\phi(\mathbf{x})|}\right)$$

$$= g(I(\mathbf{x}))|\nabla\phi(\mathbf{x})|\kappa(\mathbf{x}) + \nabla g(I(\mathbf{x}))\nabla\phi(\mathbf{x}). \tag{9.54}$$

The function $\phi(\mathbf{x}(0), 0)$ at $t = 0$ is the signed distance function, which is evolved according to (9.54). It has been shown that the choice of the initial function does not influence the result. Given its initial placement, the level set will evolve in a shortest distance curve in a Riemannian space that is defined by image attributes. The function g is

$$g(\mathbf{x}) = \frac{1}{1 + |\nabla[I(\mathbf{x}) * s(\mathbf{x})]|^p}, \tag{9.55}$$

where s is a smoothing kernel with which I is convolved and $p = 1, 2$.

The energy E_{internal} in (9.51) is a smoothness term that makes the active contour insensitive with respect to noise. In Westin et al. (2000), a variant of the geodesic active contour has been presented that can be made—based on prior knowledge—locally adaptive to enforce smoothness in some parts of the image while following image detail in other parts.

The energy E_{external} is intended to attract the geodesic active contour toward salient image features. Paragios et al. (2004) showed that using gradient vector flow (see Sect. 9.1.2) as external energy improves the speed of convergence.

9.2.8 Level Sets and the Mumford–Shah Functional

The Mumford–Shah functional describes a segmentation based on regional and boundary image attributes (Mumford and Shah 1989). Segmentation by minimizing the Mumford–Shah functional is based on reasonable generic attributes for an optimal segmentation. Hence, numerous schemes have been developed to define a segmentation for various specializations of this functional. It has been shown that level set segmentation can be defined in a way that optimizes a specific variant of the Mumford–Shah functional.

In foreground segmentation, a segmentation is a function $f_{\text{seg}}(\mathbf{x})$ which is 1 for scene elements $\mathbf{x}$ that belong to the segment and 0 otherwise. Since many functions follow this definition, additional constraints based on the desired attributes of

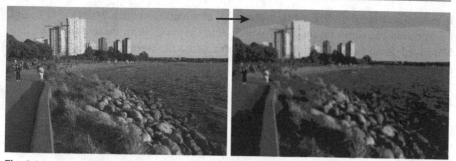

Fig. 9.31 An optimal segmentation according to the Mumford–Shah functional is a description of an image by a non-overlapping set of smooth functions with local support and minimal boundary length. It essentially creates a cartoon-like mapping of the original image with smoothed boundaries

a segment are needed. The Mumford–Shah functional

$$E(c_1, c_2, \Gamma) = \alpha \int_{\Omega_i} \left(u(\mathbf{x}) - c_1 \right)^2 d\mathbf{x} + \beta \int_{\Omega_{ei}} \left(u(\mathbf{x}) - c_2 \right)^2 d\mathbf{x} + \gamma \int_p \left| \Gamma(p) \right| dp \tag{9.56}$$

provides these constraints (Tsai et al. 2001). The equation is a specialization of the general functional of Mumford and Shah (1989) that allows for an arbitrary number of segments (see Fig. 9.31).

The first two terms of (9.56) describe the deviation of intensity $u(\mathbf{x})$ of interior elements $\mathbf{x} \in \Omega_i$ and exterior elements $\mathbf{x} \in \Omega_e$ from the expected (average) intensities c_1 and c_2 in the interior and exterior regions, respectively. Similar to the Bayesian formulation in Sect. 7.1, they ensure that the optimal segmentation separates the scene into interior and exterior elements so that they closely follow the expected characteristics of foreground and background elements.

The last term is the derivative of the curve Γ at points p along the curve. It enforces smoothness of the boundary between interior and exterior points. The effect of this term is similar to that of the internal energy terms of an active contour. It takes into account that the observable boundary in the image may be distorted by noise or may be partially missing. The parameters α, β, and γ govern the influence of the different terms on the desired optimal segmentation.

Finding a foreground segmentation requires to find a function that minimizes (9.56) given an image. Including the region attributes of (9.56) in a level set form has first been presented by Chan and Vese (1999). The method is known as *active contours without edges* since the data term controlling the level set evolution is based on region attributes and not on edges.

For separating the foreground from background, the two regions Ω_i and Ω_e have to be found. This can be conveniently expressed by a level set function $\phi(\mathbf{x})$, which is defined in the complete domain of $\mathbf{x}$, if the Heaviside function

$$H(z) = \begin{cases} 1, & z \geq 0 \\ 0, & z < 0 \end{cases} \tag{9.57}$$

is used. The foreground elements are now all elements for which $H(\phi(\mathbf{x})) = 1$, and background elements are those for which $H(\phi(\mathbf{x})) = 0$. With these definitions the Mumford–Shah functional simplifies to (now using the weighting variables λ_1, λ_2, and ν of Chan and Vese 1999)

$$E(\phi, c) = \lambda_1 \int_R \left(u(\mathbf{x}) - c_1\right)^2 H\left(\phi(\mathbf{x})\right) d\mathbf{x}$$

$$+ \lambda_2 \int_R \left(u(\mathbf{x}) - c_2\right)^2 \left(1 - H\left(\phi(\mathbf{x})\right)\right) d\mathbf{x}$$

$$+ \nu \int_R \left|\nabla H\left(\phi(\mathbf{x})\right)\right|. \tag{9.58}$$

The optimal segmentation is a function $\phi(\mathbf{x})$ that minimizes E (see Fig. 9.32 for an example). Similar to geodesic active contours, the optimal level set is computed using variational calculus (see Sect. 14.2). It is a matter of applying standard differentiation rules (and remembering that the derivative of the Heaviside function is the delta function δ) to arrive at the following Euler–Lagrange equation for the level set minimization

$$\frac{\partial E}{\partial \phi} = \delta(\mathbf{x}) \left[\lambda_1 \left(u(\mathbf{x}) - c_1\right)^2 - \lambda_2 \left(u(\mathbf{x}) - c_2\right)^2 - \nu \nabla \frac{\nabla \phi(\mathbf{x})}{|\nabla \phi(\mathbf{x})|} \right], \tag{9.59}$$

which gives the update rule

$$\frac{\partial \phi}{\partial t} = \delta(\mathbf{x}) \left[-\lambda_1 \left(u(\mathbf{x}) - c_1\right)^2 + \lambda_2 \left(u(\mathbf{x}) - c_2\right)^2 + \nu \nabla \frac{\nabla \phi(\mathbf{x})}{|\nabla \phi(\mathbf{x})|} \right]. \tag{9.60}$$

Since the Heaviside function and its derivative, the δ-function, are inherently unstable, they are replaced by a differentiable approximation such as the sigmoid function.

In (9.58), c_1 and c_2 approximate the appearance in the foreground and background region. This could be, for instance, the average intensity of the enclosed regions. If domain knowledge exists about the expected appearance in the foreground and background, this could be used as well. The two parameters λ_1 and λ_2 represent the expected reliability of the approximation by c_1 and c_2. The parameter ν enforces short and therefore smooth boundaries.

The regional terms determine the behavior of the level set. If, for instance, the level set is in the background, the variation of $(u(\mathbf{x}) - c_1)^2$ in the current foreground should be larger than that of $(u(\mathbf{x}) - c_2)^2$ in the current background. Since the two terms are minimized, the level set will move inward toward the true foreground-to-background boundary.

Sometimes, the average intensity is not a very good predictor to determine foreground or background membership of a scene element. Knowledge about the location of the segment boundary—included in active contour approaches—cannot be included in the original formulation of Chan and Vese (2001). If this information is

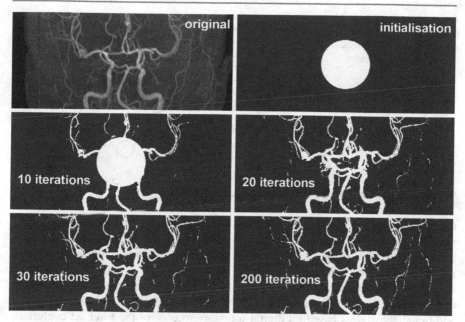

Fig. 9.32 Active contours without edges for the segmentation of vessels in a projection image: segmentation is fairly independent of the initial level set. The result is influenced by the homogeneity term. This can be seen for the smaller vessels at the periphery where the signal difference is too small for a good segmentation

present, the approach can be extended to an active geodesic regions method (Paragios 2002). Given probabilities P_{int} and P_{ext} of a scene element belonging to the interior and exterior of a segment, the level set evolution is

$$\frac{\partial \phi}{\partial t} = \alpha \left(\log \left(\frac{P_{\text{int}}}{P_{\text{ext}}} \right) \right) |\nabla \phi| + (1 - \alpha) \big(g(P_C) \kappa |\nabla \phi| + \nabla \phi \nabla g(P_C) \big), \quad (9.61)$$

where g decreases with the probability P_C of points of a curve C belonging to the true boundary.

The evolution of variational level sets will always result in the minimum if the functional to be optimized is convex (such as the one above). Hence, the result is independent from the initial level set as long as the initial boundary has nonzero length (see, e.g., Fig. 9.32). This is different to the evolution using the narrow band technique. The latter is just a local optimization of the level set function, where the global optimum may not even be the wanted segment boundary. The desirable behavior of variational level sets comes at a cost, however. The minimization can no longer be seen independently of the forces that drive the level set evolution. While it is possible to define almost arbitrary speed functions for narrow band level set evolution, adding or changing terms in variational level set requires a new optimization of the equation.

Fig. 9.33 Topology
preserving level set evolution
stops before the front moves
over non-simple points

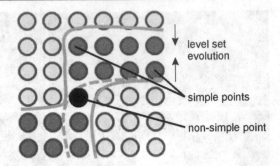

9.2.9   Topologically Constrained Level Sets

Compared to the parametrically defined active contours presented in Sect. 9.1, level
sets have the advantage that their topology may change during evolution. An initial
level set may be a simple, closed curve. This curve will split and merge during
evolution according to image properties.

This may be unwanted, if the topology of an object is known a priori. Level sets
can be adapted to prohibit such change of topology. Han et al. (2003) suggested
additional constraints based on digital topology to control the level set evolution.
Digital topology defines the closeness and connectedness for a discrete sampling of
continuous space. A connected component of a discrete scene consists of all scene
elements between which a path exists. A path exists between two scene elements s_0
and s_N if a sequence $s_0, s_1, s_2, \ldots, s_N$ exists so that every pair s_i, s_{i+1} is adjacent
and a given homogeneity criterion is true for all pairs.

Adjacency depends on the dimension of the scene. Pixels in a 2D scene can be
four-adjacent if they share a common edge, or eight-adjacent if they share a common
point. Voxels may be 6-, 18-, or 26-adjacent. Homogeneity in its simplest version
requires equal function values, but can be any other attribute that is definable on
pairs of scene elements. For topologically constrained level sets, a pair of scene
elements fulfills the homogeneity criterion, if the pair is completely inside or outside
of the boundary defined by the current 0-level set.

When adding or removing a scene element, it is of interest whether this action
changes the topology.

- Removing a scene element may split a connected component into several components.
- Adding a scene element may merge two or more components.

If a label of a scene element can be switched between foreground and background
without altering the topology, it is called a *simple point* (see Fig. 9.33). Whether a
point is simple or not changes after each label change and has to be continuously
monitored.

The speed term of the evolving level set is now supplemented by a term that prevents a front from moving into nonsimple points. The evolving front is mapped on
the discrete image after each iteration step. Subsequently, the points of the discrete
scene are classified into simple and nonsimple points. The speed is reduced to zero
if a nonsimple point is to be passed.

9.3   Concluding Remarks

Active contours fit a parameterizable model of a segment to the data by finding an optimal location for a model instance. Since the global and local constraints of the active contour are always asserted, they are particularly well suited if data alone do not provide this information.

The major difference between the two types of active contours is the representation. While an explicit representation is inherently topology-preserving and fast to optimize, implicit representations are defined independent of dimension and operate in continuous space. A preference of one of the two kinds should be given to the methodology which best fits an actual segmentation problem.

9.4   Exercises

- Sketch a segmentation problem where active contours (defined explicitly or implicitly) would be the appropriate segmentation strategy. Explain the reasons why it would be appropriate.
- What kind of information is represented by the internal energy term of an explicit active contour? What could be the possible adverse effects if this term is weighted too strongly in the equation?
- Why is it important to initialize an active contour close to the searched segment boundary?
- How can balloon forces be used for relieving the user from having to place the active contour close to its final position? Discuss the disadvantages of the strategy.
- What are the features that are used to compute the gradient in gradient vector flow?
- What would be the image properties that will cause the gradient vector flow to fail leading an active contour to the segment boundary?
- How can active contours be constructed so that topological changes are accommodated?
- How is the current segment boundary represented in the level set framework?
- Explain why it is not important how the level set function looks like.
- What is the difference for the wave propagation if represented by stationary versus dynamic level sets?
- Why is it necessary for dynamic level sets to embed the n-dimensional level set function into $(n + 1)$-dimensional space?
- What is the meaning of the speed function? Explain the three different components of the speed function.
- How is boundary smoothness represented in the level set framework?
- What is meant by an "upwind scheme" and why is it necessary to use an upwind scheme?
- What conditions have to be met for guaranteeing the stable computation of the level set evolution?
- Explain why the fast marching algorithm is less time consuming than naive computation of arrival times for stationary level set.

- What is the difference between the fast marching approach and Dijkstra's shortest path algorithm?
- Why is the narrow band technique faster than the regular propagation of a dynamic level set? What are the potential disadvantages of this technique?
- Why has using the narrow band technique also been an advantage regarding the step size of the time step compared to regular propagation of the level set function?
- What are the properties that determine the size of the band in the narrow band technique?
- What is minimized when optimizing geodesic active contours under the level set framework?
- Explain how region information can be included in level set segmentation for "active contours without edges."
- What are the assumptions that are made so that variational level sets optimize the Mumford–Shah functional?
- Why is it necessary to replace the Heaviside function for variational level sets? What are the desired properties of the function that replaces the Heavidside function?
- How can the level set evolution be modified to constrain topology? Compare this strategy with the introduction of topological variability for explicit active contours. What do the two approaches have in common?

References

Adalsteinsson D, Sethian JA (1995) A fast level set method for propagating interfaces. J Comput Phys 118(2):269–277

Caselles V, Kimmel R, Sapiro G (1997) Geodesic active contours. Int J Comput Vis, 21(1):61–79

Chan TF, Vese LA (1999) Active contours without edges. IEEE Trans Image Process 10(2):266–277

Chan TF, Vese LA (2001) A level set algorithm for minimizing the Mumford–Shah functional in image processing. In: IEEE workshop on variational and level set methods in computer vision, pp 161–168

Cohen LD (1991) On active contour models and balloons. CVGIP, Image Underst 53(2):211–218

Cohen LD, Cohen I (1993) Finite-element methods for active contour models and balloons for 2-d and 3-d images. IEEE Trans Pattern Recogn Mach Intell 15(11):1131–1147

Cohen LD, Kimmel R (1997) Global minimum for active contour models: a minimal path approach. Int J Comput Vis 24(1):57–78

Davatzikos CA, Prince JL (1995) An active contour model for mapping the cortex. IEEE Trans Med Imaging 14(2):65–80

Han X, Xu C, Prince JL (2003) A topology preserving level set method for geometric deformable models. IEEE Trans Pattern Anal Mach Intell 25(6):755–768

Honea DM, Snyder WE, Hanson KM (1999) Three-dimensional active surface approach to lymph node segmentation. Proc SPIE 3661(2):1003–1011

Ladak HM, Milner JS, Steinman DA (2000) Rapid three-dimensional segmentation of the carotid bifurcation from serial MR images. J Biomech Eng 122(1):96–99

Leventon ME, Grimson WEL, Faugeras O (2000) Statistical shape influence in geodesic active contours. In: IEEE comp soc conf computer vision and pattern recognition (CVPR'00), vol 1, pp 1316–1323

Kass M, Witkins A, Terzopoulos D (1988) Snakes: active contour models. Int J Comput Vis 1(4):321–331

Kichenassamy S, Kumar A, Olver P, Tannenbaum A, Yezzi A (1995) Gradient flows and geometric active contour models. In: 5th intl conf computer vision (ICCV'95), pp 810–817

McInerney T, Terzopoulos D (1995a) A dynamic finite element surface model for segmentation and tracking in multidimensional medical images with application to cardiac 4D image analysis. J Comput Med Imaging Graph 19(1):69–83

McInerney T, Terzopoulos D (1995b) Topologically adaptable snakes. In: Intl conf computer vision ICCV, pp 840–845

McInerney T, Terzopoulos D (2000) T-snakes: topologically adaptable snakes. Med Image Anal 4(1):73–91

Mumford D, Shah J (1989) Optimal approximations by piecewise smooth functions and associated variational problems. Commun Pure Appl Math 42(5):577–685

Neuenschwander WM, Fua P, Iverson L, Székely G, Kübler O (1997) Ziplock snakes. Int J Comput Vis 25(3):191 201

Osher S, Sethian J (1988) Fronts propagating with curvature-dependent speed—algorithms based on Hamilton–Jacobi formulations. J Comput Phys 79:12–49

Osher S, Paragios N (2003) Geometric level set methods in imaging, vision, and graphics. Springer, Berlin, 2003

Paragios N (2002) Geodesic active regions and level set methods for supervised texture segmentation. Int J Comput Vis 46(3):223–247

Paragios N (2003) A level set approach for shape-driven segmentation and tracking of the left ventricle. IEEE Trans Med Imaging 22(6):773–776

Paragios N, Mellina-Gottardo O, Ramesh V (2004) Gradient vector flow fast geodesic active contours. IEEE Trans Pattern Anal Mach Intell 26(3):402–407

Park J, Keller JM (2001) Snakes on the watershed. IEEE Trans Pattern Anal Mach Intell 23(10):1201–1205

Rousson M, Paragios N (2002) Shape priors for level set representations. In: 7th European conference on computer vision ECCV 2002. LNCS, vol 2351, pp 416–418

Sethian JA (1996) A fast marching level set method for monotonically advancing fronts. Appl Math 93(4):1591–1595

Sethian JA (1998) Level set and fast marching methods. Cambridge University Press, Cambridge

Tsai A, Yezzi A, Willsky AS (2001) Curve evolution implementation of the Mumford–Shah functional for image segmentation, denoising, interpolation, and magnification. IEEE Trans Image Process 10(8):1169–1186

Westin CF, Lorigo LM, Faugeras O, Grimson WEL, Dawson S, Norbash A, Kikinis R (2000) Segmentation by adaptive geodesic active contours. In: Medical image computing and computer-assisted intervention—MICCAI 2000. LNCS, vol 1935, pp 266–275

Xu X, Prince JL (1998) Snakes, shapes, and gradient vector flow. IEEE Trans Image Process 7(3):359–369

Registration and Normalization

10

Abstract

Information about an object from different sources can be combined if a transformation allows mapping data from one source to data of the other source. In medical imaging, the two sources are image acquisition systems. If the two sources depict the same subject, this process is called registration. If they depict different subjects, it is called normalization. The mapping is a geometric transformation that accounts for the different positioning of a patient in two image acquisition systems.

Determining a registration or normalization transformation requires redundant information in the two images, a suitable restriction of acceptable transformations, and, for iterative schemes, a criterion that rates the quality of a given transformation. Various ways to compute a registration or normalization transformation from medical images will be discussed in this chapter.

Concepts, notions and definitions introduced in this chapter

> Rigid and nonrigid registration
> Normalization
> Similarity criteria: average distance, Procrustes distance, intensity difference, correlation and covariance, stochastic and deterministic sign change, mutual information
> Analytic solution for rigid registration
> Constraints for iterative registration: elasticity, viscosity, splines, similarity of displacement vectors

Fusing information from different sources produces synergy by spatially relating data from the sources with respect to each other. Registration and normalization are the processes to find an appropriate mapping for the fusion.

Registration computes and carries out a transformation between two or more pictorial representations of the same subject. If the two scenes have the same di-

K.D. Toennies, *Guide to Medical Image Analysis*,
Advances in Computer Vision and Pattern Recognition,
DOI 10.1007/978-1-4471-2751-2_10, © Springer-Verlag London Limited 2012

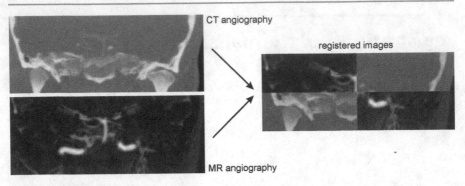

Fig. 10.1 Registration finds a transformation to map two different images of the same patient onto each other

mensionality and dimensions correspond—e.g., when comparing a 3D MRI data set with a 3D CT data set (see Fig. 10.1)—topology will often be preserved by the transformation. Hence, adjacent locations prior to registration will remain adjacent. It is a useful constraint for determining the registration transformation.

Normalization is the operation to compare images from two or more different subjects. It differs from registration in that topology is not always preserved. The use of the term normalization refers to the mapping of images of different subjects onto some common norm image. In the medical sciences it probably originates from functional imaging where normalization is routinely used for group studies. Normalization also happens, when a geometric model of shape and appearance is mapped to an image. This is also called *matching* referring to a use in general image analysis (e.g., template matching). It is used extensively to describe atlas-based segmentation (one of the first publications was R. Bajcy's work on 2D and 3D elastic matching; Bajcy et al. 1983; Bajcy and Kovacic 1989).

Registration and normalization are sometimes subsumed under the common notation registration, but different requirements and constraints justify the discrimination by name even though many normalization algorithms borrow from registration. Surveys on registration algorithms in all areas of digital image processing and analysis have been published by Brown (1992) and Zitova and Flusser (2003) (the latter is intended to be an update of the former). The two surveys may also serve as tutorials on basic requirements and characteristics in registration. The characterization of the methods used in medical applications can be found in the extensive survey of Maintz and Viergever (1998). A good introduction into numerical issues of registration is Modersitzki (2003).

Finding the appropriate transformation between two scenes f and g depends on four aspects (Brown 1992).

- The *feature space* determines features F in f and g that will be used for correspondence.
- The *similarity criterion* S defines what is meant by correspondence between two registered scenes.
- The *search space* contains all possible transformations T among which an optimal transformation is searched.

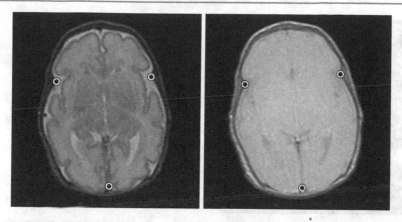

Fig. 10.2 For finding the registration transformation, redundant information must exist that defines the mapping at least at some locations (such as the landmark positions indicated in this example)

- The *search strategy* tells how—given some transformation producing some similarity—the next transformation is found.

Finding correspondence between two scenes f and g requires at least some redundancy between image features $F(f)$ and $F(g)$ so that a sufficiently large number of locations $\mathbf{x}_1$ and $\mathbf{x}_2$ in the two images exist, for which the local feature similarity $s(F(f(\mathbf{x}_1)), F(g(\mathbf{x}_2), T)$ can be defined (see Fig. 10.2). To make the search for the correct registration function a minimization task, the similarity measure is often defined such that it is low when feature locations correspond given some transformation T.

In this chapter, we will discuss techniques and their limitations to solve the problems based on registration. The concluding sections will address differences of normalization and matching methods with respect to registration.

10.1   Feature Space and Correspondence Criterion

Establishing correspondences between two scenes f and g requires finding a measure by which equivalence between locations in the two scenes is quantified. Two points in the two images are assumed to be equivalent if they have the same location with respect to some unknown patient coordinate system. The relation between the known scanner coordinate system and the patient coordinate system is influenced

- by different positioning of the patient in the scanner,
- by distortions caused by the imaging system,
- by any movements of organs due to physiology,
- by changes caused from interventions taking place between creating f and g.

Equivalent locations in the two images are assumed to have a similar appearance. This does not imply that unlike locations have different appearances. Correspondence criteria will often only apply to a subset of locations in f and g where similarity either uniquely identifies pairs of correspondent points in patient coordinates

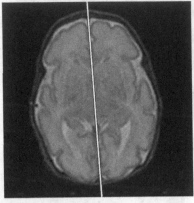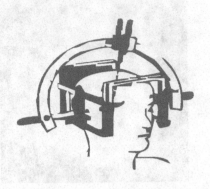

Intrinsic marker: midplane separating the two hemispheres   Extrinsic marker: stereotactic frame

Fig. 10.3 Examples for intrinsic and extrinsic markers. Markers do not have to be points but the same structure should be visible in two scenes to be registered

(this is the case for labeled landmarks) or where at least the number of possible correspondence pairs is reduced (this is the case when, e.g., landmark curves are used).

Features commonly used for measuring correspondence in medical image registration are as follows:

• Extrinsic markers;
• Intrinsic features: landmark points, curves, or regions;
• Voxel intensities or gradients.

Extrinsic or intrinsic features are *model-based features* (see Fig. 10.3), whereas voxel intensities or gradients are *image-based features* (see Fig. 10.4). Model-based features are selected intentionally according to the assumption that they provide essential information for computing the registration transformation. Using image-based features assumes that low-level operations on an image suffice for producing the necessary correspondence information. The number of locations $\mathbf{x}$ for which correspondence may be established—i.e., the domain for which local correspondence c is defined—is generally smaller in model-based registration than in image-based registration, but their accuracy is often better.

Extrinsic and intrinsic markers are assumed to be describable by a finite set of feature points that are distinguishable in the two scenes. Local correspondence may be computed only for feature points in the two scenes. A feature function F assigns the label 1 to feature points and the label 0 to all other locations in the image. Feature similarity c_c simply notes the incidence of coinciding feature points with the same label

$$c_c\big[F\big(f(\mathbf{x}_1)\big), F\big(g(\mathbf{x}_2)\big), T\big] = \begin{cases} 1, & \text{if } F(f(\mathbf{x}_1)) = F(g(T(\mathbf{x}_2))) > 0 \\ & \text{and } \mathbf{x}_1 = T(\mathbf{x}_2) \\ 0, & \text{otherwise.} \end{cases} \qquad (10.1)$$

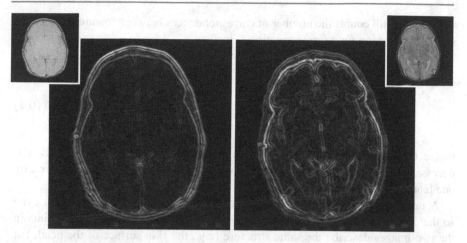

Fig. 10.4 Image-based features are generated by some filtering process from the image. Since the two images to be registered are usually not equal, image-based features do not necessarily have direct correspondence. It is assumed, however, that most features are visible in both scenes

The similarity S between scenes f and g after transforming g by some transformation T would be the inverse of the sum of local correspondences

$$S_c(F, f, g, \mathbf{x}_1, \mathbf{x}_2, T) = \left[\frac{1}{|M|} \sum_{(\mathbf{x}_1, \mathbf{x}_2) \in M} c_c \left[F(f(\mathbf{x}_1)), F(g(\mathbf{x}_2)), T \right] \right]^{-1}, \quad (10.2)$$

where M is the set of feature point pairs in f and g with $\mathbf{x}_1 = T(\mathbf{x}_2)$, and $|M|$ is the number of elements of M. Normalization by $|M|$ makes transformations T with different numbers of corresponding markers comparable to each other. Removing the normalization constant may make sense if transformations with few matching feature points shall be penalized.

The mapping is not unique (i.e., more than one transformation T may exist that minimizes S). A unique mapping is achieved if F assigns a unique non-zero label to every feature point such that corresponding features have equal labels.

The similarity criterion above counts the number of matched feature points. Its underlying assumption is that the computation of feature points is exact and a suitable transformation exists with $\mathbf{x}_1 = T(\mathbf{x}_2)$ for all feature point pairs $(\mathbf{x}_1, \mathbf{x}_2)$ of the registration transformation T.

It is possible and even likely that this is not true because the marker positions have not been determined accurately or they do not match exactly. Local correspondence can be relaxed by introducing some minimum distance ε that must not be exceeded for declaring two feature point positions to be equal:

$$c_\varepsilon \left[F(f(\mathbf{x}_1)), F(g(\mathbf{x}_2)), T \right] = \begin{cases} 1, & \text{if } F(f(\mathbf{x}_1)) = F(g(T(\mathbf{x}_2))) \\ & \qquad > 0 \wedge |\mathbf{x}_1 - T(\mathbf{x}_2)| < \varepsilon \quad (10.3) \\ 0, & \text{otherwise.} \end{cases}$$

Using c_ε still counts the number of correspondences between feature points. The similarity criterion for a transformation T is

$$S_\varepsilon(F, f, g, \mathbf{x}_1, \mathbf{x}_2, T)$$

$$= \left[\frac{1}{|M|} \sum_{M=\{(\mathbf{x}_1, \mathbf{x}_2)|\mathbf{x}_1 = CP(T(\mathbf{x}_2))\}} c_\varepsilon \big[F\big(f(\mathbf{x}_1)\big), F\big(g(\mathbf{x}_2)\big), T \big] \right]^{-1}, \quad (10.4)$$

where $CP()$ ensures that $T(\mathbf{x}_2)$ is the closest of all marker points to $\mathbf{x}_1$. This is necessary for ensuring that any feature point in f may only be mapped to exactly one feature point in g.

A unique relationship between feature points in the two scenes may not exist so that counting correspondences is not suitable. If, for instance, feature points in the two images describe the same structure (e.g., the skin surface of the head, but no specifically labeled positions on the skin surface are identified), similarity must attempt to minimize the average distance between two sets of feature points. A suitable definition for local correspondence between feature points of f and g could be the distance between two matching feature points $\mathbf{x}_1$ and $\mathbf{x}_2$ such that the transformed $\mathbf{x}_2$ is closest to $\mathbf{x}_1$:

$$c_d\big[F\big(f(\mathbf{x}_1)\big), F\big(g(\mathbf{x}_2)\big), T \big] = \begin{cases} \|\mathbf{x}_1 - T(\mathbf{x}_2)\|, & \text{if } F(f(\mathbf{x}_1)) > 0 \wedge F(g(T(\mathbf{x}_2))) \\ & \qquad > 0 \wedge \mathbf{x}_1 = CP(T(\mathbf{x}_2)) \\ 0, & \text{otherwise.} \end{cases}$$

$$(10.5)$$

The registration similarity S_d is:

$$S_d(F, f, g, \mathbf{x}_1, \mathbf{x}_2, T) = \frac{1}{|M|} \sqrt{\sum_{M=\{(\mathbf{x}_1, \mathbf{x}_2)|\mathbf{x}_1 = CP(T(\mathbf{x}_2))\}} c_d\big[F\big(f(\mathbf{x}_1)\big), F\big(g(\mathbf{x}_2)\big), T \big]}.$$

$$(10.6)$$

S_d is called the *Procrustes distance*[1] (see Fig. 10.5). Local similarity using the Procrustes distance between markers can also be used for matching markers by requiring $F(f(\mathbf{x}_1)) = F(g(T(\mathbf{x}_2))) > 0$ instead of $F(f(\mathbf{x}_1)) > 0 \wedge F(g(T(\mathbf{x}_2))) > 0$.

Similarity can be computed for feature points from extrinsic and intrinsic markers. *Extrinsic markers* are artificially attached markers to the body such as skin markers or markers on a stereotactic frame. Marker materials must be clearly visible in the two images. Appropriate materials depend on the imaging technique. Plastic, for instance, is barely visible in CT and not visible at all in MR. Any visible material that does not emit photons will not be detected by nuclear imaging techniques.

---

[1] Sometimes the square root is not taken.

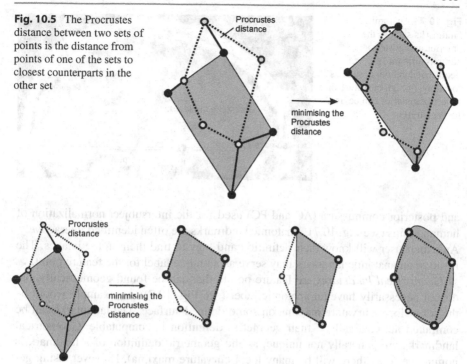

Fig. 10.5 The Procrustes distance between two sets of points is the distance from points of one of the sets to closest counterparts in the other set

Fig. 10.6 Minimizing the Procrustes distance for a set of points produces the optimal transformation only at these points. Transformations at other locations can be arbitrary unless the set of permissible transformations is suitably restricted. Any of the three regions depicted *on the right* optimize the Procrustes distance in the same way

Markers should be small for simplifying the computation of the feature point location from a segmented marker region. They should be opaque with respect to the imaging technique and produce a high-contrast signal. The accuracy with which feature point locations can be determined varies with the type of marker and the noise level and different spatial resolution of the imaging device. Hence, the computation of a registration transformation from feature point locations may be inaccurate.

A registration transformation based on matching feature point positions is valid only at these positions (see Fig. 10.6). The registration of other positions in the scene requires the space of acceptable transformations to be suitably constrained so that matching feature point positions uniquely determine a transformation for the complete image. Even for finding a rigid transformation, this can be difficult because the relation between the extrinsic markers and the patient may be nonrigid. Skin markers, for instance, may move in some nonrigid fashion with respect to the bone.

Intrinsic landmarks are feature points of an anatomical or geometrical nature. They are identifiable locations in the scenes to be registered and may be used in the same fashion as extrinsic markers. *Anatomical landmarks* are locations used in anatomy for providing spatial reference information. Examples are the anterior

Fig. 10.7 Anatomic
landmarks such as the
anterior and posterior
commissural (ac, pc) or
geometric landmarks such as
locations of high curvature on
object boundaries can be used
for registration

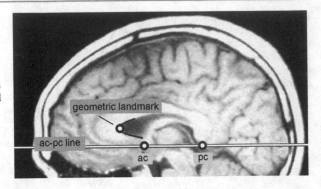

and posterior commissura (AC and PC) used for the intersubject normalization of human brains (see Fig. 10.7). Anatomic landmarks are often identified interactively. An expert user will know their definition and how to find them in the images. The name of an anatomic landmark may serve as a unique label for the feature point.

Geometrical landmarks are feature points that can be found geometrically, but do not necessarily have an anatomic label (see Fig. 10.7). An example would be the set of local curvature maxima on some defined surface. The landmarks can be computed automatically if their geometric definition is computable. Geometrical landmarks are generally not unique, as the geometric definition of a landmark is nonunique (e.g., there will be many local curvature maxima). However, using geometric features, such as SIFT, SURF, MSER, or local shape context, presented in Chap. 5 provide a rich description that allows a substantial reduction of the potential counterpart of feature locations in the other image.

Still, noise, different spatial resolution between image scenes, and other artefacts, can cause an identifiable geometric landmark in one scene not to be detected in the other scene.

Computing a registration transformation from anatomic or geometric landmarks requires similar constraints than the use of extrinsic markers. The spatial relationship between landmarks and the scenes to be registered need to be known and should be simple for inferring a scene registration transformation from landmark registration. If, for instance, the vertebra in a preoperative CT scan shall be registered with an intraoperative scan, the transformation will be rigid. If, however, some of the landmarks were on other vertebrae, the relation between the object of interest and the landmarks may no longer be rigid and too complex to be accounted for.

Inaccurate interactive depiction or automatic computation of anatomical or geometrical landmarks results in displacement errors, which affects the accuracy of the transformation between landmark positions.

Geometrical landmarks may also be curves or regions (e.g., the ridges on some surface or the surface itself; see Fig. 10.8). The mapping will be nonunique because there is no unique identification of locations within such curves or regions. Using curve or region points requires a similarity criterion such as S_d, which does not require point-to-point correspondence. The criterion needs to be adapted so that points in one scene that do not have a counterpart are not included into the similarity

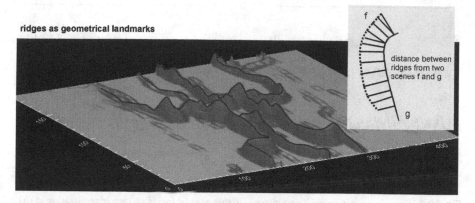

Fig. 10.8 If ridges are used as landmarks, the distance between two ridges is an average of distances of points on one ridge to closest points on the other ridge

measure. This can be done by using the ε of the c_ε measure to exclude feature points for which $|\mathbf{x}_1 - CP(T(\mathbf{x}_2))| > \varepsilon$.

Intrinsic features define the mapping for a selected subset of locations in the image similar to extrinsic features. Computing the scene registration transformation again requires a suitably constrained transformation space. However, registering two scenes does not always require equal accuracy everywhere in the scene. Often, some region of interest needs to be analyzed. Intrinsic landmarks are then placed closely to this region, which reduces adverse influences from placement inaccuracies there.

If the number of landmark locations is small, if their localization is unreliable, or if the search space for a transformation is complex, such as in non-rigid registration, landmark-based registration may not be suitable. *Image-based registration features* can provide a denser map of corresponding locations $\mathbf{x}$. Features do not require prior identification. They are computed using low-level image processing techniques. Features may not be reliable everywhere in the scene, but on average the number of reliable feature locations is larger than in landmark-based feature computation. Image-based features are not unique, though because the values of low-level features cannot serve as a unique label.

In the simplest case, intensity may serve as a feature. Using intensities requires equal objects having equal brightness in the two images. An example is the registration of two images from the same patient made at different times with the same modality under the same protocol. The local correspondence criterion $c_{\text{intensity}}$ is the intensity difference between voxel locations $\mathbf{x}$

$$c_{\text{intensity}}(\mathbf{x}, f, g; T) = \|f(\mathbf{x}) - T \circ g(\mathbf{x})\|. \qquad (10.7)$$

$T \circ g(\mathbf{x})$ indicates that function g was transformed by T prior to computing the difference. The similarity of two registered scenes is then the sum of all local correspondences. Using the intensity difference may be hampered by noise, especially if the contrast in the image is low.

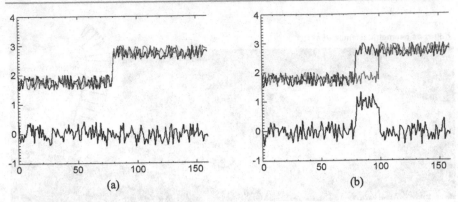

Fig. 10.9 Sign changes increase if two images (in this case 1d functions) are in registration in (**a**) compared to the non-registered images in (**b**)

Computing sign changes instead is a more stable criterion (see Fig. 10.9). The criterion was introduced by Venot and Leclerc (1984) and has been used for 2D image registration (a newer application is Maglogiannis 2004). The two images $f(\mathbf{x})$ and $T \circ g(\mathbf{x})$ are subtracted from each other to yield $d(\mathbf{x}) = f(\mathbf{x}) - T \circ g(\mathbf{x})$.

If images are in perfect registration and contain zero-mean noise, the number of sign changes between neighboring pixels in d depends only on the noise characteristics. The number of sign changes decreases if images are misregistered. A similarity criterion $S_{\text{sign\_change}}$ to be minimized that is based on sign changes is

$$S_{\text{sign\_change}}(T) = -\sum_{\mathbf{x}} \sum_{\mathbf{xn} \in Nbs(\mathbf{x})} \left| \text{sgn}(d(\mathbf{x}) - d(\mathbf{xn})) \right|, \qquad (10.8)$$

where sgn() is the signum function and $Nbs(\mathbf{x})$ contains the neighbors of $\mathbf{x}$. The authors called the criterion *stochastic sign change criterion*. It requires the images to contain noise. Its success is based on the assumption that the noise level is lower than the signal as well as that spatial frequency of noise is higher than that of the signal. High-frequency details of objects will not contribute to the registration success but lead to its deterioration. If images are noise-free, a synthetic noise-like pattern may be added to both images prior to their subtraction. This is called the *deterministic sign change criterion*.

If voxel intensities for the same object are different in the two scenes f and g, and if no simple mapping for making them equal exists, the measures above cannot be used. However, if at least some of the objects are visible in the two images, commonness between features still relates to the boundary between objects. This can be exploited in several ways.

A straightforward strategy is to use the intensity gradient as feature. Feature computation requires an extra segmentation step for identifying boundary pixels by means of the gradient properties (see Fig. 10.10). Boundary segments are treated as landmark curves or landmark regions for which the average distances between closest points are to be minimized. Gradients, however, are sensitive to noise and

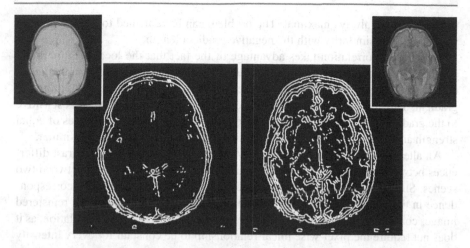

Fig. 10.10 Gradient information from the images can be exploited for segmentation if an additional edge detection step uses gradient strength for finding edges (in the case above by using the Canny edge detector)

artefacts. Artefact edges may erroneously be treated as boundary edges, localization of edges may contain displacement errors, and boundary edges may not be found in both images.

Gradient information is employed indirectly if a multiple threshold segmentation of the two images is created, which is then registered using the deterministic sign criterion. Multiple thresholds produce segments in which some of the boundaries should coincide with object boundaries. Summing sign changes over the image reduces the influence of noise and artefacts from segmentation boundaries that are not object boundaries.

If segmentation is not suitable as preprocessing step, the influence of noise at the edges can be reduced by employing a better edge model. Assuming ideal step edges, the *correlation coefficient* in a δ-neighborhood $N_\delta(\mathbf{x})$ around some location $\mathbf{x}$ can be used as local correspondence criterion c_{edge}:

$$c_{\text{edge}}(\mathbf{x}, f, g; T) = cc_\delta\big(f(x), T \circ g(x)\big)$$

$$= \frac{\frac{1}{|N_\delta(\mathbf{x})|} \sum_{\mathbf{x}_i \in N_\delta(\mathbf{x})} (f(\mathbf{x}_i) - \bar{f}(\mathbf{x}))(T \circ g(\mathbf{x}_i) - \bar{g}(\mathbf{x}_i))}{\sum_{\mathbf{x}_i \in N_\delta(\mathbf{x})} (f(\mathbf{x}_i) - \bar{f}(\mathbf{x}))^2 \sum_{\mathbf{x}_i \in N_\delta(\mathbf{x})} (T \circ g(\mathbf{x}_i) - \bar{g}(\mathbf{x}_i))^2},$$

$$(10.9)$$

where $\bar{f}(\mathbf{x})$ and $\bar{g}(\mathbf{x})$ are estimates of the expected value in f and g in $N_\delta(\mathbf{x})$. If the contrast in the two images to be registered may be reversed (i.e., a dark object in f may be bright in g) the absolute value of c_{edge} is taken. Scene similarity S_{edge} is computed by summing up voxel correspondences at all boundary locations.

If explicit edge detection has not been carried out, scene similarity may be computed by summing over all voxels in the scene. It reduces sensibility to registration errors since the correlation between two voxels with constant brightness in their neighborhood is always maximal. The problem can be remedied to some extent by weighting local similarity with the negative gradient length.

Using local correlation takes advantage of the fact that the local neighborhood parallel to an edge should be smooth while this is not true for noise. Another strategy to make use of this would be to use low pass filtering before computing the gradient. This has been done, for instance, by Bajcy et al. (1983) but it is sensitive to the gradient strength at an edge. Solutions are preferred where the edges of equal strength are mapped onto each other requiring contrast in f and g to be similar.

An alternative for using the correlation, which is not sensitive to contrast differences between f and g, is the computation of the *mutual information* between two scenes. Similar to correlation, mutual information measures brightness correspondence in the two images. It is high when brightness changes in the two registered images coincide. The measure of coincidence is less restrictive than correlation, as it does not require the pixel-wise linear relationship to be constant for every intensity level.

Mutual information $I(f, g)$ of a pair of images f and g is related their *joint entropy* $E(f, g)$ in the following way

$$I(f, g) = E(f) + E(g) - E(f, g), \tag{10.10}$$

where $E(f)$ and $E(g)$ are the entropies of f and g as defined in Sect. 4.1.2. The joint entropy $E(f, g)$ is given by

$$E(f, g) = \sum_{i=0}^{N-1} \sum_{j=0}^{N-1} p(i, j) \log_2 p(i, j). \tag{10.11}$$

The quantity $p(i, j)$ is the joint probability of intensities i and j occurring at the same location $\mathbf{x}$ in f and g. It is estimated from the normalized joint histogram of f and g. The intensity of the two images is assumed to range from 0 to $N - 1$. Mutual information measures how good intensity values in image g at some location $\mathbf{x}$ may be predicted by intensity values in image f at the same location. If the two images are in perfect registration, this predictability is at its maximum if at least some of the information in f is also depicted in g (see Fig. 10.11 for an example for translation and Fig. 10.12 for an example for rotation).

Mutual information can be used as a local correspondence criterion at any location $\mathbf{x}$ as well by computing it from some predefined neighborhood region around $\mathbf{x}$. Small local neighborhoods, however, may produce unreliable estimates of I from the underlying estimates of the probability distributions p.

If applied as a global estimate, the different domains of the two images have to be considered. If transformation T is applied to g, some locations $\mathbf{x}$ for which f is defined may become undefined for the transformed g and vice versa. Since the region in $\mathbf{x}$ for which f and g are defined changes with T, the similarity measure needs to be adapted to account for the different number of locations from which the underlying joint probabilities are estimated.

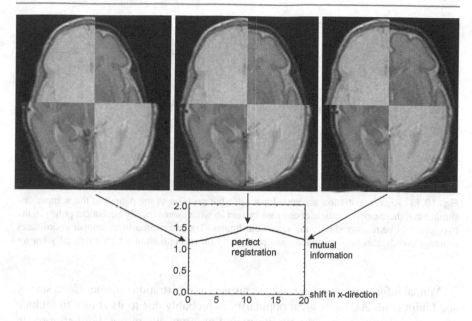

Fig. 10.11 Mutual information for differently shifted MR images (proton density and T2-weighted). Although the two images are quite dissimilar, mutual information shows a pronounced minimum, if registration is perfect

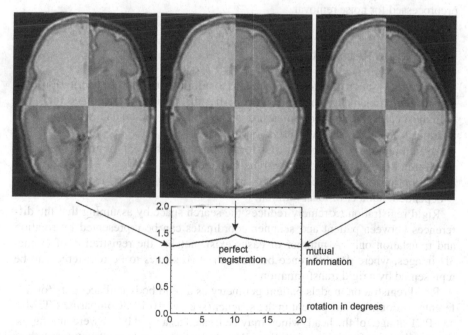

Fig. 10.12 Mutual information for differently rotated versions of the images from Fig. 10.11. Again, there is a pronounced maximum if registration is perfect

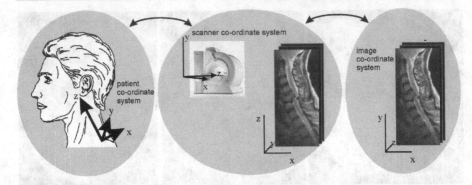

Fig. 10.13 Rigid registration accounts for a different position of the patient in the scanner, assuming that there exists a patient coordinate system in which semantically equivalent points in the two scenes to be registered have the same coordinates. Transformation from scanner coordinates in image coordinates involves scaling and potentially mirroring both of which are usually known before

Mutual information has been used in numerous registration schemes (for a survey see Pluim et al. 2003). Its great popularity is probably due to its ability to include all image information into the similarity and its simplicity of use. Furthermore, an extensive investigation about the accuracy of registration methods has found mutual information to deliver the best results (West et al. 1997; Fitzpatrick et al. 1998). Since the quality of the measure deteriorates with increasing noise, images are often preprocessed for noise removal.

10.2   Rigid Registration

Finding a registration transformation means to minimize the similarity criterion. The registration problem has a number of properties that have to be accounted for.

- In most cases, the similarity measure is an estimate based on data with noise and artefacts and a model that overly simplifies reality.
- An infinitely large number of transformations exist, but only a finite number of information pieces constrain the transformation.
- The optimization functions listed in the previous chapter have an image-dependent number of local minima.

Rigid registration extremely reduces the search space by assuming that the differences between patient and scanner coordinates can be represented by rotation and translation only. A number of cases exist, notably the registration of cranial 3D images, where the difference between the two scenes to be registered can be represented by a rigid transformation.

Rigid registration models patient geometry as a rigid body and accounts for different positioning of the patient in the scanner (see Fig. 10.13). Comparing CT, MR, and PET images of the head, which may be treated as a rigid body, were among the first applications for rigid registration. Registration of other bone structures such as the vertebrae may be represented by rigid registration as well.

Fig. 10.14 The naive registration algorithm would compute the transformation by solving a linear equation system from coordinates (x, y, z) from four pairs of landmarks $(\mathbf{p}, \mathbf{q})$

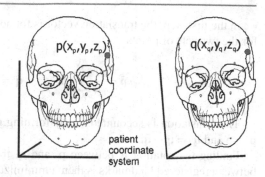

patient coordinate system

Registration usually does not account for scaling (which happens when transforming from scanner coordinates to image coordinates), as most 3D imaging devices provide information about the size of a voxel.

The unknown transformation can be described by

$$
\begin{pmatrix} y_1 \\ y_2 \\ y_3 \end{pmatrix} = \mathbf{R} \times \begin{pmatrix} x_1 \\ x_2 \\ x_3 \end{pmatrix} + \mathbf{t} \quad \text{with } \mathbf{R} = \begin{pmatrix} r_{11} & r_{21} & r_{31} \\ r_{12} & r_{22} & r_{32} \\ r_{13} & r_{23} & r_{33} \end{pmatrix} \text{ and } \mathbf{t} = \begin{pmatrix} d_1 \\ d_2 \\ d_3 \end{pmatrix},
$$

$$(10.12)$$

where $\mathbf{R}$ is a rotation matrix and $\mathbf{t}$ a translation vector. Solving the task amounts to solving linear equations with a total of 12 unknowns (9 for the rotation and 3 for the translation). A straightforward solution would be to determine pairs of four extrinsic or intrinsic markers $\{\mathbf{p}_1, \mathbf{p}_2, \mathbf{p}_3, \mathbf{p}_4\}$ and $\{\mathbf{q}_1, \mathbf{q}_2, \mathbf{q}_3, \mathbf{q}_4\}$ such that $\mathbf{p}_i$ should map onto $\mathbf{q}_i$ for $i = 1, \ldots, 4$ (see Fig. 10.14). Using the coincidence correspondence criterion c_c the registration transformation can be found by equating corresponding landmarks via the transformation in (10.12) and solving for the unknowns.

The result would be unsatisfactory because the landmark positions will not be exact. A better solution would be to require a larger number of corresponding landmarks and solving the overdetermined equation system using a minimum norm strategy. It corresponds to using the average minimum distance similarity S_d.

This would still not be satisfactory because the computed matrix $\mathbf{R}$ may not be a rotation matrix introducing unwanted shear and scaling into the registration. The nine coefficients of the rotation matrix are not independent of each other, as a rotation has only three degrees of freedom: two angles for describing an axis around which rotation takes place and the rotation angle around this axis. A matrix is a rotation matrix if it is orthonormal with a determinant of 1.

A closed-form solution for a large number of correspondence pairs of landmarks that ensures orthonormality of $\mathbf{R}$ has been presented by Arun et al. (1987). Two sets $\mathbf{p}_i$ and $\mathbf{q}_i$, $I = 1, N$ of corresponding pairs of points—called *paired landmarks*—shall be registered with respect to each other using rotation and translation. The Procrustes distance of the similarity criterion S_d is to be used for minimizing the average distance between corresponding locations after registration.

In the first step, the translation vector is found by computing the expected values for the two sets of points

$$\bar{\mathbf{p}} = \frac{1}{N}\sum_{i=1}^{N}\mathbf{p}_i, \qquad \bar{\mathbf{q}} = \frac{1}{N}\sum_{i=1}^{N}\mathbf{q}_i. \tag{10.13}$$

The translation is accounted for by forming new point sets $\mathbf{p}'$ and $\mathbf{q}'$ with $\mathbf{p}' = \mathbf{p} - \bar{\mathbf{p}}$ and $\mathbf{q}' = \mathbf{q} - \bar{\mathbf{q}}$.

Finding the rotation $\mathbf{R}$ between $\mathbf{p}'$ and $\mathbf{q}'$ that minimizes the average distance between registered landmarks is then a minimization task

$$\mathbf{R}_{\text{opt}} = \arg\min_{\mathbf{R}} \sum_{i=1}^{N} \|\mathbf{p}'_i - \mathbf{q}'_i \cdot \mathbf{R}\|^2 = \sum_{i=1}^{n} \mathbf{p}_i'^{\mathrm{T}} \cdot \mathbf{p}'_i + \mathbf{q}_i'^{\mathrm{T}} \cdot \mathbf{q}'_i - 2 \cdot \left(\mathbf{p}_i'^{\mathrm{T}} \cdot \mathbf{R} \cdot \mathbf{q}'_i\right). \tag{10.14}$$

The term $\sum_{i=1}^{N} \|\mathbf{p}'_i - \mathbf{q}'_i \cdot \mathbf{R}\|^2$ is sometimes called *fiducial registration error*. The landmarks to be matched are called *fiducial markers*.

Minimizing (10.14) means maximizing $\sum_{i=1}^{N} \mathbf{p}_i'^{\mathrm{T}} \cdot \mathbf{R} \cdot \mathbf{q}'_i$ since the other terms do not depend on $\mathbf{R}$. Arun showed that this rotation matrix can be found from a singular value decomposition of $\mathbf{D} = \mathbf{U}\boldsymbol{\Lambda}\mathbf{V}^{\mathrm{T}} = \sum_{i=1}^{N} \mathbf{p}'_i \cdot \mathbf{q}_i'^{\mathrm{T}}$. The rotation matrix is $\mathbf{R} = \mathbf{V}\mathbf{U}^{\mathrm{T}}$. The matrix is orthonormal, but may have a determinant with value -1 in which case the transformation is a rotation that is mirrored at the origin. This should be checked because it indicates severe displacement errors of landmarks or a distribution of landmarks that allows for several different mappings with similar similarity values.

Horn (1987) presented another closed-form solution for registering point sets $\mathbf{p}$ and $\mathbf{q}$ using *unit quaternions* for representing the rotation. A *quaternion* has one real and three imaginary parts and is denoted by $q = r + a \cdot i + b \cdot j + c \cdot k$ with i, j, k being the three imaginary parts. Quaternions may also be written as vectors $\mathbf{q} = (r\ a\ b\ c)$. Unit quaternions (i.e., quaternions $\mathbf{q}_r$ with $\|\mathbf{q}_r\| = 1$) have only three independent variables and can be used for representing rotations in 3D space. A 3D rotation of a vector $(x_1\ x_2\ x_3)$ in quaternion algebra requires the vector to be represented as quaternion $(0\ x_1\ x_2\ x_3)$. Rotation around a vector $\mathbf{r}$ with angle α is then

$$\begin{pmatrix} 0 \\ y_1 \\ y_2 \\ y_3 \end{pmatrix} = \begin{pmatrix} 0 \\ x_1 \\ x_2 \\ x_3 \end{pmatrix} \cdot \begin{pmatrix} \cos\alpha/2 \\ r_1\sin\alpha/2 \\ r_2\sin\alpha/2 \\ r_3\sin\alpha/2 \end{pmatrix} \cdot \begin{pmatrix} 0 \\ -x_1 \\ -x_2 \\ -x_3 \end{pmatrix}. \tag{10.15}$$

For given sets of points $\mathbf{p}'$ and $\mathbf{q}'$ that are corrected for translation and scaling, Horn showed that the optimal rotation minimizing the average displacement error has components of the eigenvector corresponding to the largest eigenvalue of a 4×4 matrix $\mathbf{Q}$ that is computed as follows:

$$\mathbf{Q}(\mathbf{S}_{pq}) = \begin{pmatrix} \text{tr}(\mathbf{S}_{pq}) & \boldsymbol{\Delta}_{pq}^{\mathrm{T}} \\ \boldsymbol{\Delta}_{pq} & \mathbf{S}_{pq} + \mathbf{S}_{pq}^{\mathrm{T}} - \text{tr}(\mathbf{S}_{pq}) \cdot \mathbf{I}_{3\times 3} \end{pmatrix}, \tag{10.16}$$

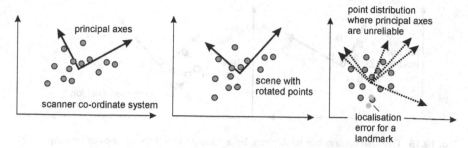

Fig. 10.15 Principal axes generated from landmarks can act as a patient coordinate system, if the landmark distribution is sufficiently anisotropic. Otherwise, the axes orientation may depend on small changes of landmark positions (which may be caused from localization errors)

where

$$S_{pq} = \begin{pmatrix} s_{11} & s_{21} & s_{31} \\ s_{12} & s_{22} & s_{32} \\ s_{13} & s_{23} & s_{33} \end{pmatrix} = \sum_{i=1}^{n} \mathbf{p}_i' \cdot \mathbf{q}_i'^{\mathrm{T}} \quad \text{and} \quad \Delta_{pq} = (s_{23} \quad s_{31} \quad s_{12})^{\mathrm{T}}, \quad (10.17)$$

and tr() is the trace of a matrix. $\mathbf{I}_{3 \times 3}$ is a 3×3 identity matrix.

The use of quaternions avoids the ambiguity of orthonormal rotation matrices that may or may not include a mirroring at the origin. It has the disadvantage that it can only be applied for 3D scenes.

The methods of Arun and Horn require paired landmarks. If this cannot be guaranteed, another strategy using principal component analysis (PCA, see Sect. 14.3) can be used for producing the average minimum distance between registered landmarks (Toennies et al. 1990). The idea is quite simple. If landmarks represent a structure of a suitably irregular shape, the origin and principal axes of the landmark distribution represent a unique patient-specific coordinate system with respect to some common world coordinate system (in this case, the scanner coordinate system, see Fig. 10.15). The registration transform is given by first translating the landmarks into the origin of the world coordinate system and then rotating them according to the principal axes.

The translation between the two systems is given as in the previously described method of Arun et al. (1987). Given a matrix of eigenvectors $\mathbf{E}_p$ and $\mathbf{E}_q$ from the PCA of the two points sets $\mathbf{p}$ and $\mathbf{q}$ the rotation is then

$$\mathbf{R}_{\mathrm{opt}} = \mathbf{E}_p \mathbf{E}_q, \quad (10.18)$$

assuming that eigenvalues in $\mathbf{\Lambda}_p$ and $\mathbf{\Lambda}_q$ correspond. This should be the case if the point distributions of $\mathbf{p}$ and $\mathbf{q}$ represent the same shape.

Using the PCA decomposition does not require paired landmarks, which makes it also applicable in cases where landmark curves or landmark surfaces shall be registered. It comes at a price, however. PCA-based registration will fail if the shape of the point distribution is approximately spherical. In such case, all three eigenval-

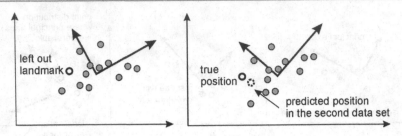

Fig. 10.16 Potential outliers can be detected by a variant of the leaving-one-out technique. The predicted position of the left-out landmark with respect to all other landmarks is measured and compared with the true position. If the difference is too large, the landmark pair is marked as potential outliers

ues will be approximately equal and orientation from eigenvectors will mainly be governed by noise and artefacts.

The strategies described above rely on two sets of corresponding points among which a transformation shall be found. If the number of points is small, noise and outliers may affect the result. If paired landmarks are to be registered, the influence of noise may be estimated by computing the average and maximum distances between corresponding points of the two data sets after registration. If the PCA is used, noise influence can be estimated from differences of corresponding eigenvalues.

Outliers (i.e., landmarks with grossly wrong locations) should also be accounted for. They may remain undetected in automatic landmark computation as their detection requires the two scenes to be registered. Outliers may be found by comparing distances between registered landmark pairs. The distance between corresponding landmarks, of which one is an outlier, should substantially vary from the distance between other pairs of landmarks. Outlier pairs should be removed.

Outlier detection for paired landmarks can also be done using a variant of the leaving-one-out technique in classification. A pair of landmarks is removed from the two landmark distributions and a registration transformation is computed without it. The resulting transformation is applied to the removed pair of landmarks and the distance between the two landmarks after registration is measured (see Fig. 10.16). It is marked for removal if the distance exceeds some threshold. After repeating this procedure for all pairs, those marked for removal are eliminated.

Outlier detection for unpaired landmarks can also be done using the leaving-one-out technique. In this case, single landmarks are removed before registration and the registration transformation is applied to this landmark. Its distance to the closest point in the other set of landmarks is computed. The landmark is marked as outlier, if the distance exceeds some maximum distance. The process is less reliable if distances between adjacent landmarks within a set of landmarks vary widely.

Outlier detection and removal should be iterated until no further outliers are detected or the number of landmarks is too small for a reliable registration.

If it is known that objects in the two scenes f and g to be registered have the same intensity (e.g., when images from the same scanner taken at different times shall be registered), rigid registration for 2D scenes may also be carried out in the frequency

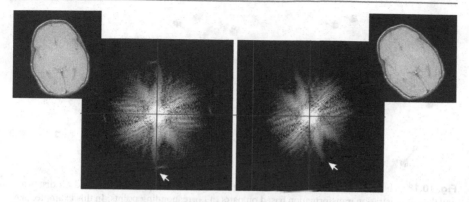

Fig. 10.17 The *image on the right* has been rotated by 20° and translated by 20 pixels in *x*-direction. Only the rotation shows up in the spectrum in frequency space

domain (Reddy and Chatterji 1996). Translating an object changes the phase but not the spectrum (amplitude) of the signal in frequency domain. The rotation around the origin in the spatial domain corresponds to a rotation in the frequency domain (see Fig. 10.17). 2D registration in frequency space thus first estimates the rotation component. The signal is transferred into polar coordinates. The rotation in Cartesian coordinates around the origin corresponds to a translation along the angular axis in polar coordinates. The rotation angle is found by 1D cross correlation along this axis. If objects have different intensities in the two images but are visible in both, the approach also works if the gradient length image instead of the intensity image is transformed.

Computing the translation is then done either by comparing phases after rotationally registering the images in the frequency domain or by just computing displacements of intensity or gradient length in the spatial domain.

The previous methods solved the registration problem in one step. They do provide an optimal solution based on the landmarks and within the model that they use. Pelizzari's registration method for registering CT, MRI, and PET images is an alternative that registers surfaces with respect to each other based on point distances (Pelizzari et al. 1989). Compared with registering patient-specific coordinate systems from the principal axes of point distributions, the method has the advantage that local point distances directly influence the result. The method requires segmentation of a surface that is visible in the scenes to be registered and which is related to the objects to be registered in a rigid fashion.

In its original version the method was applied to register cranial images using the skin surface of the head. The method is also known as *head-hat registration*. The skin of the two scenes f and g to be registered is segmented using thresholding. The skin surface of the first scene is represented by a sequence of boundary curves in slices. It is taken as "head" of the registration algorithm. The skin of the other surface (the "hat") is represented by a dense map of surface points to be fitted to the head.

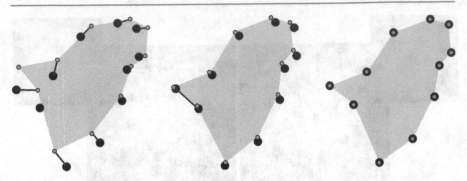

Fig. 10.18 The ICP algorithm repetitively computes point correspondences based on distances and then a registration transformation based on pairs of corresponding points. In this example, one of the correspondences is wrong at the first iteration resulting in a small registration error, which is then corrected in the second iteration where all correspondences are correct

Fitting is done iteratively using Powell's method (Press et al. 1992). Given some initial registration transformation, a new transformation is found by iteratively minimizing the distances between surface points of g to the surface f. The distances are computed by intersecting rays from points in g to the center of inertia of the surface f with f.

Powell's method is known to get stuck in local minima. Several strategies can be used to overcome this. A simple solution would be to provide a rough registration interactively. This can be done by interactively aligning 2D projections of the skin surfaces of f and g into the xy-, xz-, and yz-planes (Grimson et al. 1996). There have also been several approaches to replace Powell's method by another minimization method, which is less sensitive to the initial transformation (Xu and Dony 2004).

The *iterative closest point (ICP) algorithm* of Besl and McKay (1992) is more general than the method described above (see Fig. 10.18). Rigid registration can be applied to point sets, implicit and parametric curves and surfaces, as well as to faceted surfaces. The two scenes f and g may be surfaces or volumes. The scene f is called the data to which the model g has to be fitted. Fitting minimizes the distances of data points to the model that may be described by a variety of different representations.

Algorithms for computing the distance of a data point to the model need to be given for various model representations. If the model is a point, it is simply the Euclidian distance; if it is a cloud of points, then it is the distance to its closest point. If it is a parametric surface (e.g., a spline), distance computation depends on the type of surface. A closed-form solution may no longer exist. The distance for some implicit surfaces may be computed by inserting the point coordinates into the surface equation. For each of the measures a method has to be given to return the closest point $CP(p_i, q_j)$ in the model component q_j to a data point p_i.

Given $CP(p_i, q_j)$, an initial transformation $T^{(0)}$ has to be defined. The iterative loop proceeds as follows.

- Given a transformation $T^{(n)}$ at iteration n, this transformation is applied to the data points $\mathbf{p}_i$.
- Compute the set of all $q_i = CP(\mathbf{p}_i, T^{(n)} \circ \mathbf{q}_j)$ for the transformed data points.
- Find optimal rotation and translation of $T^{(n+1)}$ using either the method of Arun et al. (1987) or Horn (1987) above.

The algorithm terminates when the improvement in the result quality falls below some preset threshold. The quality of the result depends on the initial transformation and on the distribution of the landmark points or regions. Even though Arun et al. (1987) and Horn (1987) provided optimal solutions, this is only true for paired landmarks. The ICP algorithm iterates through different configurations of correspondence pairs and it is not guaranteed that it terminates with a correct pairing. If landmarks are distributed on some irregular surface or if the initial transformation is close to the desired result, it is less likely that the process terminates in a local minimum.

The ICP algorithm for iterative rigid registration is the most general of all registration algorithms presented so far and numerous adaptations using different similarity criteria, optimization criteria, and preprocessing routines have been published. A survey about the various adaptations can be found in Rusinkiewicz and Levoy (2001).

10.3 Registration of Projection Images to 3D Data

Although the majority of computer-assisted image analysis is carried out on data with three or more dimensions, the majority of images created in clinical routines are still projection images. Registering, say, a 2D fluoroscopy taken during a surgical intervention to a 3D x-ray CT scan from preoperative planning poses some additional problems because of the information reduction from 3D to 2D.

As there is no information about localization along the projection ray in a projection image, the registration attempts to find a projection $P(f)$ of the 3D image f such that $P(f)$ registers with the projection image g. The artificial projection $P(f)$ is called *digitally reconstructed radiograph* (DRR). All possible DRRs can be assigned to locations on a sphere. This location can be specified by two angles (θ, τ) (see Fig. 10.19). Registration has to find a location $(\theta, \tau)_{\min}$ such that $DRR((\theta, \tau)_{\min})$ produces the most similar image to g. Similarity criteria can be the Procrustes distance between landmark points or curves in $P(f)$ and g or an intensity criterion.

Using a landmark such as the curves of Lavallée and Szelinski (1995) has the advantage that it is fast. Only segmented curves or points need to be projected instead of creating the complete DRR. Furthermore, the similarity measure is independent of the appearance of a projected point. It does, however, require segmentation, which may be tedious or even impossible to integrate into the workflow of a surgical intervention.

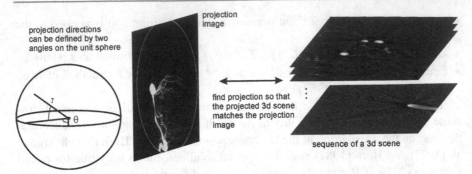

Fig. 10.19 Registration of a projection image to a 3d scene requires finding a projection of the 3d scene that matches the projection image

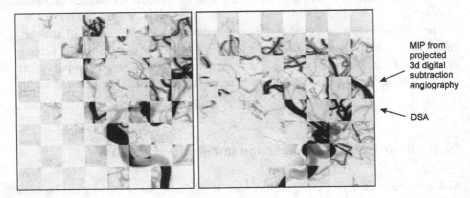

Fig. 10.20 Two views of registering 3d reconstructed DSA with projection DSA. The registration was necessary to map flow information from dynamic projection images to static 3d images (Hentschke et al. 2010)

Using similarities based on intensities such as intensity correlation, gradient correlation, mean absolute difference, or mutual information relieves the user from providing segmented scenes.[2] If the two scenes f and g are created using the same kind of measurement signal (e.g., CT and fluoroscopy), all of the criteria mentioned above should produce good results (see Fig. 10.20 for an example of registering DSA with 3D reconstructed digital angiography). However, two influences may contribute to the degradation of the criterion.

- Noise will affect gradient-based criteria more than intensity averaging criteria such as mutual information or intensity correlation.
- The depiction of surgical instruments in an intervention scenario will typically have a high contrast. As these instruments may not have been present at the preoperative scan, they are artefacts to the similarity criterion. Moreover, as they may

[2]Different similarity measures in 2d to 3d registration have been compared in Penney et al. (1998).

move during intervention, they cannot be easily accounted for by some preoperative calibration step.

If the images are from different types of acquisition systems (e.g., when comparing an MRI with a fluoroscopic image, criteria should be based on intensity edges rather than on intensities). It may still be unsuccessful if the two scenes do not possess enough common object boundaries. A pattern-based criterion, which covers the matching quality only in a region of interest, may solve this problem partially if this region is visible in the two scenes. Such a criterion was presented by Weese et al. (1997) who assumed that a segmentation in a preoperative scan—in their application it was a CT scan of the vertebrae—has been carried out that separated a structure of interest—a vertebra in their case—from the background. The DRR is created from the structure of interest. The matching criterion is applied only to this region. Given a region $(x, y) \in O$ of a projected structure and a neighborhood N_r with radius r around every pixel, the pattern intensity criterion is

$$S_{\text{pattern}} = \sum_{(x,y)\in O} \sum_{(u,v)\in N} \frac{\sigma^2}{\sigma^2 + ([P(f)(x, y) - g(x, y)] - [P(f)(u, v) - g(u, v)])^2}.$$

(10.19)

The criterion measures the amount of variation in the difference image $P(f)(x, y)$ in some neighborhood N_r. According to the authors, a neighborhood radius of three to five pixels was a good compromise between suppressing noise and saving computation time. The parameter σ^2 controls the influence of local contrast on the result. It should be higher than the noise variance and lower than the contrast between edges and texture within the structure of interest.

Creating the projection images from the 3D scene is time-consuming, although this has improved with the use of efficient light field techniques borrowed from computer graphics (Russakoff et al. 2003).

Searching the parameter space (θ, τ) may be difficult because the closeness of projection parameters does not necessarily imply similar values of the similarity criterion. This applies for the projection of curves as well as for intensity projections. On the other hand, widely different projection angles may produce similar images. This is the case when objects have a regular shape such as a sphere or when projections along opposite directions are compared. The former requires the initial guess of the projection direction to be close to the true projection direction. The latter may cause a projection direction not to be found even if the initial guess is good.

Several strategies exist to deal with this problem. A multiresolution semiexhaustive search has been applied by Cyr et al. (2000). They borrowed from aspect graph techniques used for 3D object recognition from 2D views. Projections of f are treated as aspects of f of which one registers with g. Initially, the sphere of projection direction is sampled at a coarse resolution and projections are computed for each of the sampled directions. The projection images are compared with g and directions along which projections are in good agreement with g are sampled at a finer rate. The process terminates when no further improvement is observed.

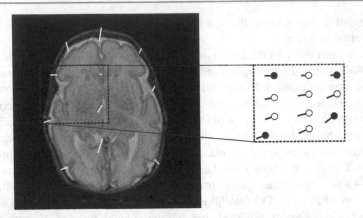

Fig. 10.21 For non-rigid registration, displacement vectors d are computed at selected locations. A smoothness constraint enforces similarity between neighboring displacement vectors and allows to interpolate displacement at locations, where no vector has been computed

Computing a matching quality based on intensity is only suitable if an assumed projection direction is close to the searched projection direction. Otherwise, the quality criterion may not hint toward the kind of change necessary for improving the registration transformation. Selecting landmarks solves this problem, but it requires their segmentation in f and g. This may be difficult for the projection image g. The solution of Cyr et al. (2000) is based on concepts of shape recognition. They use the shock graphs of segmented regions in the projection images $P(f)$ and g. A shock graph is a kind of medial axis representation where region boundaries are described by shock waves originating at the axis. A hierarchy of shocks of increasing order encodes various levels of detail of the region boundary. Similarity is computed by comparing shock graphs derived from $P(f)$ and g. It is not a simple process as it involves assigning shocks to each other in some optimal fashion and has been solved by a stochastic optimization technique similar to simulated annealing described in Sect. 14.1.

10.4   Search Space and Optimization in Nonrigid Registration

If rigidity cannot be assumed, the search space for a possible registration increases drastically. The problem is virtually unsolvable if nothing can be assumed about the transformation, except that a displacement field $\mathbf{d}(\mathbf{x})$ exists for every point $\mathbf{x}$ that maps $f(\mathbf{x})$ to its corresponding $g(\mathbf{x} + \mathbf{d}(\mathbf{x}))$. Even if some similarity criterion exists for confirming correspondence, it does not uniquely identify a displacement field. Surveys about nonrigid registration can be found in Dawant (2002) and Lester and Arridge (1999).

The necessary information for solving a nonrigid registration problem comes from the reasonable assumption that topology is preserved by the displacement field. It introduces a smoothness constraint for computing $\mathbf{d}$ (see Fig. 10.21). Various types of smoothness have been introduced.

- A linear elastic model enforces the smoothness of displacement that is proportional to the displacement (Bajcy et al. 1983; Rexilius et al. 2001).
- A viscous fluid model enforces smoothness that depends on the evolution of displacement (Lester et al. 1999).
- Registration can be modeled as free form deformation of different kinds of splines (Rueckert et al. 1999; Chui and Rangarajan 2003).
- Displacement vector similarity globally minimizes an arbitrary penalizing term for local similarity (Brox et al. 2004).

In *elastic registration* the scene is modeled as elastic surface or space that may be deformed but not cut by external forces. Deforming a scene by attraction from some external force is counteracted by forces toward the rest configuration of the elastic scene. External forces impose local similarity constraints between image f and the deformed registered image g. Elastic matching in 2D and 3D has been proposed for atlas-based segmentation by Bajcy et al. (1983) and Bajcy and Kovacic (1989) and has been used in various registration applications. The elastic model balances the image force $\mathbf{i}_{force}$ against displacement $\mathbf{d}$ depending on the gradient of the divergence of $\mathbf{d}$ and the local Laplacian ∇^2 of $\mathbf{d}$:

$$\mu \cdot \nabla^2 \mathbf{d}(\mathbf{x}) + (\mu + \beta) \cdot \nabla(\nabla \cdot \mathbf{d}(\mathbf{x})) = \mathbf{i}_{force}(\mathbf{x}). \tag{10.20}$$

The parameters μ and β are Lamé's constants representing the elasticity and stiffness with high values for μ indicating strong elasticity.

A *viscous fluid model* constrains deformation differently allowing for inhomogeneous displacement changes. It is particularly appropriate if some deformation should be varying (e.g., when a nonrigid registration should model organ displacement due to surgical intervention). In the viscous fluid model current velocity $\mathbf{v}(\mathbf{x})$ is driving the deformation

$$\mu \cdot \nabla^2 \mathbf{v}(\mathbf{x}) + (\mu + \beta) \cdot \nabla(\nabla \cdot \mathbf{v}(\mathbf{x})) = \mathbf{i}_{force}(\mathbf{x}). \tag{10.21}$$

Current velocity at some time t has to be computed from the change of displacement vectors making the computation more costly than that of the elasticity model.

Using either of the physical models has the advantage that optimization can be done by solving the differential equation iteratively. For a given displacement field and a given model, the force at every point $\mathbf{x}$ is derived from the mismatch of internal and external forces. Their difference is a vector along which a point $\mathbf{x}$ is moving. The iterative procedure is continued until equilibrium is reached.

Using *free-form deformation* employs a smoothness model given by a differentiable free-form surface or volume that may deform under an external influence from the image. Model smoothness is given by minimizing the second derivative across the surface. Image influence is a similarity criterion S such as mutual information, which is defined locally around the control points of the free-form surface or volume. Given a smoothness constraint D, the registration problem is to find a displacement field $\mathbf{d}_{min}$ so that

$$\mathbf{d}_{min} = \arg\min_{\mathbf{d}} S(f(\mathbf{x}), g(\mathbf{x} + \mathbf{d}(\mathbf{x}))) + \gamma D(\mathbf{x}). \tag{10.22}$$

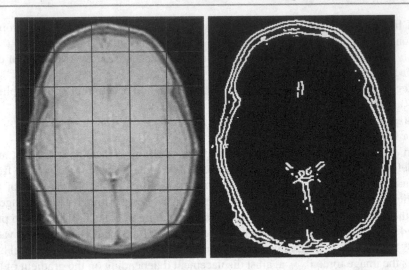

Fig. 10.22 Displacement vector computation is usually restricted to some locations such as equally sampled node locations (**a**) or feature locations (**b**)

The parameter γ governs the influence of the smoothness constraint $D(\mathbf{x})$. Minimizing the function is done iteratively starting from a good initial guess usually provided by a preceding rigid registration.

Neighborhood similarity of displacement vectors (Brox et al. 2004) does not depend on a physical model. Apart from this, it is similar to the previous strategy. It minimizes an arbitrary function penalizing nonsmoothness. This can be an interpolating function such as in the classical optical flow formulation of Horn (1986), where the square of the differences between adjacent displacements is minimized, or a strictly noninterpolating function such as (4.52) presented in Sect. 4.3.4. Optical flow techniques may be supported by local heuristics such as the block matching proposed in Ourselin et al. (2000).

In principle, displacement vectors can be computed for every point in discrete space. To speed up the process, similarity computation may be constrained to a subset of locations (see Fig. 10.22). These may either be created from a subsampling of the data (as was done in early methods like Bajcy and Kovacic 1989) or they may be selected at locations of interest such as edges. The transformation between sample locations is then predicted from sample point transformations and the particular smoothness model.

Optimizing (10.22) as well as optimization from applying a physical model suffers from the many local minima of the function as well as from the fact that the smoothness term may not adequately reflect the true displacement variation in the vicinity of some point. It is advisable to begin the registration with a rigid registration that produces an initial estimate for $\mathbf{d}_{\min}(\mathbf{x})$, which is done by most authors.

Parameters for elasticity or viscosity in the methods described above are homogeneous throughout the scene. This may be adequate if displacements are small. Additional information is needed to model inhomogeneous displacement if larger displacements between f and g are expected. This has been done for modeling displacement fields in preoperative and intraoperative MR scans in computer-assisted surgery (e.g., Lester et al. 1999; Rexilius et al. 2001; du Bois d'Aische et al. 2005) and for registering 2D images from different modalities (du Bois d'Aische et al. 2005). Information about organ boundaries can be used to assign an inhomogeneous material field as input for registration.

10.5 Normalization

Registration as described in the previous sections refers to the comparison of information of the same subject obtained from different modalities or taken at different times. Smoothness and similarity constraints imposed on the registration transformation are justified since topology can be assumed to be preserved. This is no longer true if images of different subjects are to be matched. The two main reasons necessitating intersubject matching are as follows.

- Images are taken from a group of subjects, and statistical analysis shall be carried out on variation of appearance in the images of some medically relevant feature.
- A scene f shall be mapped onto an atlas g containing model information for interpreting f.

The term normalization stems from the former. To carry out spatially resolved statistical analysis across patients, the anatomy is mapped onto some "norm anatomy," which provides a reference system. Atlas mapping can be seen as a normalization task as well with the difference that the norm is already given (the atlas) and mapping has to be found by which a scene can be mapped onto the norm anatomy.

The reasonable assumptions in registration that corresponding points exist in the two scenes, that correspondence is unique and complete, and that topology is preserved do not apply to normalization. It may even be difficult to establish what is meant by correspondence. The purpose of normalization in intersubject studies is to study functional behavior in itself and with respect to anatomy. Hence, the same function should be performed at corresponding locations in f and g. In functional brain imaging, however, which is one of the major applications of normalization, it is known that anatomy is quite different for different individuals. Defining corresponding locations by means of the morphology and appearance of anatomy is not necessarily successful. Even if there would be common architecture of anatomy in all humans, its appearance is related to the cell level which cannot be depicted by most imaging devices. Regarding the functional architecture of the brain, it has been found that correspondences at the cell level do not necessarily infer shape correspondence on the level of sulci and gyrii (Roland et al. 1997).

The normalization of human brain anatomy based on similarity of appearance usually neglects this knowledge, assuming that function and morphology coincide at a coarse level of spatial resolution. Under this assumption, normalization is a transformation into *Talairach coordinates*. The coordinate system (depicted in Fig. 10.23)—also called *stereotaxic coordinate system*—was established by Talairach and Tournoux (1988) for a normalized localization of functional Brodman

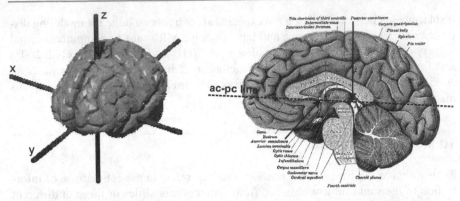

Fig. 10.23 The Talairach coordinate system is defined by the ac-pc line and the mid-sagittal plane that separates the two brain hemispheres (the *picture on the left* uses a version of plate 720 of Gray's Anatomy as published in Wikimedia under Creative Commons licence)

areas. The origin of the Talairach coordinate system is the anterior point of the brain commissura (AC point). The y-axis of the system points to the posterior point of the commissura, its x-axis from left to right, and its z-axis from the ventral to dorsal (up-down) direction. The transformation into stereotaxic coordinates can be carried out by an affine transformation for which identification of origin, axes, and length of axes are sufficient.

The Talairach transformation is only accurate at a low spatial resolution. Human brain mapping of Brodman areas using Talairach coordinates has been used for the localization of functional areas in the brain as part of stereotactic surgery planning as well as for acquiring statistical information about human brain function from PET images.

The method has been used for normalizing functional MRI images as well, however, with increased spatial resolution it is no longer deemed adequate as sole means of normalization. To improve the accuracy of normalization, three different strategies are followed.

- Probabilistic Talairach coordinates comprise the correspondence uncertainty of the affine Talairach transformation (Mazziotta et al. 1995).
- The application of nonrigid registration methods increases the range of acceptable transformations.
- ROI-based registration reduces the normalization to a region-of-interest.

The use of probabilistic coordinates acknowledges the uncertainty in the Talairach transformation, but it does not offer a solution. It will improve statistical analysis, however, if the statistical base for estimated probabilities is less biased or more reliable than data from experiments on a possibly small number of subjects.

Using nonrigid registration methods based on a smoothness model about the displacement field would truly solve the normalization problem. This is the method of choice when normalization is used for atlas-based classification and segmentation. The atlas provides a spatial label distribution, which is then mapped on the patient data (it is a kind of backward normalization).

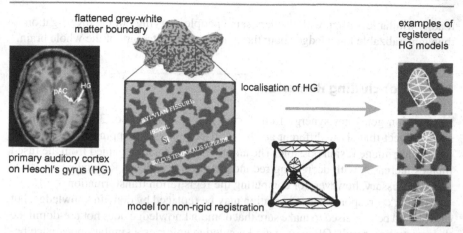

Fig. 10.24 Partial normalization of Heschl's gyrus based on non-rigid registration with a deformable model (see Engel et al. 2005)

However, nonrigid registration requires that a correspondence criterion is established and that the smoothness constraint on the displacement field reflects the true displacement characteristics. Both conditions are difficult to assert for normalization. Describing correspondence and smoothness in atlas matching is probably easier than for functional brain mapping, as the atlas consists of a relatively uniform distribution of labels. It may not matter to what location a certain boundary point in the atlas is mapped in the image as long as it is mapped on the boundary of the same object. The goal is not to map equally functioning cells onto each other, but only to assign correct labels and delineate correct boundaries. Any of the criterions based on intensities discussed in the previous sections should be sufficient, provided that the general conditions such as a good first guess are met. Hence, image analysis based on matched atlas data applied nonrigid registration techniques quite successfully (Sandor and Leahy 1997; Cootes et al. 1999).

Using nonrigid registration for normalizing functional brain images has been attempted as well and is known as brain warping (Toga 1999). The accuracy of applying a criterion that is based on image intensity and smoothness to normalize brain structures is, however, limited. The findings of Roland et al. (1997) and others suggested that model-based constraints are required since cytoarchitecture is not adequately reflected in the images. Such a model would be difficult to create in view of the still limited knowledge about the functional architecture of the brain. Hence, the third strategy is to restrict normalization to a region of interest for which such a model might be easier to establish and use. ROI-based normalization is often carried out on surface maps of the boundary between gray matter and white matter because surfaces may be displayed for letting the user enter the model knowledge interactively. The methods for the automatic finding of functional regions of interest have been published as well (Engel et al. 2005; see Fig. 10.24). The advantage of selecting a region of interest is that expert knowledge about a single region is often more readily available—often with the very same people carrying out the investigation—than generalizable knowledge about the functional architecture of the whole brain.

10.6   Concluding Remarks

Registration generates synergy from fusing two or more 2D or 3D images of the same subject that show different attributes. It computes a mapping transformation for making image fusion possible. The amount of information gained from the fused images increases with decreasing redundancy between them. Redundant information is necessary, however, for computing the registration transformation.

Missing correspondence information may be replaced by domain knowledge, but care should be exercised to make sure that domain knowledge does not pre-dominate the registration result. Often, domain knowledge enforces a similar appearance between registered images. Hence, the result may look visually pleasing, but does not reflect the true spatial relation between locations in the two registered scenes.

The reliance of a good registration on sufficient and trustworthy redundant information between the two scenes to be registered has resulted in several attempts to combine segmentation with registration. If the same segment has been identified in the fixed and the moving image, it provides ample redundancy for registration. On the other hand, combining registered images may improve the information necessary to carry out the segmentation. For optimizing registration transformation and segmentation simultaneously, a probability is maximized to create a specific segmentation result given a transformation.

The problem is formulated as an MRF to represent domain knowledge about the expected spatial continuity for each image and between registered locations. Examples can be found in Flach et al. (2002), who described their approach from an application perspective, and in Wyatt and Noble (2003) and Pohl et al. (2006), who developed generic models that are then demonstrated by means of specific applications. The last two papers discussed the performance of the strategy and the validity of incorporated a priori knowledge as well as the potential dependencies between a priori knowledge, optimization performance, and quality of the results.

10.7   Exercises

- Consider registering CT and MR images of the head from the same patient. What kind of registration transformation would be necessary? What similarity criterion could be used and what could be used to evaluate it on the data?
- How can similarity between curves be measured if the curves are used for measuring the correspondence of the two scenes to be registered?
- Why is it unwise to assume that landmarks are in perfect correspondence after successful registration? Please give a similarity criterion that allows relaxing this condition.
- What is meant by the Procrustes distance and how is it computed?

- What are the advantages of using anatomical landmarks instead of geometrical landmarks? What are the disadvantages?
- Why should a rigid registration transform not be computed by taking the minimum number of corresponding points and solving the associated linear equation system?
- What is the advantage of using quaternions for computing a rigid registration transformation? What is a disadvantage?
- How can point correspondence be created from two sets of landmarks of which pairwise correspondence is not known? What are the assumptions that have to be met so that this approach is successful?
- How can a rigid registration be computed from two sets of landmarks without requiring their pairwise correspondence? When and why does this method fail?
- Describe a method to detect outliers for landmark-based registration.
- What feature describes the mutual information criterion? How does it differ from the stochastic sign change criterion?
- What kind of constraints can be used for making nonrigid registration solveable? What assumption is made about the data by these constraints? Describe a situation where this assumption is not true.
- How can the iterative nonrigid registration be initialized with a good guess?
- What is the result of a registration of a projection image (such as an x ray) with a 3D scene?
- Usually, registering a projection image with a 3D scene requires a good initial guess. What could be the reasons for this?
- What is the goal of normalization? How does it differ from registration?
- Which problem may arise if a nonrigid registration technique is applied for a normalization task? How could this problem be dealt with?

References

Arun KS, Huang TS, Blostein SD (1987) Least-squares fitting of two 3-D point sets. IEEE Trans Pattern Anal Mach Intell 9(5):698–700

Bajcy R, Lieberson R, Reivich M (1983) A computerized system for the elastic matching of deformed radiographic images to idealized atlas images. J Comput Assist Tomogr 7(4):618–625

Bajcy R, Kovacic S (1989) Multiresolution elastic matching. Comput Vis Graph Image Process 46(1):1–21

Besl PJ, McKay ND (1992) A method for registration of 3-d shapes. IEEE Trans Pattern Anal Mach Intell 14(2):239–256

Brown LF (1992) A survey of image registration techniques. ACM Comput Surv 24(4):325–376

Brox T, Bruhn A, Papenberg N, Weickert J (2004) High accuracy optical flow estimation based on a theory for warping. In: Proc 8th Europ conf computer vision, ECCV 2004. LNCS, vol 3024, pp 25–36

Chui H, Rangarajan A (2003) A new point matching algorithm for non-rigid registration. Comput Vis Image Underst 89:114–141

Cootes TF, Beeston C, Edwards GJ, Taylor CJ (1999) A unified framework for atlas matching using active appearance models. In: Proc 16th intl conf information processing in medical imaging IPMI'99. LNCS, vol 1613, pp 322–333

Cyr CM, Kamal AF, Sebastian TB, Kimia BB (2000) 2d-3d registration based on shape matching. In: IEEE workshop math methods in biomedical image analysis, pp 198–203

Dawant B (2002) Nonrigid registration of medical images: purpose and methods, a short survey. In: Proc IEEE intl symp biomedical imaging, pp 465–468

du Bois d'Aische A, Craene MD, Geets X, Gregoire V, Macq B, Warfield SK (2005) Efficient multi-modal dense field non-rigid registration: alignment of histological and section images. Med Image Anal 9(6):538–546

Engel K, Brechmann A, Toennies KD (2005) A two-level dynamic model for the representation and recognition of cortical folding patterns. In: IEEE intl conf image processing, ICIP2005, vol I, pp 297–300

Fitzpatrick JM, West JB, Maurer CR Jr (1998) Predicting error in rigid-body point-based registration. IEEE Trans Med Imaging 17(5):694–702

Flach B, Kask E, Schlesinger D, Skulish A (2002) Unifying registration and segmentation for multi-sensor images. In: Pattern recognition 2002. LNCS, vol 2449, pp 190–197

Grimson WEL, Ettinger GJ, White SJ, Lozano-Pérez T, Wells WM III, Kikinis R (1996) An automatic registration method for frameless stereotaxy, image guided surgery, and enhanced reality visualization. IEEE Trans Med Imaging 15(2):129–140

Hentschke CM, Serowy S, Janiga G, Rose G, Toennies KD (2010) Estimating blood flow by reprojection of 2d-DSA to 3d-RA data sets for blood flow simulations. Int J Comput Assisted Radiol Surg 5(1):342–343

Horn BKP (1986) Robot vision. MIT Press, Cambridge

Horn BKP (1987) Closed form solution of absolute orientation using unit quaternions. J Opt Soc Am A 4:629–642

Lavallée S, Szelinski R (1995) Recovering the position and orientation of free-form objects from image contours using 3d distance maps. IEEE Trans Pattern Anal Mach Intell 17(4):378–390

Lester H, Arridge SR (1999) A survey of hierarchical non-linear medical image registration. Pattern Recognit 32(1):129–149

Lester H, Arridge SR, Jansons KM, Lemieux L, Hajnal JV, Oatridge A (1999) Non-linear registration with the variable viscosity fluid algorithm. In: Proc 16th intl conf information processing in medical imaging, IPMI'99. LNCS, vol 1613, pp 238–251

Maglogiannis I (2004) Automatic segmentation and registration of dermatological images. J Math Model Anal 2(3):277–294

Maintz JBA, Viergever MA (1998) A survey of medical image registration. Med Image Anal 2(1):1–36

Mazziotta JC, Toga AW, Evans A, Fox P, Lancaster J (1995) A probabilistic atlas of the human brain: theory and rationale for its development. Neuroimage 2(2):89–101

Modersitzki J (2003) Numerical methods for image registration. Oxford University Press, London

Ourselin S, Roche A, Prima S, Ayache N (2000) Block matching: a general framework to improve robustness of rigid registration of medical images. In: Medical image computing and computer-assisted intervention—MICCAI 2000. LNCS, vol 1935

Pelizzari CA, Chen GT, Spelbring DR, Weichselbaum RR, Chen CT (1989) Accurate three-dimensional registration of CT, PET, and/or MR images of the brain. J Comput Assist Tomogr 13(1):20–26

Penney GP, Weese J, Little JA, Desmedt P, Hill DLG, Hawkes DJ (1998) A comparison of similarity measures for use in 2-d–3-d medical image registration. IEEE Trans Med Imaging 17(4):586–595

Pluim JBW, Maintz JBA, Viergever MA (2003) Mutual-information based registration of medical images: a survey. IEEE Trans Med Imaging 22(8):986–1004

Pohl KM, Fisher J, Grimson WEL, Kikinis R, Wells WM (2006) A Bayesian model for joint segmentation and registration. NeuroImage 31:228–239

Press WH, Flannery BP, Teukolsky SA, Vetterling WT (1992) Numerical recipes in C: the art of scientific computing, 2nd edn. Cambridge University Press, Cambridge

Reddy BS, Chatterji BN (1996) An FFT-based technique for translation, rotation, and scale-invariant image registration. IEEE Trans Image Process 5(8):1266–1271

Rexilius J, Warfield SK, Guttmann CRG, Wei X, Benson R, Wolfson L, Shenton M, Handels H, Kikinis K (2001) A novel nonrigid registration algorithm and applications. In: Proc 4th intl conf medical image computing and computer-assisted intervention—MICCAI 2001. LNCS, vol 2208, pp 923–931

Roland PE, Geyer S, Amunts K, Schormann T, Schleicher A, Malikovic A, Zilles K (1997) Cytoarchitectural maps of the human brain in standard anatomical space. Hum Brain Mapp 5:222–227

Rueckert D, Sonoda LI, Hayes C, Hill DLG, Leach MO, Hawkes DJ (1999) Nonrigid registration using free-form deformations: application to breast MR images. IEEE Trans Med Imaging 18(8):712–721

Rusinkiewicz S, Levoy M (2001) Efficient variants of the ICP algorithm. In: 3rd intl conf 3-d imaging and modelling (3DIM'01), pp 145–152

Russakoff DB, Rohlfing T, Maurer CR Jr (2003) Fast intensity-based 2d-3d image registration of clinical data using light fields. In: Proc 9th intl conf computer vision (ICCV2003), pp 416–422

Sandor S, Leahy R (1997) Surface-based labelling of cortical anatomy using a deformable atlas. IEEE Trans Med Imaging 16(1):41–54

Talairach J, Tournoux P (1988) Co-planar stereotaxic atlas of the human brain: 3-dimensional proportional system—an approach to cerebral imaging. Thieme, Stuttgart

Toga AW (1999) Brain warping. Academic Press, San Diego

Toennies KD, Udupa JK, Herman GT, Wornum IL III, Buchman SR (1990) Registration of 3-d objects and surfaces. IEEE Comput Graph Appl 10(3):52–62

Venot A, Leclerc V (1984) Automated correction of patient motion and gray values prior to subtraction in digitized angiography. IEEE Trans Med Imaging 3(4):179–186

Weese J, Penney GP, Buzug TM, Fassnacht C, Lorenz C (1997) 2D/3D registration of pre-operative CT images and intra-operative X-ray projections for image guided surgery. In: Proc intl symp computer assisted radiology and surgery (CARS97), pp 833–838

West J, Fitzpatrick JM et al (1997) Comparison and evaluation of retrospective intermodality brain image registration techniques. J Comput Assist Tomogr 21(4):554–568

Wyatt PP, Noble JA (2003) MAP MRF joint segmentation and registration of medical images. Med Image Anal 7:539–552

Xu X, Dony RD (2004) Differential evolution with Powell's direction set method in medical image registration. IEEE Int Symp Biomed Imaging I:732–735

Zitova B, Flusser J (2003) Image registration methods: a survey. Image Vis Comput 21(11):977–1000

Detection and Segmentation by Shape and Appearance

11

Abstract

Object detection in medical image analysis can be modeled as a search for an object model in the image. The model describes attributes such as shape and the appearance of the object. The search consists of fitting instances of the model to the data. A quality-of-fit measure determines whether one or several objects have been found.

Generating the model for a structure of interest can be difficult. It has to include knowledge about the acceptable variation of attributes within an object class while remaining suitably discriminative.

Several techniques to generate and use object models will be presented in this chapter. Information about acceptable object variation in these models is either generated from training or it is part of the model prototype.

Concepts, notions and definitions introduced in this chapter

> Representation of shape and appearance
> Template matching and Hough transform
> Quadrics and superellipsoids
> Medial axis representation
> Active shape and active appearance models
> Mass spring models
> Finite element models

Instances of an object may be searched explicitly if a model of the object's outline or appearance exists. The search may be carried out automatically. Found instances are reported together with a quality of fit between model representation and data. User interaction may be allowed or required for model creation as well as for the correction of search results. Ideally, a model is defined such that interaction supporting the search can be incorporated into the model.

K.D. Toennies, *Guide to Medical Image Analysis*,
Advances in Computer Vision and Pattern Recognition,
DOI 10.1007/978-1-4471-2751-2_11, © Springer-Verlag London Limited 2012

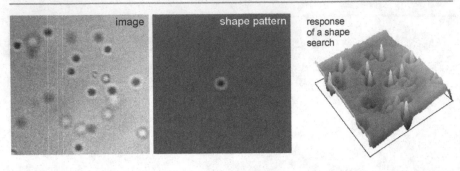

Fig. 11.1 A shape pattern as model can be used to search for possible occurrences of this pattern in an image by placing an instance of this pattern at arbitrary positions in the image an comparing the correlation of the pattern with the local appearance at this location

The power of a model to describe variants of a class of objects increases with the number of degrees of freedom that exist for describing shape or appearance. Parameters need to be specified, however, before the model can be used for searching object instances. For simplicity, we will call all these models *shape models*. It should be understood that shape comprises the outline of a figure as well as the expected appearance of the region that is enclosed by the outline.

A model in the engineering sciences abstracts or approximates a real-world entity. Its purpose is to describe or simulate this entity in a more accessible fashion. In image processing and computer vision the use of the term model is similar, although its purpose is slightly different. It is used for searching, detecting, or identifying objects depicted in an image. Models in computer vision share some similarities with the geometric models used in computed geometry and computer-aided design. In computer-aided geometry, a *model* is a system of rules and entities to describe rigid or nonrigid objects. A *representation* is a specific way to describe such a model. An instance of a model representation (or short: *model instance*) is a parameterized representation. We will use the term *shape model* to describe a model and its representation and *model instance* to describe a specific instance.

A shape model is a powerful constraint for foreground segmentation as well. Fitting model instances to the data singles out locations where a foreground object of known outline and appearance may be found (see Fig. 11.1). The accuracy with which this happens depends on the kind of model. Simple models only report a potential site of an object instance and make a rough approximation of its actual shape. A postprocessing step is needed for segmentation that uses this as a spatial constraint for a local boundary search. More advanced models include shape variation and may deliver a fairly accurate description of the true object boundary. Using such a model is sometimes the only automatic way to achieve a segmentation since noise or missing or false boundaries in the data can make it impossible to generate a data-driven delineation of object boundaries.

11.1   Shape Models

Using shape models has a long history in image analysis. They help to search instances of a class of objects described by shape, and they support the classification of
segments based on outline and appearance attributes. Surveys on deformable shape
models in image analysis are found in Terzopoulos and Fleischer (1988) and Cheung
et al. (2002).

The two different goals do not necessarily lead to the same kind of model.

- If object instances are searched, regions containing the shape need to be separated
  from those that do not. The number of different object instances is unknown. The
  data need to be expressed in terms of the model. A *quality-of-fit measure* (*QoF*)
  rates the correspondence between model instance and data. It guides the search
  and decides on acceptable deviations in the data from predictions by the model.
  Stopping criteria are required to decide whether a search has been successful
  (*shape detection*) and to decide to which extent the model instance is similar to
  the instance in the image (*shape deviation*). The two criteria may be different.
- If an object shall be classified by means of its shape, a descriptor of a detected
  object instance is generated. The perceived similarity within classes should map
  to the represented similarity in the descriptor. The model and instances of its
  representation do not need to describe the exact shape or appearance of the object
  as long as the representation suffices for differentiation between shape classes.

Some models and representations such as the *active shape model* (ASM) (Cootes
and Taylor 1992) may be applicable for both of the two purposes. However, most
models may be categorized into one of the two classes listed above.

Within this chapter, we will focus on the first kind and its use for segmentation
and object detection. Object recognition that can also be carried out using a shape
model will be discussed only briefly. Object recognition techniques in general are
surveyed in Edelman (1997). The review in Riesenhuber and Poggio (2000) contains
a brief description of the underlying theories for model-based object recognition.

There is potential for confusion in the use of the terms *segmentation* and *registration* when discussing the use of shape models. Using a shape model in segmentation
requires the model instance to be registered with an object instance in the image.
The registered model instance segments the scene because it provides an estimate
of the object's boundary. Hence, registration is the method to find an object instance
in the scene resulting in a foreground segmentation if the detection has been suc
cessful. Shape models used for the search and delineation of object boundaries will
be discussed in this chapter under the term segmentation.

For successful shape matching, attributes of an object instance in an image should
be characteristic to make it different from other regions in the image. The shape representation needs to describe these characteristics and permissible ranges of variation. Shape representations do this in different ways.

- A constant shape representation (such as the one in Fig. 11.1) describes the expected appearance of an object instance. The locations of object instances are
  found by correlating the representation with the image. Object variation is captured by the correlation measure. The criteria for shape detection and shape deviation are not separable since both have an impact on the correlation. Segmentation

Fig. 11.2 A variable shape
representation includes
(constrained) variation of the
object shape

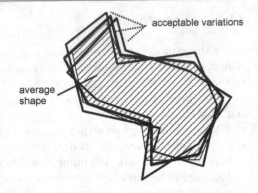

requires postprocessing since the representation has usually too few parameters
for exactly representing the object's outline. Models of this kind are presented in
Sect. 11.2.

• A deformable representation includes some or all of the object-specific variation (see Fig. 11.2). Representations of such models can differentiate between
the foreground and background with potentially arbitrary accuracy. Deformable
models and representations may be differentiated by the way variation is represented.

– *Implicit models* describe objects as functions of the domain in which the image is defined. Variation is implicitly given by the variation of the function
parameters. It enables an arbitrarily exact adaptation of the function to the object's shape and appearance, given that the parameter set of the function is rich
enough. Implicit models will be described in Sect. 11.3.

– *Explicit models* describe objects by a finite number of object details. Variation
is defined explicitly on these details and is directly related to variation in the
object's appearance. It may be difficult to find a finite number of attributes that
capture object appearance and its variation sufficiently well. Various kinds of
explicit models will be described in Sects. 11.4 through 11.6.

From a Bayesian point of view, shape representations are estimates of the a priori
term in the Bayesian equation. The estimate is particularly simple for a constant
representation. The a priori probability of an object instance is 1 for objects that
have a similar appearance and boundary than the model instance. The threshold for
similarity is user-specified. Otherwise the probability is 0.

A better approximation of the a priori term is achieved by a deformable shape
representation. Shape deformation incurs a cost that should be closely related to
the usually unknown probabilities. Several strategies exist for establishing the link
between the cost of variation and a priori probability. For the ASMs described in
Sect. 11.5 this is straightforward because probability distributions are learned from
samples. Proper training of the distribution, however, may require too many samples. Separating shape variation in a predefined high-level part and a trainable low-
level part is a strategy for keeping probability distributions simple. An example for
this is the medial axis representation (Sect. 11.4) where only local variation needs
to be trained from the samples. Variation may also be derived from the composition

Fig. 11.3 Geon theory states that the semantics of a depicted structure mainly stems from the decomposition of it into its constituent parts

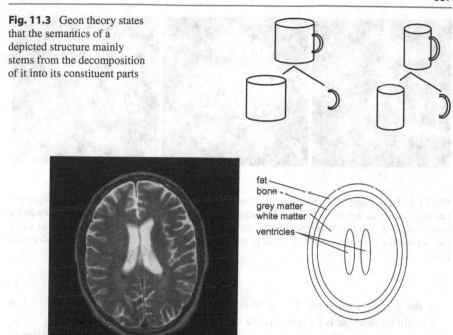

Fig. 11.4 Application of a shape decomposition strategy: providing a simplified structure of expected image content will enable identification of structures based on their configuration. The model does not have to be accurate as long as the spatial relationship between shape components is correct

of a shape model from simple subunits without further training. This is the case for physically based shape models such as a *finite element model* (FEM, Sect. 11.6).

All strategies for acquiring a priori knowledge need to deal with the problem that sufficient reliable information is seldom present. Again, there are a number of ways to deal with this.

- *Shape decomposition*: This strategy relates to the Geon theory (Biederman 1985; Rivlin et al. 1995) (see Fig. 11.3) and the fact that objects are often recognized based on context (Toussaint 1978). In short, the theory states that objects are recognized by their composition rather than by the deformation of the constituting components. In consequence, a proper, user-defined decomposition of a shape into subunits provides a representation with few parameters that are easy to estimate (see Fig. 11.4 for an example).
- *Scale space*: This relates to a theory that different levels of importance for object features are assumed to be represented at different levels of spatial resolution (e.g., Mokhtarian and Mackworth 1986; Jackway and Deriche 1996 for an application for shape detection and Lindeberg 1994 for an introduction and review). The shape representation is scaled and applied to an image that is scaled accordingly. Examples for scale space operators are the Gaussian pyramid (see Fig. 11.5)

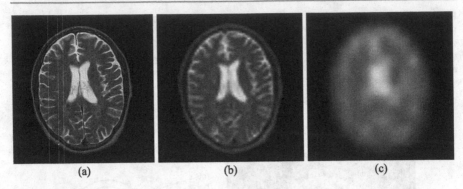

    (a)   (b)   (c)

Fig. 11.5 Three stages of a multi-scale representation (up-sampled to the original size). Representation of semantics will be different at different scales. In this example, the fact that the ventricles consist of a left and a right ventricle is representable only at scales depicted in (**a**) and (**b**) while the fact that the ventricles are in the center of the brain is representable at the lowest scale depicted in (**c**)

or the wavelet transform. The segmentation at a given resolution may be used as domain knowledge for a subsequent segmentation at a higher resolution.

- *Shape hierarchy*: The strategy is also rooted in the Geon theory. It is similar to shape decomposition and may be combined with it. The underlying assumption is the idea of a semantic scale space (i.e., that shape components can be ordered in a way that the most important shape attributes are described at the highest level). Less important detail may be neglected for segmentation. Defining semantic scales requires user intervention since specifying importance is highly application-dependent and requires high-level knowledge.

Some or all of these strategies have been employed by most of the representations being described in the following sections.

11.2   Simple Models

If shape can be described by few parameters with values in a finite range, finding an object instance can be done by sampling the parameter space and evaluating a quality-of-fit measure. Two often-used models are rigid templates and the Hough transform.

11.2.1 Template matching

A rigid *template* $t(\mathbf{x})$ is defined on a domain $0 \leq \mathbf{x} \leq \mathbf{x}_{\max}$. Values of t describe the outline and appearance of an object in an image $f(\mathbf{x})$ by assuming that a QoF measure $d_{\text{QoF}}(f(\mathbf{x}), t(\mathbf{x} + \Delta\mathbf{x}))$ exists that is minimal if an object instance can be

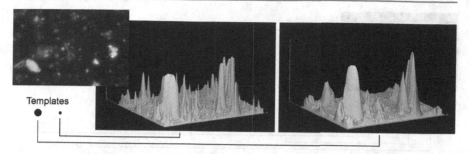

Fig. 11.6 Template matching with two different circular templates: the smaller template generates strong responses for the small objects in the image while the larger template generates the strongest response for the *large object on the lower left in the original image* although its shape is not circular

found at position $\Delta \mathbf{x}$ in f. Often-used quality-of-fit measures are the mean square distance

$$d_{\mathrm{MSD}}(f, t, \Delta \mathbf{x}) = \sqrt{\sum_{\{\mathbf{x}|0 \le \mathbf{x} \le x_{\max}\}} \left(f(\mathbf{x} + \Delta \mathbf{x}) - t(\mathbf{x})\right)^2} \qquad (11.1)$$

or the correlation coefficient

$$d_{\mathrm{corr}}(f, t, \Delta \mathbf{x}) = 1 - \frac{\sigma_{f,t}}{\sigma_f^2 \sigma_t^2}$$

$$= 1 - \frac{\sum_{\{x|0 \le x \le x_{\max}\}} (f(\mathbf{x} + \Delta \mathbf{x}) - \bar{f})(t(\mathbf{x}) - \bar{t})}{\sum_{\{\mathbf{x}|0 \le x \le x_{\max}\}} (f(\mathbf{x} + \Delta \mathbf{x}) - \bar{f})^2 \sum_{\{\mathbf{x}|0 \le x \le x_{\max}\}} (t(\mathbf{x}) - \bar{t})^2},$$

$$(11.2)$$

where $\bar{f}$ is the expected value of f in the region overlapped by the template and $\bar{t}$ is the expected value of the template (see Fig. 11.6 for an example).

The QoF function in (11.1) requires the intensities of f and t to be equal if the template overlaps an object instance. The QoF function in (11.2) only requires the template intensities to be linearly correlated to the intensities of an object instance in f. If covariance d_{cov} is used instead of correlation, template matching can be computed quickly in the frequency domain

$$d_{\mathrm{cov}}(f, t, \Delta \mathbf{x}) = \mathbf{FT}^{-1}\left(\mathbf{FT}(f) \cdot \left(\mathbf{FT}(t)\right)^*\right)(\Delta \mathbf{x}), \qquad (11.3)$$

where $\mathbf{FT}$ and $\mathbf{FT}^{-1}$ are the Fourier transform and its inverse and $\mathbf{FT}(t)^*$ is the conjugate complex of $\mathbf{FT}(t)$. The method requires t to be defined over the domain of f. Since the template domain is usually much smaller, unknown values for t outside its original domain are filled with zeros and the template is created such that its expected value is $\bar{t} = 0$. The difference between the zeros in the template and the true intensities in f degrade the matching result.

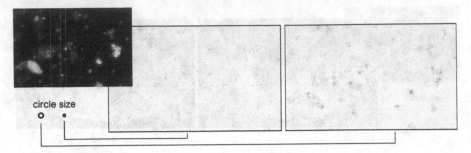

circle size

Fig. 11.7 The Hough transform for circles votes for circles of a given size

Template matching assumes that exact outline, appearance, orientation, and scale of an object are known. Small variations may be tolerated as long as the response of the QoF function in the background regions is still different from that of a true match. Defining the threshold can be difficult.

Variation of an object's orientation and scale quickly degrades the QoF measure. In this case, a bank of templates at different scales and orientations needs to be applied to the scene. The result of the matching is the optimum response from all these templates.

Template matching may be accelerated by introducing a multiscale strategy. Templates are applied first at a coarser resolution. The acceptance of potential object sites is generous at this stage and serves to restrict the search space at finer resolutions.

11.2.2 Hough Transform

The *Hough transform* already introduced in Sect. 5.2 can be extended to arbitrarily parameterizable boundaries without changing the principles of the method. A particularly simple variant is the search for circular objects (Davies 1998). The parametric equation is

$$r\,(c_1, c_2) = (x_1 - x_{c1})^2 + (x_2 - x_{c2})^2 . \tag{11.4}$$

The 3D parameter space (c_1, c_2, r) requires every edge point to vote for all centers and radii of circles containing this edge point as a boundary point. If the radius is known, the problem becomes 2D with every edge point voting for potential circle centers (see Fig. 11.7).

With increasing dimension of parameter space the average number of votes per accumulator cell may become so small that the voting result is no longer reliable. If too many parameters are required to describe a shape or if no parametric description of the shape exists, the parametric Hough transform can be replaced by the *generalized Hough transform* (GHT), which uses lookup tables to represent shape instead of an analytic equation. A review of the different ways to compute the GHT can be found in Kassim et al. (1999).

Fig. 11.8 Tabulation of (r, α) values with respect to ϕ: If the shape is concave, there may be several entries for the same value of ϕ

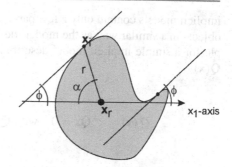

For the GHT, an arbitrary reference point $\mathbf{x}_r = (\mathbf{x}_{r,1}\ \mathbf{x}_{r,2})$ is chosen that represents a 2D shape described by boundary points $\mathbf{X} = \{\mathbf{x}_1, \mathbf{x}_2, \ldots, \mathbf{x}_N\}$ with coordinates $\mathbf{x}_i = (x_{i,1}\ x_{i,2})$. The spatial relation of each boundary point to the reference point is given by

$$x_{r,1} = x_{i,1} + r_i \sin\alpha_i, \qquad x_{r,2} = x_{i,2} + r_i \cos\alpha_i, \tag{11.5}$$

where α_i is the angle of a line from $\mathbf{x}_i$ to $\mathbf{x}_r$ with the $\mathbf{x}_1$-axis (see Fig. 11.8). A boundary point is characterized by its orientation as given by the angle ϕ of the tangent at $\mathbf{x}_i$ with the $\mathbf{x}_1$-axis. Pairs $(\mathbf{r}, \alpha)$ are now tabulated with respect to ϕ.

For carrying out the Hough transform in an edge image, first the angle ϕ of the gradient with the $\mathbf{x}_2$ axis is computed. This angle corresponds to the angle between the edge tangent and $\mathbf{x}_1$ axis. Then, $(\mathbf{r}, \alpha)$-values corresponding to this angle are taken from the $\mathbf{r}$-table and are used to compute the potential locations of reference points. The edge point votes for all these locations. There will be more than one entry in the $\mathbf{r}$-table for a given angle ϕ if the shape of the model is concave.

The GHT, as described above, is actually a special case of the GHT since the orientation and scale of the shape need to be known. If the rotation around some angle θ and scaling are unknown, the dimension of the Hough space is increased by these two variables. A vote for an edge at location $(x_{i,1}x_{i,2})$ is given for the cells $H(x_{r,1}, x_{r,2}, \theta, s)$, fulfilling

$$x_{r,1} = x_{i,1} + s \cdot r_i(x_{i,1}\cos\theta + x_{i,2}\sin\theta),$$
$$x_{r,2} = x_{i,2} + s \cdot r_i(-x_{i,1}\sin\theta + x_{i,2}\cos\theta). \tag{11.6}$$

The angle α of the orientation of the edge gradient is no longer needed because the rotation between the model and object instance in the image is unknown.

11.3 Implicit Models

An implicit model is a function $m(\mathbf{x}) = 0$ of image space describing the outline of object instances that it may contain. Implicit models are commonly restricted to boundary descriptions, although appearance models are possible as well. Simple implicit models contain only a few parameters restricting the range of representable objects in a similar way as the models described in the previous sections. An example for a simple implicit model describing object boundaries in 3D is the *quadric* $\mathbf{Q(x)}$

$$Q\left(\mathbf{x}\right) = \mathbf{x}^T \mathbf{Q x} = 0 \quad \text{with } \mathbf{Q} = \begin{pmatrix} a & e & f & g \\ e & b & h & j \\ f & h & c & k \\ g & j & k & d \end{pmatrix}, \tag{11.7}$$

where $\mathbf{x} = (x_1 \ x_2 \ x_3 \ 1)$ is represented in homogeneous coordinates and $\mathbf{Q}$ is the parameter matrix of the quadratic equation

$$ax_1^2 + bx_2^2 + cx_3^2 + 2ex_1x_2 + 2fx_1x_3 + 2hx_2x_3 + 2gx_1 + 2jx_2 + 2kx_3 + d^2 = 0. \tag{11.8}$$

A quadric may describe a large number of regular boundaries, which are all symmetric with respect to the origin of the coordinate system. Used as a shape model, parameter ranges describe the expected object shapes.

Fitting requires a QoF measure that connects the model with the data. Since the model describes boundaries, the QoF measures the probability of locations $\mathbf{x}$ of being boundary points for which $\mathbf{Q(x)} = 0$ holds. This can be done by computing the average gradient strength in an image weighted by the inverse distance to the boundary $\mathbf{Q(x)} = 0$:

$$QOF\left(Q_i\right) = \sum_{\mathbf{x} \in D(\mathbf{x})} \frac{\nabla f\left(\mathbf{x}\right)}{\left|Q_i\left(\mathbf{x}\right)\right|^n + 1}, \tag{11.9}$$

where $D(x)$ is the domain of $\mathbf{x}$ and n controls how the quality decreases with increasing distance to the expected boundary. Optimization may be carried out by gradient ascent in parameter space that includes transformation parameters and the shape parameters of the quadric.

A different implicit representation are the *superellipsoids* presented by Barr (1992), which are defined by

$$\left(|x_1|^{\frac{2}{e}} + |x_2|^{\frac{2}{e}}\right)^{\frac{e}{k}} + |x_3|^{\frac{2}{k}} = 1. \tag{11.10}$$

For $e = k = 1$, (11.10) describes a sphere that is inscribed in a cube with sides parallel to the axes of the coordinate system. Increasing the value of parameters e and k creates soft edges parallel to these axes (Fig. 11.9 shows several variants that can be created by varying e and k). The curvature of edges increases with n ($k \rightarrow \infty$ lets the boundaries approach the enclosing cube). The ratio e/k determines the ratio of curvatures parallel to and orthogonal to the x_3-axis. Using the superellipsoid equation, scaling along the three axes has to be determined from optimizing the QoF measure.

Fig. 11.9 Various shapes can be generated by varying the two parameters of the super ellipsoid equation

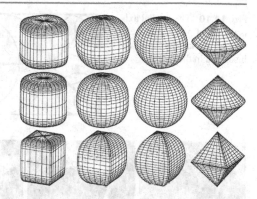

Implicit shape representations as simple as the ones described above are not suited for describing the rather intricate shapes of many anatomic objects. Hence, the representation is either combined with an explicit shape model, which uses the fitted implicit model for initialization, or it is replaced by a model offering more degrees of freedom for shape variation.

Complex shapes can be constructed by combining superellipsoids (Chevalier et al. 2001), but this is probably more appropriate if artificial objects shall be represented. For biological structures, the implicit model can be combined with an explicit model by adding free-form deformations of an adapted superellipsoid (Terzopoulos and Metaxas 1991; Bardinet et al. 2003; Gong et al. 2004). First, a superellipsoid is fitted to the data. The resulting shape is then enclosed by a box that is aligned with the axes of the fitted superellipsoid. Control points $\mathbf{p}_{i,j,k}$ for a spline representation of the ellipsoidal surface are defined on the box surface

$$\mathbf{f}(u, v, w) = \sum_{i,j,k} \mathbf{p}_{i,j,k} B_i(u) B_j(v) B_k(w), \tag{11.11}$$

where points $\mathbf{f}(u, v, w)$ are surface locations on the superellipsoid. The location and number of control points may be changed in a subsequent optimization process that adapts the model instance to potential surface locations in the image.

11.4   The Medial Axis Representation

Using the *medial axis* of an object for shape representation is motivated by investigations about carriers of semantics in shape (Blum 1967). The notion of a shape descriptor consisting of a supporting curve-like structure in the center of a shape that may possibly contain branches was among others adopted from research results in human vision by D. Marr (1983). He claimed that humans recognize the nature and shape of a 3D figure from supporting center curves, their branches, and a hypothesis about circles with varying radius perpendicular to the center curves. Circle radii are derived from the apparent radii of the visible silhouette of the figure. Hence, a suitable representation of shape that efficiently separates important shape features

Fig. 11.10 The medial axis is the set of points that are centers of maximal *circles* inscribed in the figure

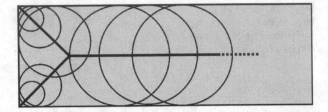

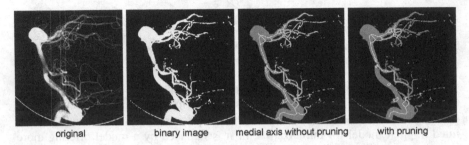

original   binary image   medial axis without pruning   with pruning

Fig. 11.11 Computation of the medial axis from a binary image. Pruning attempts to remove small branches from the axis but may also remove much of the central axis

from negligible features, noise, and artefacts should be a representation by a graph of curves with varying radii (called generalized cylinders, see Binford 1987).

11.4.1 Computation of the Medial Axis Transform

The *medial axis transform* presented by Blum (1967) creates such a curve from a given shape. It provides the means to analyze given shapes and to synthesize new shapes. The medial axis is computed from local data information, yet resulting in a high-level representation of relevant shape detail. This is, of course, only true in cases where the desired high-level shape description is buried in the outline of the object in question. A major part of the research regarding medial axis-based representations has been devoted to establishing such a relationship between an object outline and a meaningful medial axis (see, e.g., Giblin and Kimia 2004).

The medial axis consists of a set of points that are centers of maximal hyperspheres (circles for 2D shapes, spheres for 3D shapes) filling a bounded object (see Fig. 11.10). A hypersphere is maximal if it is fully contained in the object and if no hypersphere with the same center exists that has a larger radius and is still fully contained in the object. The point set forms connected curves if objects are defined in continuous space. For discrete space objects, several approximations of the medial axis transform exist that use various definitions of connectivity between pixels or voxels and various distance metrics.

The computation of the medial axis is done by a thinning algorithm (see Fig. 11.11; for a discussion of thinning algorithms see Lam et al. 1992). These algorithms initially treat the complete figure as the medial axis. Scene elements (pixels or voxels) are then iteratively removed until no element can be removed without violating the connectivity constraint. A simple thinning algorithm is the iterative application of a series of hit-or-miss operators.

A *hit-or-miss operator* (HOM operator) finds the known figures in an image by combining morphological erosion on a binary image with one on the inverse image. The two erosion operators model the shape of the figure and its background. The HOM operator combines the result of these two operations by a Boolean "and" and returns locations where the figure on the expected background are found in the scene.

Thinning by the hit-or-miss operator is carried out by searching boundary elements in the scene that can be removed without disconnecting the remaining figure. Boundary elements can be grouped by their angle with respect to the image coordinate system. Eight different types $(0°, 45°, 90°, \ldots, 315°)$ exist. The two HOM operators for $0°$ and $45°$ boundary elements in the usual notation for such operators[1] are

$$\begin{pmatrix} 0 & 0 & 0 \\ X & 1 & X \\ 1 & 1 & 1 \end{pmatrix} \quad \text{and} \quad \begin{pmatrix} 0 & 0 & X \\ 0 & 1 & 1 \\ X & 1 & 1 \end{pmatrix}.$$

The remaining HOM operators are generated by rotating these two operators by multiples of $90°$.

Thinning is carried out by applying all eight operators to the binary image, marking elements found by the HOM operator and removing them. The process ends when no further elements can be removed. The remaining elements are the medial axis (sometimes also called the *skeleton*) of the figure. A distance transform is applied to the original image. Distances at medial axis elements are the radii of the maximal hyperspheres centered at those elements.

11.4.2 Shape Representation by Medial Axes

The medial axis does not always describe the shape appropriately for object detection. The main problem stems from the fact that every intrusion or protrusion of the boundary spawns a new branch of the medial axis system. Although some of these branches may be important shape attributes, others represent detail pertaining to a specific object instance, but not to the object class in general.

There are several ways to deal with this. The application of the multiscale theory is one of these ways (Pizer et al. 1987). Medial axes are created in scale space (e.g., computed on images of a Gaussian pyramid). If scale space correlates with

---

[1]The notation is the usual shorthand notation for HOM operators combining the two structuring elements in a single operator. The '0's represent the erosion structuring element that is applied to the inverted binary image and the '1' represent the erosion structuring element that is applied to the original binary image.

the importance of the figure detail, the scale space representation can be used for shape analysis. If figure details, which are relevant for the intended application, manifest themselves at a known scale, the medial axis at this scale will be chosen for representation. The strategy often helps to separate noise effects from true shape details.

The hierarchy induced by scale space does not always coincide with a semantic hierarchy. Spatial scale for some detail of an object may vary within an object. If, for instance, the palm and fingers of the hand are assumed to be at the same level of a semantic hierarchy, a higher spatial resolution may be required to represent the fingers than the hand. In such a case, it is more appropriate to define a semantic scale space by imposing hierarchy levels by the user, as has been suggested recently for using a medial axis representation (called *m-rep*) in segmentation and registration (Pizer et al. 1999; Joshi et al. 2002). The authors suggested that a hierarchy of representations is to be created that consists of four different levels.

1. *Object level*: Primitives at this level are subfigures. Each subfigure has its own medial axis representation. It may interact with other subfigures by changing the relative position, orientation, or scale with respect to each other. Subfigures are ordered hierarchically and represented as an acyclic, directed graph. Relations may be differentiated into those between subfigures at the same level (typically different details of a shape or group of shapes) and those between a (sub)figure and its descendent child figures (typically the relationship between two subsequent levels in the scale space defined by the subfigure hierarchy).

2. *Figural level*: Primitives at this level are medial axis representations describing the specific shape of a subfigure.

3. *Medial axis primitive level*: Interactions between elements of the medial axis are represented at this level. The medial axis representation consists of a sequence of nodes representing a sampling of the medial axis. Nodes are attributed with their positional relation to neighboring axis nodes, and with the orientation and distance to their two closest boundary points of the subfigure that they represent.

4. *Boundary primitive level*: The medial axis primitives are meant to represent the shape variation of a class of shapes. The position of boundary points of an actual object instance may differ from this because of influences from data acquisition or within-class shape variation.

If the m-rep is applied to segmentation, it provides domain knowledge. Deviation of a model instance m from the expected shape is permitted, but incurs a penalty $C(m)$. The penalty term is assumed to be related to the a priori likelihood of the model to take this particular shape. The authors of the m-rep present a geometric term for estimating C, but claim that replacing this by a trained probability distribution is possible.

$C(m)$ is combined with a cost term $C(x, m)$ related to the likelihood of obtaining an image x given the model instance m. In Joshi et al. (2002), this is again a geometric term based on the distance between the expected and data appearances. If nodes are boundary nodes this is related to the gradient length in the image.

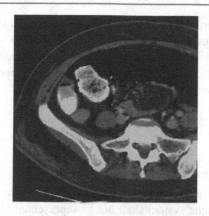
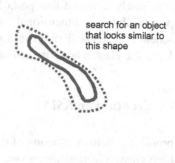

search for an object
that looks similar to
this shape

Fig. 11.12 Principle of an active shape model: a shape and acceptable variation taken from a sufficiently large training data set is used to find instances of the object in an image

Segmentation using an m-rep is carried out by placing the model in the image and letting it deform to maximize $C(m) + C(x, m)$. It produces a MAP estimate of an optimal segmentation if $C(m)$ and $C(x, m)$ are assumed to be the logarithms of the a priori probability $P(m)$ and the likelihood function $P(x|m)$, respectively.

11.5   Active Shape and Active Appearance Models

The *active shape model* (ASM) represents the shape of an object by an expected shape and permissible variations (see Fig. 11.12). It was presented by Cootes and Taylor (1992) and Cootes et al. (1995) and has found numerous applications since then. It is a *point distribution model* (PDM) representing the attributes of boundary points. The distribution is estimated from feature vectors of sample instances. The concept is simple and very attractive. Variation is directly related to the Bayesian formulation of image segmentation. Observed variation from a training phase is used to predict variation for unknown objects.

An active shape model describes a K-dimensional shape that is represented by L boundary points in a *shape feature vector* $\mathbf{s} = (s_0, s_1, \ldots, s_N) = (x_{1,1} x_{1,2}, \ldots, x_{1,L} x_{2,1} x_{2,2}, \ldots, x_{2,L}, \ldots, x_{K,1}, \ldots, x_{K,L})$, where $x_{k,l}$ is the kth component of the lth boundary point $\mathbf{x}_l$. Elements of the shape vector are treated as random variables. The density function for each random variable is assumed to be Gaussian with unknown mean and variance.

The concept can be easily applied to any dimension K. However, increasing the dimension of the shape vector will require more samples in feature space to compute a reliable estimate of the distribution. The dimension of feature space is large, even for 2D objects. An outline in 2D that is represented by 50 boundary points spans a 100-dimensional feature space. If the features were truly independent, it would require a very large number of samples for computing reliable estimates for the mean and variance of the Gaussians than is usually available.[2] Fortunately, it can be safely assumed that point locations are highly correlated. Samples will occupy a much lower-dimensional subspace. Decorrelating the data using principal component analysis will result in a small number of uncorrelated components of which parameters can be estimated independently of each other.

11.5.1 Creating an ASM

The probability density function of the ASM is meant to reflect deformation within an object class. The position or orientation of an object instance in some external reference system such as a world coordinate system shall not be represented. This would only make sense if this reference system is somehow object-specific (such as a patient coordinate system). Training from samples hence requires the proper alignment of training shapes.

Computing the density functions of an active shape model from training samples consists of several steps.

- In *landmark selection*, a number of points on the object boundary are to be identified in all samples. Cootes and Taylor (1995) suggested a hierarchy of landmarks.
  - *Primary landmarks* are anatomical landmarks (see Fig. 11.13a). The semantic equivalence between different exemplars of the training set is assured. However, it may be difficult to detect primary landmark locations based on local image characteristics.
  - *Secondary landmarks* are locations of extrema of some local image features such as curvature (see Fig. 11.13b). Since they are defined on local image features, it is possible to detect them automatically. However, semantic equivalence cannot be assured. A secondary landmark may not even be present in all data sets of the training data. Hence, the validity of the assumption needs to be tested that a secondary landmark indicates semantically equivalent locations in different exemplars of the training data.
  - *Tertiary landmarks* are equally spaced landmarks that fill the gap between uniquely identifiable primary or secondary landmarks (see Fig. 11.14). Their purpose is to represent the curvature properties of regions without other landmarks.
- Landmarks are *aligned* with respect to a common, shape-specific coordinate system by minimizing distances between corresponding landmarks.
- The estimated covariance matrix is *decorrelated* by applying the PCA transform. New, uncorrelated features $s' = \Phi s$ are generated from the matrix Φ containing the eigenvectors of the covariance matrix.

---

[2]A rule of thumb borrowed from statistical pattern recognition for estimating likelihood functions from samples predict for a 100-dimensional feature space that at least 2^{100} samples would be needed.

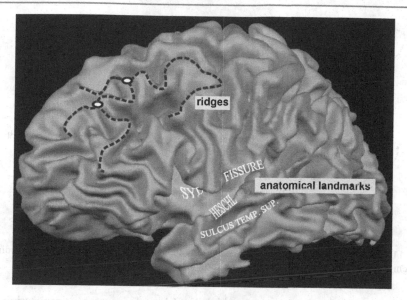

Fig. 11.13 Primary landmarks are named anatomical locations, while secondary landmarks are geometrically identifiable locations such ridge intersections

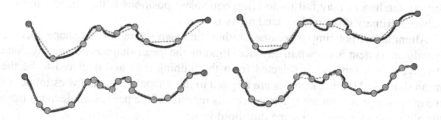

Fig. 11.14 Tertiary landmarks are used to represent curvature of the shape boundary. Sampling may depend on local curvature (*left*) or it may be an even sampling (*right*)

- The feature space is reduced by removing the axes for which the corresponding eigenvalues indicate the insignificant feature variance. The selection of significant *modes of variation* is commonly done by thresholding the accumulated variance. Modes are kept as long as the sum of variances is below some percentage of the total variance in the training data.

Several aspects should be kept in mind when creating the probabilistic shape model. They can influence the performance since landmark selection assumes that a set of semantically equivalent locations can be identified on each shape. Apart from the fact that it is difficult to define what is meant by semantic equivalence, it is often impossible to find a sufficient number of them. Interactive landmark selection requires human interaction, which is seldom feasible in a medical environment. Consequently, landmark detection is based on local attributes such as curvature (Brett

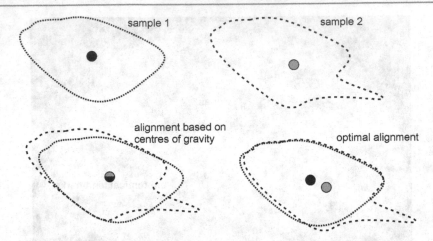

Fig. 11.15 Alignment based on invalid assumptions about the object-specific intrinsic coordinate system may lead to wrongly estimated shape variation

and Taylor 1999) or by introducing high-level knowledge such as registering the shape with an atlas containing known landmarks (Frangi et al. 2001). Geometric shape features such as the ones described in Chap. 5 could be used as well. These attributes may not always capture the full meaning of semantic equivalence. Using tertiary landmarks may fail to describe equivalent positions if the shape variation between primary or secondary landmarks is large.

Alignment is not simple because neither the mean shape nor the shape specific coordinate system is known in advance. Finding the mean shape is commonly done iteratively. A sample s_0 is selected from the training data and declared to be the mean shape $\bar{s}$. All other samples are aligned to this shape. Then, a new estimate for the mean shape is computed. The process is repeated if the new mean deviates from the old mean by more than some threshold value.

The transformation between the world and shape coordinate systems is assumed to be rigid. Hence, shapes are translated with their center of gravity into the center of gravity of the mean shape. A rotation is then searched that minimizes the Procrustes distance $\|s - \bar{s}\|$. For taking scaling into account, Cootes et al. (1995) suggested to normalize all shape vectors s such that $\|s\| = 1$.

The problems from alignment arise when the assumptions about the mean shape and the transformation are not true (see Fig. 11.15). Using centers of gravity for finding the translation vector implies that these centers of gravity are semantic landmarks. It may not be true if object instances of a class vary widely. Accounting for scaling, whether by normalization of the shape vector or by other means, may be inappropriate as well, if part of the scaling is due to object-specific variation. Hence, often some of the variation in the model will be due to alignment errors.

The often-limited number of samples for training from which the probability distribution is estimated may decrease the significance of the estimate. As pointed out above, the relatively small number of samples used for training is justified by the assumption that the actual number of uncorrelated components describing shape variation is much smaller than the number of elements in the shape vector. This is certainly true, but it is unknown how many uncorrelated components (modes) describe the shape variation. It is computed from a covariance estimate from a few samples in the original, high-dimensional space.

The representation of the density functions by a multivariate Gaussian may not approximate reality very well. It implicitly assumes that the local variation is Gaussian—which may be true as it is mainly influenced by noise—and that global shape variation can be represented as sum of spatially distributed Gaussians with different variances. This may not be true if the variation between different object parts has deterministic components. Employing a decomposition strategy solves this problem at the expense of user-supplied knowledge. The shape is decomposed into a group of subshapes that are represented as ASM. Relations between subshapes such as relative orientation and scale are defined and modeled as a high-level ASM (Al-Zubi and Toennies 2003).

11.5.2   Using ASMs for Segmentation

The ASM approach is useful for image segmentation because many of the problems listed above relate to classification issues rather than to matching issues. Deforming an ASM instance that is placed in the vicinity of some object instance so that it takes its most probable shape will often deliver a good approximation of the true boundary even though the a priori probability of the deformed ASM instance in the image may not reflect the true a priori probability.

Using an ASM in segmentation requires a method to align and deform the shape such that it fits a potential shape instance in the image. Given a truncated $M \times N$ matrix Φ' consisting of the first M eigenvectors (i.e., the first M modes of variation) of Φ, boundary points of a shape are approximated by

$$\tilde{s}(\mathbf{b}) = \bar{s} + \Phi'\mathbf{b}, \tag{11.12}$$

where $\mathbf{b}$ is a feature vector that describes deviation from the mean shape $\bar{s}$. Since modes are uncorrelated, the a priori probability to belong to a shape class can be approximated from multiplying the underlying feature probabilities

$$P_s(\mathbf{b}) \approx \prod_{i=1}^{M} \frac{1}{2\pi\sigma_i} \exp\left(-\frac{b_i}{\sigma_i^2}\right). \tag{11.13}$$

Given potential boundary points in a scene (e.g., from edge detection), the objective is to find transformation parameters and values for $\mathbf{b}$ that maximize this probability given the data information.

The search for pose parameters is independent of the search for shape features $\mathbf{b}$ since transformation parameters were excluded during generation of the ASM. Hence, the mean shape with $\mathbf{b} = \mathbf{0}$ is registered with the image using a rigid registration algorithm (see Chap. 10 and Fig. 11.16).

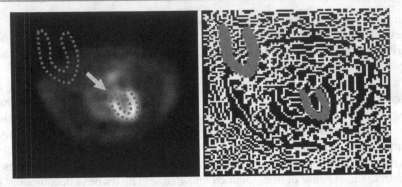

Fig. 11.16 The first step of segmentation with an ASM is to register the shape model with the data accounting for attributes not captured by the ASM such as position, orientation and scale of the model instance

Fig. 11.17 Local deformation is done after the average shape has been registered

The result is a pose estimate $\mathbf{T}$ for which a deformation vector $\mathbf{b}$ is computed that minimizes $\log P_{\mathbf{sT}}(\mathbf{b}) + \log P_{\mathbf{sT}}(f|\mathbf{b})$ given the data (see Fig. 11.17). The log-likelihood function $\log P_{\mathbf{sT}}(f|\mathbf{b})$ can be computed by summing likelihoods of boundary points belonging to the true boundary. Similar to optimization for m-reps, this can be done by measuring the gradient length at presumed boundary locations. The deformed shape is used as a new estimate for computing the next pose estimate. The process is repeated until convergence.

11.5.3 The Active Appearance Model

The ASM can be extended to an *active appearance model* (AAM) comprising intensity and texture information at points of the PDM (Cootes et al. 1998). A shape vector $\mathbf{s}$, which after decorrelation is reduced to $M_{\mathbf{s}}$ modes of variation from a mean shape $\bar{\mathbf{s}}$, is concatenated with an appearance vector $\mathbf{a}$. The latter may contain intensity or texture values for each point of the PDM being measured in the vicinity of the corresponding point.

Appearances are initially trained separately from shape features. They are decorrelated as well resulting in M_a modes describing appearance variation. The two aspects of an object are then combined by

$$\hat{\mathbf{b}} = \begin{pmatrix} \mathbf{b}_a \mathbf{W}_a \\ \mathbf{b}_s \end{pmatrix}, \tag{11.14}$$

where $\mathbf{W}_a$ is a diagonal matrix which may contain weights to rate the importance of appearance features. The resulting feature vector is decorrelated again to remove any linear correlation that may exist between shape and appearance features. This results in the final feature vector $\mathbf{b}$ that represents mode variations for integrated shape and appearance. The AAM is matched with the image in a similar way than the ASM.

11.6 Physically Based Shape Models

It has been noted by the authors of the ASM that the amount of training data is sometimes insufficient for providing a reliable estimate for the shape model. They suggested to apply an FEM for generating sufficient samples from its deformation (Cootes and Taylor 1995). As the number of training samples increases, the influence of the FEM part should decrease. FEMs are an example of a physically based *deformable shape model* (DSM) in its own right. The main difference to ASMs is that deformation is not trained but uses domain knowledge.

A DSM is a nonrigid, explicit model with a priori constrained shape variation. Physically based constraints have been presented (e.g., by Terzopoulos et al. 1987 and Pentland and Sclaroff 1991) and have been used in modeling anatomical objects (e.g., by Hamarneh et al. 2001). It should be noted that using a DSM for computer vision purposes poses two problems that do not exist, if it is used for simulation of a true physical entity such as, for example, the modeling of cloth described in Provot (1995).

- If used for the search of object instances, a DSM needs to be attracted by image features. Attraction forces have to be defined based on the image data. They can be thought of as a gravitational force in some strange world. The developer of such a model needs to ensure that the behavior of a model instance in this world is still perceived as being somewhat natural.
- If model deformation shall capture variation between different object instances, this needs to be parameterized as part of the model based on domain knowledge. Parameterization may be difficult because variation among shapes of the same class is not caused by a physically induced deformation (consider a model of a person: shape differences of different persons are not due to some force exerted on a basic shape).

In view of the inaccuracies to be expected in model parameterization, applying a DSM for registering a model instance with an object instance requires sufficient redundancy between the model and data. Inaccuracies in the model are then overridden by data information. This is required for any deformation model. It can never be assured that a model with a finite number of elements, components, or parameters captures all details that characterize an object in an image. Even if these details were captured, their exact description by the model representation cannot be guaranteed.

If DSMs are so difficult to use, it is fair to ask why it should be used at all. A major reason is that such models allow the explicit specification of shape variation of an object without prior training. It restricts the efficient use[3] of such a model to those objects whose variation is mainly described by decomposition into simpler model components. Adding the ability for variation without training is difficult—as it would be for a statistical model as well—but in a first approximation it can be done by overly relaxing variation constraints (for a statistical model this would translate into assuming a flat distribution function). Low image forces would cause large object deformations. Such a model is successful if the image information is "strong" enough to counteract overly relaxed variation constraints.

Some user involvement will always be necessary because user input extends the generalization ability of the model. A fully automatically acting model requires definition and parameterization that describes shape and appearance variation of all possible object instances completely and unambiguously. If this were possible at all, such a representation would be very specific to some application.

User involvement, as in all vision applications, should not merely accept or correct a result. Each interaction can be interpreted as additional information to the a priori knowledge about the object and should be included into the model.

The correction of a wrong result as well as training or teaching the model can be very straightforward in a DSM. A physically based DSM, despite the strangeness of the world of forces created by an image, reacts in a way that is familiar to the viewer. If a result is not satisfactory or if the behavior while searching for the result is not correct, this familiarity allows the user to pinpoint elements of the model that should behave differently.

11.6.1 Mass Spring Models

A mass spring model is a DSM that receives its shape by physical constraints from springs between mass points [used, for instance, for shape modeling in surgical simulation (Paloc et al. 2002) or for searching object instances in an image (Bergner et al. 2004), see Fig. 11.18a]. The DSM can be represented as a graph. Nodes with coordinates specified by vectors $\mathbf{n}_i$ are assumed to have masses m_i. Its edges are represented by springs $\mathbf{s}_{ij}$ connecting two mass points $\mathbf{n}_i$ and $\mathbf{n}_j$. The model—if placed in an image—moves toward an object of interest while keeping its shape controlled by external forces $\mathbf{f}_i^{\text{ext}}$ and internal forces $\mathbf{f}_i^{\text{int}}$. External forces attract the

---

[3]Each of the models presented here can be essentially extended such that it can replace any of the other models. However, each of the models has been built with some idea about the objects to be described and the way necessary knowledge is to be gathered. It works most efficiently if objects or scenes to which it is applied follow this idea.

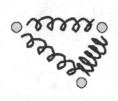

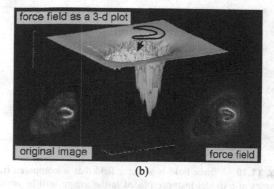

(a) (b)

Fig. 11.18 (a) A mass-spring model consists of masses connected by springs. (b) Placed in an image, masses are attracted by image forces while springs are responsible for controlling the shape deformation

model toward image features while internal forces act between nodes and cause the model to retain its shape and size.

The net force acting on every node $\mathbf{n}_i$ is a weighted combination of external and internal forces

$$\mathbf{f}_i = \alpha \mathbf{f}_i^{\text{ext}} + (1 - \alpha) \mathbf{f}_i^{\text{int}}. \tag{11.15}$$

The weight $0 \leq \alpha \leq 1$ indicates the importance of shape preservation and it is application-dependent. The behavior of a model instance over time t can be computed if node locations are made dependent on t. At time $t = 0$, every node has an initial location $\mathbf{n}_i(0)$ with velocity $\mathbf{v}_i(0) = 0$. Usually, initial node locations are set in such a way that internal forces are zero. The shape described by such a configuration is the *prototype* of the model instance and represents the average shape of the object instance in the scene.

Given node locations $\mathbf{n}_i(t)$ and velocities $\mathbf{v}_i(t)$, node locations at time $t + \Delta t$ are

$$\mathbf{n}_i(t + \Delta t) = \mathbf{n}_i(t) + \Delta t \cdot \mathbf{v}_i(t). \tag{11.16}$$

Acceleration $\mathbf{a}_i$ at node $\mathbf{n}_i$ is computed from node mass m_i and force $\mathbf{f}_i$ as $\mathbf{a}_i = \mathbf{f}_i / m_i$. New velocities can now be computed:

$$\mathbf{v}_i(t + \Delta t) = \mathbf{v}_i(t) + \Delta t \cdot \mathbf{a}_i(t). \tag{11.17}$$

The time step Δt is application-specific. Small time steps increase the accuracy of the approximation of the differential equation. They also increase the number of iterations needed for the model to approach the object of interest.

To prevent oscillations, the acceleration of nodes may be multiplied by a damping factor d which decreases with time t such as $d(t) = \exp(-\Delta t)$.

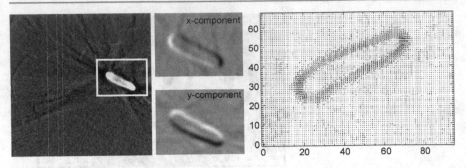

Fig. 11.19 A force field is a vector field that is computed from the gradient of image features. Masses of a model instance placed in the image will be attracted in direction of the force field vectors

External forces are directed toward attraction points in an image. They may be thought of as gravitational forces toward inert masses. Attraction forces acting on a node of the DSM should decrease with the increasing distance of the node from the attraction point (see Fig. 11.18b).

Every location **x** in an image may attract a model instance. Whether and to which extent it will be attracted by a particular location in the image depends on the image attribute $a(\mathbf{x})$ at this location. The length of the intensity gradient can be such an attribute, if the model nodes shall be attracted by the object boundaries.

The force acting at **x** can be precomputed by convolving $a(\mathbf{x})$ with a force kernel, of which the magnitude increases with decreasing distance, for example,

$$k(\mathbf{x}) = \begin{cases} \frac{w}{\|\mathbf{x}\|^2}, & \text{if } \|\mathbf{x}\| \neq 0 \\ 0, & \text{otherwise.} \end{cases} \qquad (11.18)$$

The value of w is a scale factor. The force vector for the external force $\mathbf{f}^{\text{ext}}$ exerted at location **x** is computed by convolving the force kernel with the attribute map and taking the gradient

$$\mathbf{f}^{\text{ext}}(\mathbf{x}) = \nabla\big(a(\mathbf{x})^*k(\mathbf{x})\big). \qquad (11.19)$$

The gradient vector field presented by Kichenassamy et al. (1995) and Xu and Prince (1998) detailed in Sect. 9.1.2 could be used as well.

The vector field can be precomputed for every attribute field. The external force that pulls a node $\mathbf{n}_i$ is now (see Fig. 11.19)

$$\mathbf{f}_i^{\text{ext}} = \mathbf{f}^{\text{ext}}(n_i). \qquad (11.20)$$

If a model instance is placed into a scene, each node will start to move toward its attractors. Since a moving mass possesses kinetic energy, it will pass the main attraction zone and will move away from it until the external forces start acting against the kinetic forces pulling the mass back toward the object.

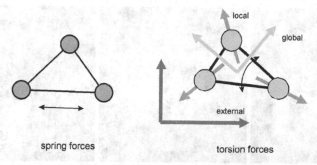

local
global
external
spring forces
torsion forces

Fig. 11.20 Spring forces and torsion forces govern the behavior of a mass-spring model. Spring forces act along the springs. They mainly restrict the change of scale. Torsion forces are angular forces with respect to a local, global or external coordinate system and restrict the deformation of the model instance

Moving further than the attraction point is intentional as it enables the model instance to find potentially better suited locations in the image. The damping factor mentioned above will cause the model instance to reach equilibrium after some oscillations.

Two kinds of internal forces govern the behavior of a stable mass-spring model: *spring forces* and *torsion forces* (see Fig. 11.20). The former mainly controls size changes of the model (Terzopoulos et al. 1987) and the latter restricts shape variation (Dornheim et al. 2005).

For computing spring forces, a rest length s_{ij}^0 needs to be assigned to each spring s_{ij}. It is the length of a spring if the shape model takes its prototypical shape. If the distance between two nodes $\mathbf{n}_i$ and $\mathbf{n}_j$ along the spring s_{ij} deviates from the rest length, it creates a spring force $\mathbf{f}_{ij}^s$ acting in the direction of s_{ij} (this is under the assumption that $m_i = 1$ for each mass point)

$$\mathbf{f}_{ij}^s = \left[k_{ij}\left(s_{ij}^0 - \|\mathbf{n}_i - \mathbf{n}_j\|\right)\right]\frac{s_{ij}}{\|s_{ij}\|}. \tag{11.21}$$

The parameter k_{ij} is the spring constant that describes the spring's stiffness. An effective net force acting on a node $\mathbf{n}_i$ is a sum of forces from all $K(i)$ springs $s_{ik}, k = 1, K(i)$ that are connected to $\mathbf{n}_i$:

$$\mathbf{f}_i^s = \sum_{k=1}^{K(i)} \mathbf{f}_{ik}^s. \tag{11.22}$$

Mass-spring models using spring forces to control the model shape do not necessarily prevent deformations. A mass-spring model usually has many stable states of which the prototype shape is just one. Hence, the kinetic energy of a moving model may cause a model instance to converge to any of the other stable states. Adding stabilizing and almost rigid springs can solve this problem, but will result in a heavily connected model whose behavior will not be easily predictable.

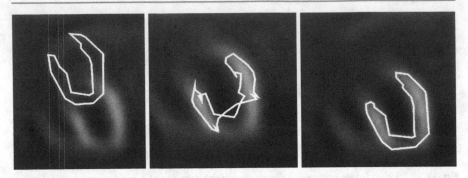

Fig. 11.21 Model deformation without and with torsion forces (based on the work of Dornheim et al. 2005)

Stiffness control can be explicitly added as an additional force to the node network. The force inhibits the relative rotation between nodes and controls the spatial relationship between all springs connected to a single node. It is called *torsion force* and restricts the twisting movement by rotating nodes into the rest location (see Fig. 11.21). This local force is implicitly defined by the shape prototype.

The introduction of the torsion force reduces the number of stable states of the model to just the one that corresponds to the prototype shape. To compute and apply the torsion force, springs connected to a node $\mathbf{n}_i$ need to be defined in a node coordinate system that may be one of three kinds (see Fig. 11.20).

- A fixed *external coordinate system* keeps the orientation of the model stable. This is simply the world coordinate system that is assigned to every node.
- A *global model coordinate system* keeps the shape of the object stable but allows for object rotations. It needs to be rotated appropriately after each iteration.
- A *local point coordinate system* has similar properties as a global model coordinate system, but allows for local variation of acceptable twisting of the model instance. It is computed from spring directions that are incident to a mass point.

Given a node coordinate system, a spring vector $\mathbf{s}_{ij}$ in world coordinates can also be represented as a vector $\mathbf{s}_{ij}^i$ in the node coordinates of node $\mathbf{n}_i$. If the model has its prototypical shape, all spring directions in node coordinates attain their rest directions $\mathbf{s}_{ij}^{i,0}$. If the shape is deformed, actual spring directions $\mathbf{s}_{ij}^i$ may vary from their rest directions. The torsion force acting on node $\mathbf{n}_i$ is then a rotational force relative to the node $\mathbf{n}_j$ that attempts to rotate spring $\mathbf{s}_{ij}$ around $\mathbf{n}_j$ back to its rest orientation. It is defined as

$$\mathbf{f}_{ij}^t = t_{ij} \cdot \frac{\Delta \mathbf{s}_{ij}^i}{\|\Delta \mathbf{s}_{ij}^i\|}, \tag{11.23}$$

where t_{ij} depends on the angle between rest position and actual position of the spring and $\Delta \mathbf{s}_{ij}^i$ determines the direction of the force. The value of t_{ij} is

$$t_{ik} = t_i \cdot \angle\left(\mathbf{s}_{ik}^i, \mathbf{s}_{ik}^{i,0}\right). \tag{11.24}$$

The factor t_i is a torsion constant governing the local stiffness at node $\mathbf{n}_i$. The direction in which the force is acting is given by

$$\Delta s_{ij}^i = s_{ij}^{i,0} - s_{ij}^i \left(\frac{s_{ij}^i \bullet s_{ij}^{i,0}}{\|s_{ij}^i\| \cdot \|s_{ij}^{i,0}\|} \right), \tag{11.25}$$

where "$\bullet$" is the inner product.

To compute node displacement due to torsion, the sum of torsion forces of all springs $k = 1, K(i)$ that are connected to $\mathbf{n}_i$ has to be computed:

$$\mathbf{f}_i^t = \sum_{k=1}^{K(i)} \mathbf{f}_{ik}^0. \tag{11.26}$$

Since $s_{ij}^{i,0}$ remains constant with respect to the local coordinate system of node $\mathbf{n}_i$, but varies with respect to the world coordinate system, it has to be computed after each iteration. The rotation of the node coordinate system with respect to the world coordinate system can be determined by averaging the rotations caused by all springs that are connected to this node. Combining spring forces and torsion forces results in an effective internal force $\mathbf{f}_i^{\text{int}}$ acting on each node i:

$$\mathbf{f}_i^{\text{int}} = (1 - \beta) \mathbf{f}_i^s + \beta \mathbf{f}_i^t. \tag{11.27}$$

The factor β with $0 \le \beta \le 1$ governs the relative influence of spring and torsion forces.

External forces attracting a model instance to object boundaries create a complex world of attractions because nonzero intensity gradients exist almost everywhere in the image. A model instance may only be attracted to the "correct" location (i.e., by the object instance in a search) if it is placed close to this location. For automatic segmentation by a DSM the most likely location of the object instance needs to be determined beforehand.

If the shape or appearance of other objects differs substantially from that of the object instance a correlation measure between the average model instance and image may be used. Otherwise, a stochastic search may be enacted where model instances are placed at several locations in the image. Decisions as to whether such an instance has found an object will be based on a quality-of-fit measure of the fitted model instance. This could be, for instance, the magnitude of the sum of internal forces in the model (i.e., a deformation cost) or the magnitude of the sum of external forces (i.e., the support by the image), or a combination of the two. Successful candidates of the stochastic search may spawn new model instances in their vicinity until the average QoF of the population of model instances no longer increases.

Fig. 11.22 A mass-spring model transfers forces only along springs, while an FEM is a continuous space model where forces are defined everywhere in the elements

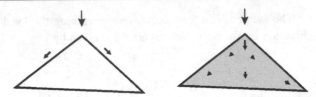

11.6.2 Finite Element Models

Finite element models (FEMs, see, e.g., Zienkiewics et al. 2005; Petyt 1998 for an introductory treatment) are an alternative way to solve the equilibrium problem when placing a deformable shape model instance into an image and letting it deform according to external forces (Sclaroff and Pentland 1995). The conceptual difference between a mass-spring model and an FEM is that the FEM is a continuous space model that may be defined for each location **x** in the model whereas the mass-spring model is only defined at the mass points (see Fig. 11.22).

Finite element models are often used in the material sciences. They approximate the behavior of a continuous physical entity by means of a finite number of elements. Each element is bounded by nodes. The behavior of the represented entity under the influence of forces is reduced to the influence at these nodes. Elements of an FEM may be 1D, 2D, or 3D and they may be embedded in 2D or 3D space. It should be kept in mind that the FEM controls the degrees of freedom of shape deformation only within its elements. If, for instance, the boundary of a 3D object is represented by a 2D FEM, this restricts the shape of the bounded object only in a very indirect fashion.[4] However, if the dimensionality of the elements equals that of the space in which they are embedded, the FEM represents physical behavior at any location **x** in a bounded region covered by the elements. Shape deformation is controlled by the decomposition into elements and their physical attributes.

FEMs have been used to represent a deformable object boundary (Delingette et al. 1992; Mandal et al. 1998) and to describe deformable object shapes (Ferrant et al. 2000; Engel and Toennies 2010). The former is a topological constraint restricting the number of closed boundaries, while the latter constrains object shapes. We will restrict our discussion to FEMs constraining the object shape.

Given an element of the FEM and external forces acting on it, it deforms until the potential energy of the element (strain and stress) and external forces balance. Strain and stress within the element are interpolated by *shape functions* such that they result in a continuous displacement field for this element (see Fig. 11.23). Interpolation guarantees that displacement at node locations does not depend on other nodes. This is necessary for a continuous displacement field of a mesh of connected elements.

---

[4]A FEM may be defined in a similar fashion than the mass-spring model by letting 1D springs being the elements. In such case, a bounded 2D or 3D object may be represented by a dense mesh of springs restricting shape variation.

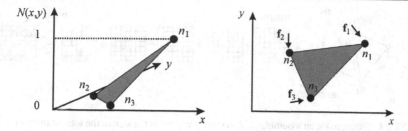

Fig. 11.23 (a) Shape functions $N(x, y)$ describe the influence of forces acting at some node on all other places in the element. The example in (a) shows a linear shape function for node n_1. (b) The deformation of the element is then computed from the influence of forces acting on all nodes

Potential energy usually describes the element as an elastically deformable object. This imposes a smoothness constraint on element deformation. Together with the continuity of a displacement field, it ensures a kind of stability of the shape representation that is similar to that achieved by torsion forces in the mass-spring model.

The following is a more detailed explanation of this application using a triangular grid as example. A triangular grid would be appropriate to represent shape and its variations of a 2D figure. The triangle as basic element of this FEM consists of three bounding nodes $\mathbf{n}_1$, $\mathbf{n}_2$, $\mathbf{n}_3$ with coordinates $(x_{i,1}, x_{i,2})$, $i = 1, 3$. A force acting on a node $\mathbf{n}_i$ is represented by a 2D vector $\mathbf{f}_i = (f_{2i}, f_{2i+1})$. It causes displacement of $\mathbf{n}_i$ by $\mathbf{u}_i = (u_{2i}, u_{2i+1})$ until internal forces from elasticity of the material and stress caused by the deformation balance the external force.[5] This can be expressed by the following relationship for an element e:

$$\mathbf{u}^{(e)} \mathbf{K}^{(e)} + \mathbf{f}^{(e)} = 0. \tag{11.28}$$

The (e) customarily indicates that we are talking about a single element of an FEM.

The matrix $\mathbf{K}^{(e)}$ is called a stiffness matrix. It summarizes material-specific elasticity and stress components. The equation above only defines a displacement for nodes. Displacement for all other locations within the element is interpolated using shape functions $\boldsymbol{\phi}(\mathbf{x})$ for which $\boldsymbol{\phi}(\mathbf{n}_i) = \mathbf{u}_i$ must be true.

If finite elements are combined to a mesh, a common stiffness matrix has to be assembled from the element matrices. The following two conditions must hold for the assemblage of any two elements of a mesh to keep displacements within the mesh continuous.

1. The displacements at a common node of two elements must be the same for each element.

---

[5]Node values and force values of all nodes of an element (and later of the complete FEM mesh) are combined in a single vector. Hence, values for a node with index i in 2D have indices $2i$ and $2i + 1$ in the displacement vector $\mathbf{u}$ and the external force vector $\mathbf{f}$.

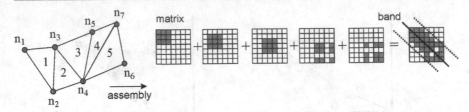

Fig. 11.24 Example for an assemblage. A common matrix of the size of the total number of nodes is created and entries from the element matrices are set at the appropriate positions in the common matrix

2. The sum of all forces exerted from elements meeting at a common node must balance the external force at this node.

The two conditions can be guaranteed by the following, simple assemblage step. If the components of all N nodes in an assembled mesh are indexed from 1 to $2N$ and node features of an element e of this mesh have indices $n_1, n_2, \ldots, n_6$ with a corresponding 6×6 stiffness matrix $\mathbf{K}^{(e)}$, an extended stiffness matrix $\mathbf{K}^{(\text{ext})}$ of size $2N \times 2N$ is created with

$$K_{k,l}^{(\text{ext})} = \begin{cases} K_{i,j}^{(e)} & \text{if } k = n_i \wedge l = n_j \wedge i, j = 1, 2, 3, 4, 5, 6, \\ 0 & \text{otherwise.} \end{cases} \tag{11.29}$$

This is done for all element matrices (see Fig. 11.24). The extended matrices are added. The result is an assembled stiffness matrix $\mathbf{K}$ for the mesh[6] fulfilling the two conditions above.

The displacement of nodes of an FEM mesh requires the solution of the linear equation system $\mathbf{uK} = \mathbf{f}$ for the displacement vector $\mathbf{u}$. Additional constraints are needed, however, because the mesh may still freely move in the 2D space. These constraints are called *essential boundary conditions* and *natural boundary conditions* in the FEM literature. Essential boundary conditions restrict the displacement vector $\mathbf{u}$ (e.g., by stating that $(u_{2i}, u_{2i+1}) = 0$ for some nodes $\mathbf{n}_i$). Natural boundary conditions restrict the force vector. Given a sufficiently constrained problem, the displacement of an FEM mesh under an external force can be computed by solving the linear equation system for $\mathbf{u}$.

So far, the FEM is static. The concept is extended to include dynamics for modeling external image forces attracting a model instance to depicted objects (see Fig. 11.25). The influence of external forces depends on the current placement of the model in the scene. Since it changes while the model instance moves, displacement $\mathbf{u}$ and forces $\mathbf{f}$ are made time-dependent. External forces in the dynamic FEM attract

---

[6]This kind of assemblage becomes costly for the sparse matrix $\mathbf{K}$ if N is large. Faster methods to carry out this operation exist but the operation itself stays the same. For application in medical image analysis, however, the size of N is usually small (i.e., $N \ll 100.000$) and model creation does not happen often.

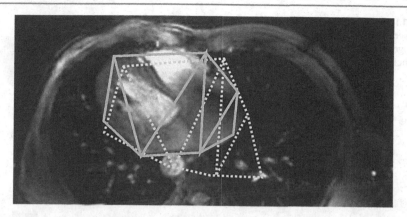

Fig. 11.25 A dynamic FEM deforms depending on external image forces towards the sought object

the nodes to image regions of relevance, and are balanced against the topology-preserving internal mesh forces. This is represented by the linear dynamic model

$$\mathbf{M}\ddot{\mathbf{u}}(t) + \mathbf{D}\dot{\mathbf{u}}(t) + \mathbf{K}\mathbf{u}(t) + \mathbf{f}(t) = 0. \tag{11.30}$$

The nodal displacements $\mathbf{u}(t)$ depend on time t. The terms $\dot{\mathbf{u}}$ and $\ddot{\mathbf{u}}$ are the first and second derivatives of the displacement with respect to time (i.e., velocity and acceleration). Acceleration depends on a mass-specific inertia represented by the mass matrix $\mathbf{M}$. The matrix $\mathbf{D}$ models velocity-dependent damping.[7] If the viscosity of the modeled material is unknown, the damping matrix $\mathbf{D}$ can be taken as *Raleigh damping* $\mathbf{D} = \alpha\mathbf{M} + \beta\mathbf{K}$. $\mathbf{K}$ is the stiffness matrix already known from static FEMs.

The mass and stiffness matrices restrict the variation of the DSM. Hence, these material properties encode the domain knowledge about the object variance. Using an FEM to describe intersubject variation of organs and structures does not require the description of a specific material since this is not a simulation that describes real deformation processes. Material properties represent an abstract deformation concept.

Stiffness $\mathbf{K}^{(e)}$ of an element e is computed from the following:

- a stress matrix $\mathbf{B}^{(e)}$,
- an elasticity matrix $\mathbf{C}^{(e)}$,
- the element thickness k,
- the area A of the element.

For an element of constant thickness (which is usually assumed when using finite elements in object detection and segmentation) stiffness is

$$\mathbf{K}^{(e)} = kA\big(\mathbf{B}^{(e)}\big)^{\mathrm{T}}\mathbf{C}^{(e)}\mathbf{B}^{(e)}. \tag{11.31}$$

---

[7]A dynamic system can be modeled without damping but damping prevents oscillation.

Fig. 11.26 The Poisson ratio
n describes the deformation
orthogonal to the direction of
the incident force

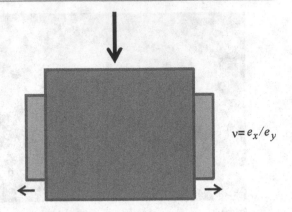

$$v = e_x/e_y$$

Stress represents the deformation under (initial) forces such as a shrinking due to a change in temperature. The influence of stress can be computed for arbitrary directions by a stress tensor that describes translation and shearing forces. For a 2D element, this is

$$\varepsilon = S\mathbf{u} = \begin{bmatrix} \frac{\partial}{\partial x} & 0 \\ 0 & \frac{\partial}{\partial y} \\ \frac{\partial}{\partial y} & \frac{\partial}{\partial x} \end{bmatrix} \begin{pmatrix} u \\ v \end{pmatrix} \approx S\mathbf{N}\tilde{u}^{(e)} = \mathbf{B}^{(e)}\tilde{u}^{(e)}. \tag{11.32}$$

Hence, the stress matrix results from the shape functions in $\mathbf{N}$ and the shape of the elements. Since shape functions are usually fixed and simple when using FEM to model a DSM, the component is not used to vary deformation constraints for the DSM. This is different for elasticity. Elasticity describes the deformation of the element under some external force. For a linear-elastic homogeneous body, elasticity can be described by the elasticity modulus E and the Poisson ratio v. It is

$$\mathbf{C}^{(e)} = \frac{E}{1 - v^2} \begin{bmatrix} 1 & v & 0 \\ v & 1 & 0 \\ 0 & 0 & (1-v)/2 \end{bmatrix}. \tag{11.33}$$

The Poisson ratio is the ratio $v = -e/e_\perp$ by which an object expands or shrinks orthogonal to the direction of the impacting force (see Fig. 11.26). In other words, it tells how much of the acting force is transferred sideways. The Poisson ratio may vary between -1 and 0.5. It is positive for most materials (a negative Poisson ratio would mean that a force causing a shrinking in one direction would also cause shrinking in directions orthogonal to it).

The elasticity modulus E describes how much permanent deformation is caused by an acting force. A sufficient description for isotropic materials is the use of Young's modulus, which is a single scalar value and assumes that the deformation is independent of the direction in which the force acts on the material.

The mass matrix $\mathbf{M}$ is the second component that describes the behavior of the FEM. It describes the inertia of the system with respect to external forces. The mass matrix $\mathbf{M}^{(e)}$ of an element e depends on the material density ρ and the shape functions $\mathbf{N}$

$$m_{i,j} = \int_{\Omega_e} \mathbf{N}_i^T \rho \mathbf{N}_j \, d\Omega_e. \tag{11.34}$$

The mass matrix for a 2D element with area A, thickness k, material density ρ, and linear shape functions is

$$\mathbf{M}^{(e)} = \frac{\rho k A}{12} \begin{pmatrix} 2 & 0 & 1 & 0 & 1 & 0 \\ 0 & 2 & 0 & 1 & 0 & 1 \\ 1 & 0 & 2 & 0 & 1 & 0 \\ 0 & 1 & 0 & 2 & 0 & 1 \\ 1 & 0 & 1 & 0 & 2 & 0 \\ 0 & 1 & 0 & 1 & 0 & 2 \end{pmatrix}. \tag{11.35}$$

Given mass, damping, and stiffness matrices concatenated from their respective element matrices, external forces cause the model to move and deform. The global force vector $\mathbf{f}(t)$ contains dynamic loads that attract the FEM toward image features. Similar to the use of mass-spring models for segmentation and registration, these features need to be attributes $a(\mathbf{x})$ that are correlated to features of sought objects. Examples are the image gradient or image intensity. The external force at time t exerted on nodes $\mathbf{n}_i$, $i = 1, \ldots, N$ with current position $\mathbf{x}_i(t)$ is

$$\mathbf{f}_i(\mathbf{x}, t) = \lambda(t) \nabla a[\mathbf{x}(t)], \tag{11.36}$$

where $\lambda(t)$ is a weighting factor that prevents oscillation similarly to the damping factor in a mass-spring model.

Dynamic displacement can be computed by solving the system of partial differential equations iteratively, given that initial displacement and displacement speed are known. A standard solution technique is the *Newmark-β algorithm*. The general principles behind this algorithm are as follows.

- Differentials are approximated by differences in a sequence $\mathbf{u}_1, \mathbf{u}_2, \ldots, \mathbf{u}_n$, $\mathbf{u}_{n+1}, \ldots$ that are Δt apart.
- The state of the system at time t_{n+1} is given by a Taylor approximation of $\mathbf{u}$ at time t_{n+1}.
- The remainder term of the Taylor series is replaced by a weighted difference between differentials at t_n and t_{n+1} (the weight is the name-giving β).
- The second derivative of $\mathbf{u}$ is computed first, then it is used to compute the first derivative, which in turn is used to compute $\mathbf{u}$ at time t_{n+1}.

To derive the Newmark-β algorithm we follow the argumentation of Zienkiewics et al. (2005) and start with a simplified FEM without mass matrix $\mathbf{M}$ (which describes a so-called transient field used, e.g., to describe heat conduction). The solu-

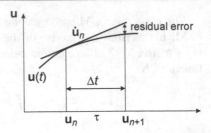

Fig. 11.27 The finite difference solution is inherently instable, as it extrapolates the displacement $\mathbf{u}_{n+1}$ from known values $\mathbf{u}_n$ at time t_n

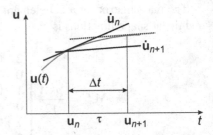

Fig. 11.28 Using derivatives at time t_n and t_{n+1} produces a more stable solution for estimating $\mathbf{u}_{n+1}$

tion will then be extended to a complete FEM without detailed derivation. A transient field is given by

$$\mathbf{D}\dot{\mathbf{u}}(t) + \mathbf{K}\mathbf{u}(t) + \mathbf{f}(t) = 0. \tag{11.37}$$

Approximating $\mathbf{u}$ by a Taylor approximation (see Fig. 11.27) results in the finite difference solution $\mathbf{u}_{n+1} = \mathbf{u}_n + \Delta t \cdot \dot{\mathbf{u}}_n$. However, this extrapolates the function based on an extrapolation of the derivative. The error from omitting the remainder term of the Taylor series is not accounted for. If the function $\mathbf{u}(t)$ is sufficiently differentiable, a ratio between $\dot{\mathbf{u}}_n$ and $\dot{\mathbf{u}}_{n+1}$ exists that exactly represents the average derivative between t_n and t_{n+1}. Hence, interpolation of this value produces a more stable solution than extrapolating from t_n (see Fig. 11.28). The value of $\mathbf{u}_{n+1}$ is now approximated by

$$\mathbf{u}_{n+1} = \mathbf{u}_n + \Delta t \big[(1 - \beta)\dot{\mathbf{u}}_n + \beta \dot{\mathbf{u}}_{n+1} \big], \tag{11.38}$$

where β is a weighting parameter that has to be set. Approximating (11.37) results in

$$\mathbf{D}\dot{\mathbf{u}}_{n+1} + \mathbf{K}\mathbf{u}_{n+1} + \mathbf{f}_{n+1} = 0,$$
$$\mathbf{K}\mathbf{u}_{n+1} = \mathbf{K}\big(\mathbf{u}_n + \Delta t \big[(1 - \beta)\dot{\mathbf{u}}_n + \beta \dot{\mathbf{u}}_{n+1}\big]\big) \tag{11.39}$$
$$\Rightarrow \quad \mathbf{D}\dot{\mathbf{u}}_{n+1} + \mathbf{K}\big(\mathbf{u}_n + \Delta t \big[(1 - \beta)\dot{\mathbf{u}}_n + \beta \dot{\mathbf{u}}_{n+1}\big]\big) + \mathbf{f}_{n+1} = 0.$$

Except for $\mathbf{f}_{n+1}$, $\dot{\mathbf{u}}_{n+1}$ only depends on quantities that are known at time t_n. If $\mathbf{f}_{n+1}$ is approximated by forward differencing, $\mathbf{u}_{n+1}$ is given by rearranging the terms and resolving for $\dot{\mathbf{u}}_{n+1}$:

$$\dot{\mathbf{u}}_{n+1} = -\left(\mathbf{D} + \Delta t \beta \mathbf{K}\right)^{-1} \big[\mathbf{K}\big(\mathbf{u}_n + \Delta t (1 - \beta)\dot{\mathbf{u}}_n\big) + \mathbf{f}_{n+1} \big]. \tag{11.40}$$

From $\dot{\mathbf{u}}_{n+1}$ the value for $\mathbf{u}_{n+1}$ can be computed based on (11.38).

The system is not self-starting (i.e., $\mathbf{D}\dot{\mathbf{u}}_0 + \mathbf{K}\mathbf{u}_0 + \mathbf{f}_0 = 0$ needs to be guaranteed). The values of the external forces $\mathbf{f}_{n+1}$ need to be computable (e.g., by another Taylor approximation).

The choice of β influences the behavior of the algorithm. Choosing $\beta = 0$ results in a finite difference approximation. In the absence of domain knowledge $\beta = 0.5$ is a usual choice. Since the stability of the solution cannot be guaranteed without knowledge about the difference between the chosen β and the unknown optimal β, the time step Δt should be rather small.

The Newmark-β algorithm can be extended to FEMs with mass matrix. The derivation strategy is the same except for the fact that the expression gets longer. The resulting scheme for computing $\mathbf{u}$ and its derivatives at time t_{n+1} is

$$\ddot{\mathbf{u}}_{n+1} = \mathbf{A}^{-1}\left(\mathbf{D}\left[\dot{\mathbf{u}}_n + (1 - \beta_1)\Delta t\ddot{\mathbf{u}}_n\right] + \mathbf{K}\left[\mathbf{u}_n + \Delta t\dot{\mathbf{u}}_n\right.\right.$$

$$\left.\left. + \frac{1}{2}(1 - \beta_2)\Delta t^2\ddot{\mathbf{u}}_n\right] + \mathbf{f}_{n+1}\right), \tag{11.41}$$

with

$$\mathbf{A} = \mathbf{M} + \beta_1\Delta t\mathbf{D} + \frac{1}{2}\beta_2\Delta t^2\mathbf{K}, \tag{11.42}$$

$$\dot{\mathbf{u}}_{n+1} = \dot{\mathbf{u}}_n + (1 - \beta_1)\Delta t\ddot{\mathbf{u}}_n + \beta_1\Delta t\ddot{\mathbf{u}}_{n+1}, \tag{11.43}$$

$$\mathbf{u}_{n+1} = \mathbf{u}_n + \Delta t\dot{\mathbf{u}}_n + \frac{1}{2}(1 - \beta_2)\Delta t^2\ddot{\mathbf{u}}_n + \frac{1}{2}\beta_2\Delta t^2\ddot{\mathbf{u}}_{n+1}. \tag{11.44}$$

An alternative to the direct solution is to decouple the equations by transforming it from the space of displacements $\mathbf{u}$ into the space of *free vibration modes* $\mathbf{v}$. Free vibration modes are the solution of a free vibration problem without damping. In such a case

$$\mathbf{M}\ddot{\mathbf{u}}(t) + \mathbf{K}\mathbf{u}(t) = 0 \tag{11.45}$$

for $t > 0$. The equation system describes the observed motion of an FEM mesh that is put into motion by an impulse at $t = 0$. Being a homogeneous linear differential equation system, solutions must be a sum of weighted periodic functions (see Fig. 11.29):

$$\mathbf{u}(t) = \sum_{j=1}^{2N}\mathbf{v}_j\exp(i\omega_j t). \tag{11.46}$$

Replacing $\mathbf{u}(t)$ in (11.45) by (11.46) and computing the second derivative $\ddot{\mathbf{u}}$ results in

Fig. 11.29 Free vibration of an FEM

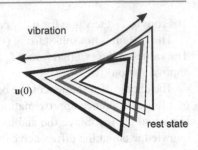

$$\mathbf{M} \sum_{j=1}^{2N} -\omega_i^2 \mathbf{v}_j \exp(i\omega_j t) + \mathbf{K} \sum_{j=1}^{2N} \mathbf{v}_j \exp(i\omega_j t) = 0$$

$$\Leftrightarrow \quad \sum_{j=1}^{2N} \mathbf{K} \mathbf{v}_j \exp(i\omega_j t) = \sum_{j=1}^{2N} -\omega_i^2 \mathbf{M} \mathbf{v}_j \exp(i\omega_j t). \tag{11.47}$$

Comparing factors on both sides and noting that the periodic term $\exp(i\omega_i t)$ is always nonzero, it can be seen that $2N$ solutions of pairs $(\omega, \mathbf{v})$ to the following equation

$$\mathbf{K}\mathbf{v} = \omega^2 \mathbf{M}\mathbf{v} \quad \Leftrightarrow \quad \mathbf{M}^{-1}\mathbf{K}\mathbf{v} = \omega^2 \mathbf{v} \tag{11.48}$$

are searched. Hence, the $2N$ solutions are the eigenvectors of $\mathbf{M}^{-1}\mathbf{K}$ and the corresponding eigenvalues ω^2.

This does not only solve the free vibration problem of (11.45). It also provides the means to solve (11.30) by a set of decoupled partial differential equations, if Raleigh damping $\mathbf{D} = \alpha\mathbf{M} + \beta\mathbf{K}$ is assumed. In this case, diagonalization of $\mathbf{M}$ and $\mathbf{K}$ also diagonalizes all linear combinations.

The equation is transformed into the space of vibration modes. A matrix $\boldsymbol{\Omega}$, containing eigenvectors that are normalized such that $\boldsymbol{\Omega}^{\mathrm{T}}\mathbf{M}\boldsymbol{\Omega} = \mathbf{I}$, is created. Eigenvalues ω_i^2 are the values of a diagonal matrix $\boldsymbol{\Lambda}$. Transformation in the vibration modes produces a new system of decoupled equations

$$\hat{\mathbf{M}}\ddot{\mathbf{v}}(t) + \hat{\mathbf{D}}\dot{\mathbf{v}}(t) + \hat{\mathbf{K}}\mathbf{v}(t) = \mathbf{Q}(t), \tag{11.49}$$

with the diagonal matrices

$$\hat{\mathbf{M}} = \boldsymbol{\Omega}^{\mathrm{T}}\mathbf{M}\boldsymbol{\Omega} = \mathbf{I}, \tag{11.50}$$

$$\hat{\mathbf{K}} = \boldsymbol{\Omega}^{\mathrm{T}}\mathbf{K}\boldsymbol{\Omega} = \boldsymbol{\Lambda}, \tag{11.51}$$

$$\hat{\mathbf{D}} = \alpha\mathbf{I} + \beta\boldsymbol{\Lambda}, \tag{11.52}$$

and the transformed force vector $\mathbf{Q}(t) = \boldsymbol{\Omega}^{\mathrm{T}}\mathbf{f}(t)$.

The now decoupled equations can be brought in the following standard form for differential equations

$$\ddot{v}_i + 2\omega_i \varsigma_i \dot{v}_i + \omega_i^2 v_i + f_i = 0 \tag{11.53}$$

by dividing each equation by the transformed mass factor $\hat{m}_i$ and letting

$$2\omega_i \varsigma_i = \frac{\hat{c}_i}{\hat{m}_i}, \qquad \omega_i^2 = \frac{\hat{k}_i}{\hat{m}_i}, \qquad f_i = -\frac{q_i}{\hat{m}_i}. \tag{11.54}$$

The analytical solution for this differential equation is

$$y_i(t) = \exp(-\xi_i \omega_i t) \left[\frac{\dot{y}_i(0) + \xi_i \omega_i y_i(0)}{\bar{\omega}_j} \sin \bar{\omega}_i t + y_i(0) \cos \bar{\omega}_i t \right]$$
$$+ \frac{1}{\bar{\omega}_i} \int_0^t \exp\left(-\xi_i \omega_i(t - \tau)\right) \sin \bar{\omega}_i(t - \tau) f_i(\tau) \, d\tau, \tag{11.55}$$

with

$$\bar{\omega}_j = \omega_j \sqrt{1 - \xi_j^2} \quad (\xi \text{ is a damping constant}) \tag{11.56}$$

and initial conditions $y_i(0) = \mathbf{v}_i^T \mathbf{M} \mathbf{u}_i(0)$ and $\dot{y}_i(0) = \mathbf{v}_i^T \mathbf{D} \dot{\mathbf{u}}_i(0)$.

The solution does not contain derivatives and the approximation of the integrals can be done using numerically stable methods. Hence, this solution is preferred if instabilities can be expected because computing time constraints require long time intervals or if the system is meant to be simulated over a long time.

The representation of the deformation by a set of uncorrelated modes of vibrations is similar to the representation of shape variation by uncorrelated modes of variation in ASMs (Sect. 11.5.1). The major difference is that *variation modes* are derived from trained variation, whereas *vibration modes* result from material properties and decomposition of a shape.

Material properties are often set constant throughout the figure described by the FEM. As already mentioned earlier, the FEM can be combined with an ASM (Cootes and Taylor 1995). A shape model is constructed as an FEM that "produces" training data for an ASM. Thus, the modes of variation of the initial model are actually modes of the vibration of the FEM. If the model is used for some application, each confirmed segmentation result is considered to be a training sample. The FEM behavior is gradually replaced by the trained statistics of an ASM.

Vibration modes are object-specific symmetries that represent the intrinsic properties of the object. This was used by Sclaroff and Pentland (1995) to create an object-specific intrinsic coordinate system for registering instances of the same object class. Vibration modes are ordered according to their variance (the eigenvalues) and separated into three groups. The lowest-variance modes represent rigid transformations (since the largest total displacement from a given external force is that by a rigid transformation). In the case of 2D models these are the first three modes representing translation in x and y as well as rotation around the origin. They do not carry information about object-specific deformation.[8] The next lowest set of modes is then used to represent intrinsic object-class variation. Vibration modes with high eigenvalues are not considered. Most likely they are severely influenced by inaccuracies from model generation.

The differences between two shapes that are represented by different deformations of the same FEM can now be modeled by modal displacement in the truncated eigenspace (i.e., without the rigid transformation components and low-order modes). The corresponding locations for producing the match in the original space can be reconstructed by projecting the modal amplitudes back using the truncated matrix of eigenvectors.

Similar to ASMs, the deformation in modal amplitudes provides an estimate of the similarity of an object instance with the model. In object detection, the quality of fit of an FEM instance is defined by the deformation. Together with a data term that rates the local appearance in the vicinity of an FEM instance in the image, a weighted QoF measure can be computed.

This can be used for a stochastic search and detection algorithm. FEM instances are placed with arbitrary pose parameters into the image. They are allowed to deform and displace under image forces. The QoF is computed after the instance no longer moves. Pose parameters of the best fitting instances are varied and the process is repeated until the average quality-of-fit of the population no longer improves. Instances with QoF values exceeding some threshold are then detections of object instances. In conjunction with a hierarchical model (see below), this approach has been shown to be very successful for object detection of single objects (Engel and Toennies 2010) or an unknown number of objects (Engel and Toennies 2009).

In classification, a similar strategy is employed. Instead of using a single model, FEMs for different classes are used for the search. Classification is then done by comparing the QoF values of different FEMs.

Almost any kind of shape variation under external forces can be modeled by appropriately varying the material attributes of the underlying physical model, but this puts a heavy burden on the developer of the model. Furthermore, the model has to be adapted for every object class. Hence, the original objective for introducing a physically based model—to replace training by a less costly procedure—is no longer achieved.

If the expected shape variation is too complex, a solution is to resort to shape hierarchies (Engel and Toennies 2010). Similarly to a hierarchical ASM described in Sect. 11.5.1, a shape is decomposed into subunits. Each subunit is modeled by an FEM mesh. Relationships among subunits are modeled by a higher-level FEM. This FEM describes subunits by a number of nodes that are sufficient to represent relationships among subunits (see Fig. 11.30).

---

[8]These modes are not contained in an ASM, since influence from rotation and translation is removed during normalization of the training data.

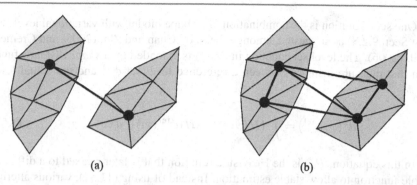

(a)   (b)

Fig. 11.30 Different kinds of second-layer FEMs represent different kinds of spatial relationships between components (a: distance, b: approximate parallelism)

If, for instance, two subunits are related to each other by an expected average distance between them, a single node per subunit is sufficient to represent the location of the subunit. If the relationships are more complex (e.g., if subunits are supposed to be nearly parallel to each other with an expected distance between them) this can be represented as well. High-level nodes representing subunits are related to the FEM representation at the lower level via essential boundary conditions (i.e., the low-level FEM restricts the displacement of its high-level representation).

11.7 Shape Priors

Shape models, such as ASM or other deformable models, may be used for segmentation if part of the data knowledge is misleading. Ideally, the boundary of a fitted model instance already sits on the segment boundary (see Heimann et al. 2006 and Okada et al. 2007 for two different uses of an active shape model to segment the liver in CT). However, the result may be unsatisfactory. Delineation of the object boundary can be inaccurate in locations where the data are reliable. A shape model will have just as many degrees of freedom as are necessary to describe the object characteristics. Object detail may not be representable with sufficient accuracy. Increasing the number of adaptable parameters is not a good solution since the restriction is intentional to train or set shape variation from limited information. A more flexible deformable model may be able to adapt to the object boundary, but it fails to fulfill the original goal for using a shape model. The model is no longer able to predict object shape and adapts to image detail irrespective of whether this detail is reliable or not.

The solution to this dilemma lies in separating the two issues into two steps. The result of fitting a model instance to the data is used as a priori information for a subsequent segmentation by a method that is not driven by shape. This will have little effect in locations, where data are unreliable, but it will drive the segment boundary from its shape-based estimate toward the true boundary in a region where strong and reliable boundary information is present in the data.

One such solution is the combination of a shape model with variational level sets (see Sect. 9.2.8) as suggested, among others, by Chan and Zhu (2005) and Cremers et al. (2006). The level set equation in (9.57) is extended by a *shape distance* function that measure distance between a reference level set ϕ^{ref} and the actual level set ϕ

$$d^2\left(\phi, \phi^{\text{ref}}\right) = \int_{\Omega} \left(H\left(\phi(\mathbf{x})\right) - H\left(\phi^{\text{ref}}(\mathbf{x})\right)\right)^2 dx. \tag{11.57}$$

In this equation, $H()$ is the Heaviside function that is later relaxed to a differentiable function to allow stable estimation. Instead of using (11.57), various alternatives are listed by Cremers et al. (2006) that make the measure independent of the size of the region Ω.

The reference level set is generated by a signed distance transform from a shape instance that estimates the object of interest (this could be a fitted ASM instance or any other suitable deformable model). It also initializes the level set evolution since it is already a good first guess of the final segmentation. The level set evolution will now fit the level set to features in the data while deviations from the reference shape will be penalized. It will leave the initial boundary estimate unchanged in regions where there is no data support, while it will guide the level set to the true boundary in locations where image intensity indicates that the current boundary estimate does not agree with the data.

The shape distance term is weighted against the other terms in the level set equation. The weight reflects assumptions about the reliability of the shape prior and the data information. Shape priors for a level set computation are particularly useful when parts of the boundary are missing because of poor contrast between the object and background. The intensity terms of the variational level set will then be either of little use, since intensities in foreground and background overlap, or they will result in segmentation errors because part of the background is assumed to be the foreground. The shape prior will add just the missing information, as it has been shown, for instance, for liver segmentation in MRI (Gloger et al. 2011).

Shape information can also be added to graph cut segmentation (Vu and Manjunath 2008; Freedman and Zhang 2005). To make shape distance exploitable to graph cuts, the shape deviation penalty has to be assigned to pixel sites. This is realized in Freedman and Zhang (2005) by generating an unsigned distance function $\bar{\phi}$ of the reference shape and by using this to adapt the n-link energy of Boykov et al. (2001), see Sect. 8.1.2, by a shape distance (see Fig. 11.31)

$$d^2(\mathbf{p}, \mathbf{q}) = \bar{\phi}\left(\frac{\mathbf{p} + \mathbf{q}}{2}\right). \tag{11.58}$$

Similar to (11.57), this term needs to be weighted against the other terms in the equation, which in this case is the n-link energy $B_{\mathbf{p},\mathbf{q}}$ that decreases with the increasing gradient between the two pixels $\mathbf{p}$ and $\mathbf{q}$. The effects will be similar to the application of shape priors in level set segmentation. In the absence of strong gradients, the boundary will be defined by the shape prior.

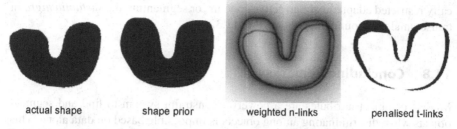

actual shape   shape prior   weighted n-links   penalised t-links

Fig. 11.31 The difference between shape prior and actual shape may be integrated into a graph cut algorithm by weighting the n-links between neighboring pixels or by penalizing t-links between pixels and source or sink node

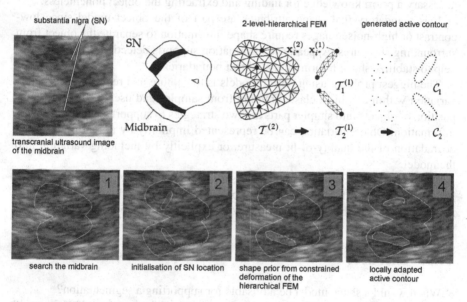

substantia nigra (SN)   2-level-hierarchical FEM   generated active contour

SN

Midbrain

transcranial ultrasound image
of the midbrain

search the midbrain   initialisation of SN location   shape prior from constrained   locally adapted
                                                          deformation of the   active contour
                                                          hierarchical FEM

Fig. 11.32 Shape priors can be used in data with very strong artefacts if the final segmentation method (active contours in this case) is optimized only locally (Engel and Toennies 2008)

In Vu and Manjunath (2008) an overlap difference between actual shape and reference shape has been used as shape distance. The shape prior predicts whether a pixel belongs to the foreground or to the background. A weighted penalty is added to each t-link that depends on whether pixels should be foreground or background (see Fig. 11.31). This will increase the cost of the cut when the difference between reference shape and the produced segmentation gets larger.

If artefacts in images are too strong, global optimization based on the shape prior may fail since the data contain too many false object boundaries. Using a shape instance as prior still makes sense since it can initialize a local search for the segment boundary. This was done by Engel and Toennies (2008), who used a shape model to detect an object of interest using a global shape search followed by a locally restricted adaptation of an active contour for segmenting the *sustantia nigra* in transcranial ultrasound images (see Fig. 11.32).

11.8   Concluding Remarks

Models of object attributes are a powerful constraint system to find and segment objects when discriminating among objects is impossible based on data alone. This may be the case if the data are severely distorted by artefacts (e.g., in an ultrasound) or if adjacent, different objects have the same intensity in the image (which is the case for many soft tissues in MR or CT images). The object model introduces the necessary a priori knowledge for finding and extracting the object nonetheless.

It is mandatory that shape attributes are part of the object model since low-contrast or high-noise images require shape information to separate the object from surrounding structures. Appearance information supports detection and it may also help to stabilize shape information at object boundaries.

The biggest problem using object models is to capture and represent acceptable variation within an object class. Training from samples and user-specified decomposition of objects into simpler parts are two strategies to support acquisition of this information. Object variation can be represented implicitly by accepting a certain degradation of the quality-of-fit measure, or explicitly by including variation into the model.

Although a shape model can be necessary to produce a segmentation at all, restrictions of its deformation may require postprocessing that allows a fitting of segment boundaries to the data at locations where image information is reliable.

11.9   Exercises

• When would a shape model be advisable for supporting a segmentation?
• How is an active shape model used if an object is to be segmented? How could one deal with the fact that the ASM probably would not represent enough shape detail for the segment delineation?
• How could template matching be used to estimate the kidney position (of a healthy kidney) in MRI? Please explain what information is needed and how it could be gathered and represented by the template.
• Assume that the Hough transform is used to find the spherical microorganisms in Fig. 11.7. What would be a strategy to differentiate between bad fits (but microorganisms are found) and wrong detections? Please explain under which assumption your criterion works.
• How could the GHT be used to find the typical shape of the ventricles in Fig. 11.4, given that some shape and size variance has to be expected?
• What is the difference between using normalized cross correlation (see (11.2)) and covariance (see (11.3)) for template matching? What would be a situation where (11.2) should be preferred?

- Why does the medial axis transform not always represent major shape attributes properly? With what kind of strategy can the problem be solved?
- What is the advantage of the hierarchical structure of the medial axis representation? Please explain how the domain knowledge for each of the levels can be acquired if the m-rep were used to detect vertebrae in CT image sequences.
- How is variability encoded in an ASM and how is this information acquired?
- Why could it produce problems when training data for a 2D ASM consisting of 50 boundary points consists of 100 samples?
- What kinds of landmarks are used for representing an ASM? What kind of information about the shape is encoded by the different types of landmarks?
- What influence on the trained ASM does it have when the alignment of the training samples was incorrect? What is the influence if landmark positions are inexact?
- Please explain how alignment is carried out? Under which assumptions will this alignment be successful?
- Why can it safely be assumed that the true dimension of the feature space of an ASM is much lower than the number of degrees of freedom given by the boundary points?
- Why should the dimensionality be further reduced than the dimension that is spanned by the features from the samples?
- What are the stages necessary to fit an ASM to the image?
- How can the ASM be extended to carry appearance information? Why is shape and appearance first trained separately?
- How is shape variability represented by a mass-spring model? How can this variability be changed if necessary?
- What is the purpose of introducing torsion forces in the mass-spring model?
- How is a mass-spring model fitted to the data? How is the influence from the data represented?
- What is the difference of a shape representation by a mass-spring model and a finite element model?
- How can appearance information be represented in a mass-spring-model or a finite element model?
- What role do Poisson ratio and elasticity modulus play when defining a finite element model for detecting objects in an image?
- What is meant with natural and essential boundary conditions of a finite element model? Why are such conditions needed?
- What is the advantage of computing free vibration modes for an FEM when computing the motion of a dynamic finite element model? When would it be preferred instead of a direct computation of the displacement?
- How can the transformation into free vibration modes be used to compute a quality-of-fit measure?
- What are the similarities and what are the differences between vibration modes of finite element models and variation modes of ASMs?
- How can finite element models be used to support training of an ASM? Why can this be assumed to be successful (what does it say about the data)?

References

Al-Zubi S, Toennies KD (2003) Generalizing the active shape model by integrating structural knowledge to recognize hand drawn sketches. In: Proc CAIP 2003. LNCS, vol 2756, pp 320–328

Bardinet E, Cohen LD, Ayache N (2003) Tracking medical 3D data with a parametric deformable model. In: Proc IEEE intl symp computer vision, pp 299–304

Barr AH (1992) Rigid physically based superquadrics. In: Kirk D (ed) Graphics gems III. Academic Press, San Diego, pp 137–159

Bergner S, Al-Zubi S, Toennies KD (2004) Deformable structural models. In: Proc IEEE intl conf image processing ICIP, pp 1875–1878

Biederman I (1985) Human image understanding: recent research and a theory. Comput Vis Graph Image Process 32:29–73

Binford T (1987) Generalized cylinder representation. In: Encyclopedia of artificial intelligence. Wiley, New York, pp 321–323

Blum H (1967) A transformation for extracting new descriptors of shape. In: Proc symp models for the perception of speech and visual form, pp 362–380

Boykov Y, Veksler O, Zabih R (2001) Fast approximate energy minimization via graph cuts. IEEE Trans Pattern Anal Mach Intell 23(11):1222–1239

Brett AD, Taylor CJ (1999) A framework for automated landmark generation for automated 3d statistical model construction. In: Proc 16th intl conf information processing in medical imaging IPMI'99. LNCS, vol 1613, pp 376–381

Chan T, Zhu W (2005) Level set based shape prior segmentation. In: Intl conf computer vision and pattern recognition, pp 1164–1170

Cheung KW, Yeung DY, Chin RT (2002) On deformable models for visual pattern recognition. Pattern Recognit 35(7):1507–1526

Chevalier L, Jaillet F, Baskurt A (2001) 3D shape coding with superquadrics. In: Proc IEEE intl conf image processing ICIP, II, pp 93–96

Cootes TF, Taylor CJ (1992) Active shape models—'smart snakes'. In: Proc British machine vision conference.

Cootes TF, Taylor CJ (1995) Combining point distribution models with shape models based on finite-element analysis. Image Vis Comput 13(5):403–409

Cootes TF, Taylor CJ, Cooper DH, Graham J (1995) Active shape models—their training and application. Comput Vis Image Underst 61(1):38–59

Cootes TF, Edwards GJ, Taylor CJ (1998) Active appearance models. In: 5th European conference on computer vision, ECCV1998. LNCS, vol 1407, pp 484–498

Cremers D, Osher SJ, Soatto S (2006) Kernel density estimation and intrinsic alignment for shape priors in level set segmentation. Int J Comput Vis 69(3):335–351

Davies ER (1998) A modified Hough scheme for general circle location. Pattern Recognit 7(1):37–43

Delingette H, Hebert M, Ikeuchi K (1992) Shape representation and image segmentation using deformable surfaces. Image Vis Comput 10(3):132–145

Dornheim L, Toennies KD, Dornheim J (2005) Stable dyaminc 3d shape models. In: IEEE intl conf image processing ICIP, III, pp 1276–1279

Edelman S (1997) Computational theories in object recognition. Trends Cogn Sci 1:296–304

Engel K, Toennies KD (2008) Segmentation of the midbrain in transcranial sonographies using a two-component deformable model. In: 12th ann conf medical image understanding and analysis, pp 3–7

Engel K, Toennies KD (2009) Hierarchical vibrations: a structural decomposition approach for image analysis. In: Energy minimization methods in computer vision and pattern recognition. LNCS, vol 5681, pp 317–330

Engel K, Toennies KD (2010) Hierarchical vibrations for part-based recognition of complex objects. Pattern Recognit 43(8):2681–2691

Engel K, Toennies KD, Brechmann A (2011) Part-based localisation and segmentation of landmark-related auditory cortical regions. Pattern Recognit 44(9):2017–2033

Ferrant M, Macq B, Nabavi A, Warfield SK (2000) Deformable modeling for characterizing biomedical shape changes. In: 9th intl conf discrete geometry for computer imagery, DGCI 2000. LNCS, vol 1953, pp 235–248

Frangi AF, Rueckert D, Schnabel J, Niessen WJ (2001) Automatic 3d ASM construction via atlas-based landmarking and volumetric elastic registration. In: Proc 17th intl conf information processing in medical imaging, IPMI 2001. LNCS, vol 2082, pp 78–91

Freedman D, Zhang T (2005) Interactive graph cut based segmentation with shape priors. In: IEEE comp society conf on computer vision and pattern recognition (CVPR 2005), vol 1, pp 755–762

Giblin P, Kimia BB (2004) A formal classification of 3d medial axis points and their local geometry. IEEE Trans Pattern Recogn Mach Intell 26(2):238–251

Gloger O, Toennies KD, Kuehn JP (2011) Fully automatic liver volumetry using 3d level set segmentation for differentiated liver tissue types in multiple contrast MR datasets. In: Image analysis. LNCS, vol 6688, pp 512–523

Gong L, Pathak SD, Haynor DR, Cho PS, Kim Y (2004) Parametric shape modeling using deformable superellipses for prostate segmentation. IEEE Trans Med Imaging 23(3):340–349

Hamarneh G, McInerney T, Terzopoulos D (2001) Deformable organisms for automatic medical image analysis. In: Medical image computing and computer-assisted intervention, MICCAI 2001. LNCS, vol 2208, pp 66–76

Heimann T, Wolf I, Meinzer HP (2006) Active shape models for a fully automated 3d segmentation of the liver—an evaluation on clinical data. In: Medical image computing and computer-assisted intervention, MICCAI 2006. LNCS, vol 4191, pp 41–48

Jackway PT, Deriche M (1996) Scale-space properties of the multiscale morphological dilation-erosion. IEEE Trans Pattern Anal Mach Intell 18(1):38–51

Joshi S, Pizer SM, Fletcher PT, Yushkevich P, Thall A, Marron JS (2002) Multiscale deformable model segmentation and statistical shape analysis using medial descriptions. IEEE Trans Med Imaging 21(5):538–550

Kassim AA, Tan T, Tan KH (1999) A comparative study of efficient generalised Hough transform techniques. Image Vis Comput 17(10):737–748

Kichenassamy S, Kumar A, Olver P, Tannenbaum A, Yezzi A (1995) Gradient flows and geometric active contour models. In: 5th intl conf computer vision (ICCV'95), pp 810–817

Lam L, Lee SW, Suen CY (1992) Thinning methodologies—a comprehensive survey. IEEE Trans Pattern Anal Mach Intell 14(9):869–885

Lindeberg T (1994) Scale-space theory: a basic tool for analysing structures at different scales. J Appl Stat 21(2):225–270

Mandal C, Vemuri BC, Qin H (1998) A new dynamic FEM-based subdivision surface model for shape recovery and tracking in medical images. In: Medical image computing and computer-assisted intervention, MICCAI'98. LNCS, vol 1496, pp 753–760

Marr D (1983) Vision. Henry Holt & Company, New York

McInerney T, Terzopoulos D (1996) Deformable models in medical image analysis. Med Image Anal 1(2):91–108

Mokhtarian F, Mackworth A (1986) Scale-based description and recognition of planar curves and two-dimensional objects. IEEE Trans Pattern Anal Mach Intell 8(1):34–43

Okada T, Shimada R, Sato Y, Hori M, Yokota K, Nakamoto M, Chen YW, Nakamura H, Tamura S (2007) Automated segmentation of the liver from 3d CT images using probabilistic atlas and multi-level statistical shape model. In: Medical image computing and computer-assisted intervention, MICCAI 2007. LNCS, vol 4791, pp 86–93

Paloc C, Bello F, Kitney R, Darzi A (2002) Online multiresolution volumetric mass spring model for real time soft tissue deformation. In: Proc 5th intl conf medical image computing and computer-assisted intervention, MICCAI 2002. LNCS, vol 2489, pp 219–226

Pentland AP, Sclaroff S (1991) Closed-form solutions for physically-based modeling and reconstruction. IEEE Trans Pattern Anal Mach Intell 13(7):715–729

Petyt M (1998) Introduction to finite element vibration analysis. Cambridge University Press, Cambridge

Pizer SM, Oliver WR, Bloomberg SH (1987) Hierarchical shape description via the multiresolution symmetric axis transforms. IEEE Trans Pattern Anal Mach Intell 9(4):505–511

Pizer SM, Fritsch DS, Yushkevich PA, Johnson VE, Chaney EL (1999) Segmentation, registration, and measurement of shape variation via image object shape. IEEE Trans Med Imaging 18(10):851–865

Provot X (1995) Deformation constraints in a mass model to describe rigid cloth behaviour. In: Graphics interface, pp 147–154

Riesenhuber M, Poggio T (2000) Models of object recognition. Nat Neurosci Suppl 3:1190–1204

Rivlin E, Dickinson SJ, Rosenfeld A (1995) Recognition by functional parts. Comput Vis Image Underst 62(2):164–176

Sclaroff S, Pentland AP (1995) Modal matching for correspondence and recognition. IEEE Trans Pattern Anal Mach Intell 17(6):545–561

Terzopoulos D, Platt J, Barr A, Fleischer K (1987) Elastically deformable models. Proc SIGGRAPH Comput Graph 21(4):205–214

Terzopoulos D, Fleischer K (1988) Deformable models. Vis Comput 4(6):306–331

Terzopoulos D, Metaxas D (1991) Dynamic 3D models with local and global deformations: deformable superquadrics. IEEE Trans Pattern Anal Mach Intell 13(7):703–714

Toussaint GT (1978) The use of context in pattern recognition. Pattern Recognit 10(3):189–204

Vu N, Manjunath BS (2008) Shape prior segmentation of multiple objects with graph cuts. In: IEEE comp society conf on computer vision and pattern recognition (CVPR 2008), pp 1–8

Xu C, Prince JL (1998) Snakes, shapes, and gradient vector flow. IEEE Trans Image Process 7(3):359–369

Zienkiewics OC, Taylor RL, Zhu JZ (2005) The finite element method: its basis & fundamentals, 6th edn. Elsevier, Amsterdam

Classification and Clustering

12

Abstract

Assigning semantics to segments is required if segmentation has not been combined with object detection. Classification is then based on evaluating segment attributes such as shape and appearance. The dimension of feature space is often high (>10) and the number of samples to train a classifier or to deduce a clustering is low. Methods are different compared to classification or clustering of pixels or voxels. For the most part, likelihood functions are not estimated and the classification criterion is directly based on the training data.

Feature reduction techniques, classifiers, and clustering methods that focus on analysis in sparse feature spaces are the topic of this chapter. These methods complement the methodology presented in Chap. 7.

Concepts, notions and definitions introduced in this chapter

> Feature reduction: PCA, ICA, Fisher's discriminant analysis
> Distance-based classification: minimum distance classifier, kNN classifier
> Decision boundaries: linear decision boundaries, backpropagation networks, support vector machines
> Discriminant functions
> Agglomerative clustering
> Fuzzy clustering

Structures of interest in an image may be divided into different classes based on their segment properties. In medical image analysis, classification and segmentation sometimes mix since class membership may also be assigned based on pixel attributes (see Chap. 7). *Classification* discussed in this chapter relates to the assignment of class membership to samples—which could be segments— based on their features. The major difference to classification integrated in segmentation is that the number of samples is often smaller and the number of features per sample is often larger. This has consequences for the classification strategy. If pixels are treated as

K.D. Toennies, *Guide to Medical Image Analysis*,
Advances in Computer Vision and Pattern Recognition,
DOI 10.1007/978-1-4471-2751-2_12, © Springer-Verlag London Limited 2012

samples, their large number and the low dimension of feature space result in a fairly accurate estimate of underlying probabilities. Training becomes more difficult when the dimensionality of feature space is high and few training samples exist. Classification resorts to strategies that do not estimate the probability distribution functions for the complete feature space but

- compute a posteriori probabilities only for those feature values of samples to be classified, or
- compute the boundary at which two a posteriori probability functions have the same values (i.e., the boundary where class label assignment changes).

This will be discussed in the following sections. It will be followed by a treatment of clustering techniques that merely detect patterns in the data that may be influential for classification. Often clustering is a first step to analyze the significance of features.

12.1   Features and Feature Space

A segment may be characterized by different types of attributes that make up the feature space.

- Average gray values or—as it is the case of some MR images—a vector of average gray values from different channels represent a (possibly known) relationship between measurement and membership to an object class.
- Second- or higher-order statistics such as gray level variance within the segment represent possible object-specific variations of the measurement value within an object class or object-specific measurement artefacts.
- Texture features of the gray level distribution in the segment represent tissue characteristics. They may also be important attributes for differentiating between different states of an organ's class (such as healthy organs versus pathologic variations).
- Shape features such as size and elongation of a segment, or ASM mode variation may typify a segment as well. If the segment represents the complete object (and not a part of it), shape features may help to determine the type of object.

The first three types of features may be reliable, even if the segment comprises only a part of the object to be classified as long as it is mainly located within the object. Shape features are only reliable if the segment boundary closely follows the object boundary.

In general, any feature that contributes to the characterization of a segment may be included in the feature vector. Not all of the features may be necessary and some redundancy will be included in such a representation.

12.1.1 Linear Decorrelation of Features

Features $f_1, \ldots, f_N$ of a vector $\mathbf{f} = (f_1 f_2, \ldots, f_N)$ in N-dimensional feature space are initially assumed to be independent of each other. The dimensionality of feature space is often much higher than the two or three dimensions that can easily be

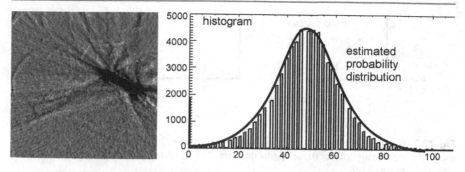

Fig. 12.1 If the number of samples per feature is high, it is easy to reliably estimate a probability distribution from samples

Fig. 12.2 It is difficult to approximate an unknown distribution from samples if the histogram shows few occurrences in a high-dimensional feature space

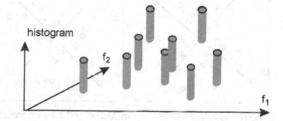

rendered by some visualization technique. Thus, interactive techniques that display a feature distribution of samples and ask the user to identify classes based on visible clustering are difficult to implement. Sample distributions in feature space can be projected on 2D subspaces and then displayed, but assessing distributions in N dimensions from a series of 2D projections is very difficult for $N \gg 2$.

The high dimensionality of feature space complicates automatic classification as well because most techniques rely on applying the Bayesian Theorem. The necessary probability distributions are often not known in advance and need to be estimated from classified samples. This training of the classifier requires a certain density of sample distribution for delivering reliable estimates (see Fig. 12.1).

For a given number of samples in the training database the density decreases with the increasing number of feature dimensions. In such a case, estimates from a feature histogram may be difficult to generate (see Fig. 12.2). However, initial feature selection often accumulates all computable attributes of a segment that may contribute to the identification of the object class. The initial assumption of uncorrelated features may not be true.[1]

---

[1]Consider, for instance, Haralick's texture features from the co-occurrence matrix. Many of the features measure quantities which may behave similar for a class of segments. The same may be true for shape features. E.g., the size of a segment may be closely related to its elongatedness if segments are cells in a microscopic image of two types of which the small ones are mostly circular while the larger ones are not.

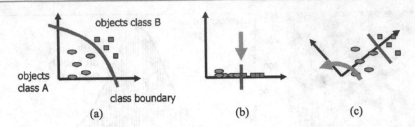

Fig. 12.3 Feature reduction from original space (**a**) can be done by simply removing features with the least discriminative power (**b**) or by first de-correlating the data and then apply reduction in the de-correlated space (**c**)

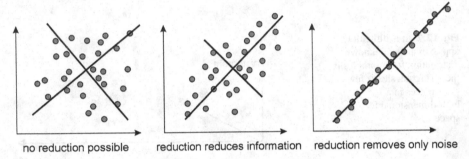

Fig. 12.4 PCA produces an axis system that decorrelates the data. It is oriented along the data distribution in feature space. Features of this new coordinate system may be removed, if projection on the remaining axes produces only a small error

The simplest way to reduce the dimensionality of the feature space is a repeated removal of features that produces the least increase of the classification error. Feature reduction is more efficient if features are decorrelated first and the dimension of feature space is reduced afterward (see Fig. 12.3).

Linear decorrelation and subsequent feature reduction can be carried out by *principal component analysis* (*PCA*) in feature space (see Sect. 14.3, a detailed treatment can be found in Abdi and Williams 2010). If features are correlated, the distribution of samples in feature space actually occupies a lower-dimensional subspace. The PCA produces an orthogonal transformation in feature space such that all covariance values between features are zero. Coordinate axes after transformation are aligned or orthogonal to this subspace (see Fig. 12.4). Features corresponding to orthogonal axes to the subspace can be identified and removed.

12.1.2   Linear Discriminant Analysis

Using PCA for feature reduction can be tricky because the decomposition does not tell anything about class separability after reduction. This would require knowledge on class membership from a set of classified training samples. A simple strategy is

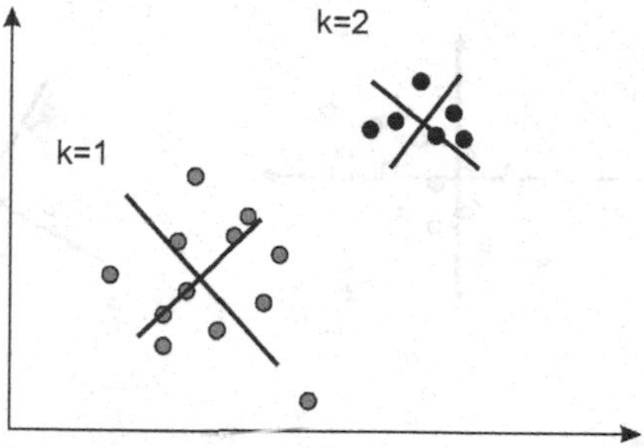

Fig. 12.5 The within-class scatter matrix is computed from adding co-variance matrices of the different classes weighted by their a priori probability

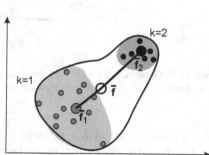

Fig. 12.6 The between-class scatter matrix is computed from the vectors from class centers $\bar{\mathbf{f}}_i$ to the center $\bar{\mathbf{f}}$ of all classes

to select features such that the within-class scatter is minimized and the between-class scatter is maximized for some distribution of samples in feature space. The technique is known as *linear discriminant analysis* (LDA) or *Fisher's discriminant analysis* (Fisher 1936).

The *within-class scatter matrix* $\boldsymbol{\Sigma}_W$ is defined as (see Fig. 12.5)

$$\boldsymbol{\Sigma}_W = \sum_{k=1}^{K} P(k) \cdot \boldsymbol{\Sigma}_k, \qquad (12.1)$$

where $P(k)$ is the a priori probability of a sample belonging to class k and $\boldsymbol{\Sigma}_k$ is the covariance matrix for the distribution of samples of class k in feature space. The a priori probabilities can be estimated from the ratio of samples belonging to class k to the number of all samples. The covariance matrix can be estimated as above, but now including only feature values of samples of class k.

The *between-class scatter matrix* $\boldsymbol{\Sigma}_B$ is defined as (see Fig. 12.6)

$$\boldsymbol{\Sigma}_B = \sum_{k=1}^{K} P(k)(\bar{\mathbf{f}}_k - \bar{\mathbf{f}})(\bar{\mathbf{f}}_k - \bar{\mathbf{f}})^{\mathrm{T}}, \qquad \mathbf{f} = \sum_{k=1}^{K} P(k)\mathbf{f}_k. \qquad (12.2)$$

It measures the scatter of average feature vectors $\bar{\mathbf{f}}_k$ for the different classes k with respect to the average feature vector $\mathbf{f}$ of the whole data set.

Feature reduction should produce new features $\mathbf{f}'$ with improved class separability by maximizing the between-class scatter and minimizing the within-class scatter. A new set of orthogonal feature axes is selected so that the combined variances of

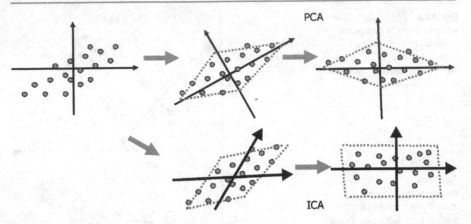

Fig. 12.7 Opposed to PCA, ICA produces a system of linear independent features. No prediction about the value of one feature can be made based on the value of another feature

Σ_B and the inverse of Σ_W given by the sum of diagonal elements of their product $\mathrm{tr}(\Sigma_W^{-1}\Sigma_B)$ (the *trace* of the matrix) are maximal. Hence, using a similar argumentation than for computing the PCA, eigenvectors, and eigenvalues of $\Sigma_W^{-1}\Sigma_B$ are computed. Eigenvectors are the new basis onto which features $\mathbf{f}$ are projected yielding $\mathbf{f}'$. Features with large eigenvalues are selected for subsequent classification.

12.1.3 Independent Component Analysis

Transformation in feature space, as discussed above, mainly attempts to reduce redundancy in the data for the purpose of assigning classes to samples. Sometimes, however, each sample may contain a mixture of two or more components. No class assignment is desired. Instead, the ratio of this mixture shall be determined. This scenario may arise, for example, in time signal analysis describing organ function. Functional units are often much smaller than the image resolution and information carriers would be subpixels. As they cannot be measured, analysis attempts to decompose the measured signal into its unknown components. This is possible if the different components are independent and some additional assumptions hold. The procedure is called *independent component analysis (ICA)* (Hyvärinen and Oja 2000; Hyvärinen et al. 2009), see Fig. 12.7.

As opposed to PCA, a closed-form solution for computing the independent components does not exist. ICA methods are iterative optimization methods that are not guaranteed to find the global optimum. Independent component analysis assumes that

- a feature vector $\mathbf{f}$ consists of a number of independent components $\mathbf{f}_{c1}, \ldots, \mathbf{f}_{cn}$,
- the number of components is known,
- their distribution is non-Gaussian.

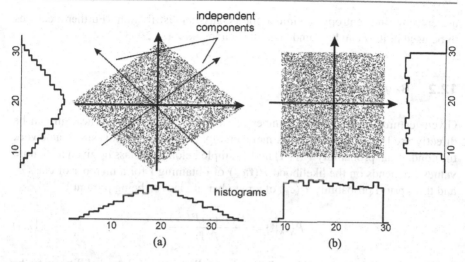

Fig. 12.8 The distribution of dependent components (**a**) resembles a Gaussian, whereas truly independent data (**b**) does not

The procedure consists of two steps. First, independent components are computed from the feature distribution in some data set. Then, each feature vector is projected on the independent components to determine the composition in every sample.

The computation of independent components from observed feature values f_i is done by finding feature axes f' that minimize the Gaussianity of the decomposed data set. The underlying assumption is a general observation about probability. A probability distribution of some stochastic process approaches a Gaussian distribution if the number of independent causes for the process increases.[2] In reverse, a distribution is less Gaussian, if it consists of fewer independent components (see Fig. 12.8). ICA estimates Gaussianity of the current set of axes and rotates one of the axes so that Gaussianity is minimized. This process is repeated until convergence. Gaussianity can be measured, for instance, by computing the absolute value of *kurtosis excess* γ_2 (Hyvärinen and Oja 2000)

$$\gamma_2 = \frac{E((f - \bar{f})^4)}{E((f - \bar{f})^2)^2} - 3, \tag{12.3}$$

which measures the peakedness of a distribution. A distribution with high peak is called leptokurtic and has values of $\gamma_2 < 0$, one with a flat peak is called platykurtic with $\gamma_2 > 0$. The Gaussian distribution is mesokurtic with $\gamma_2 = 0$. Maximizing $|\gamma_2|$ therefore minimizes Gaussianity. Another option for computing Gaussianity is to

---

[2]The central limit theorem states that the probability density function of a sum of independent random variables having the same but unknown distribution characteristics will approximately be a Gaussian function, if the variance for each variable is finite.

use entropy since entropy is minimal for a Gaussian distribution. (Further measures to be used in ICA can be found, e.g., in Blanco and Zazo 2003.)

12.2 Bayesian Classifier

Given features of a sufficient number of samples, the Bayesian Theorem can be directly used for computing class membership. Stated in the Bayesian framework the conditional probability $P(c_k|\mathbf{f})$ that a sample belongs to class c_k given its feature values $\mathbf{f}$ depends on the likelihood $P(\mathbf{f}|c_k)$ of obtaining $\mathbf{f}$ for a member of class c_k and the a priori probability $P(c_k)$ of a member of class c_k being present:

$$P(c_k|\mathbf{f}) = \frac{P(f|c_k)P(c_k)}{P(\mathbf{f})}. \tag{12.4}$$

The normalizing probability $P(\mathbf{f})$, also called marginal probability, may be dropped for classification since $P(\mathbf{f})$ is independent of c_k. The classification of a sample with feature vector $\mathbf{f}$ requires to choose the class c_{opt} with

$$c_{\mathrm{opt}} = \arg\max_{c_k} P(c_k|\mathbf{f}) = \arg\max_{c_k} P(f|c_k)P(c_k). \tag{12.5}$$

The likelihood function and the a priori probability have to be estimated from training data or specified using expert knowledge.

The normalized multidimensional histogram of binned feature values generated from classified training samples may be used as estimate for $P(\mathbf{f}|c_k)$. A rule of thumb says that the number b of bins along an axis in N-dimensional feature space should relate to the number of available samples M by

$$b = M^{\frac{1}{N+1}}. \tag{12.6}$$

Even if feature space is reduced, the number of classified samples may still not be adequate for a reliable estimate of the likelihood function.

Various techniques exist for constraining the range of possible likelihood functions without being overly restrictive. If the number of classified samples is rather large, it can be assumed that every sample represents the expected value of a Gaussian distribution of known variance in feature space. This corresponds to convolving the histogram with a Gaussian kernel with zero mean and this variance. This is a special case of a *kernel density estimator* (Rosenblatt 1956; Sarle 1994), which computes a likelihood function $f_h(x)$ from samples x_i, $I = 1, \ldots, N$ that are drawn from this distribution by convolving the samples with a kernel function K

$$f_h(x) = \frac{1}{nh} \sum_{i=1}^{n} K\left(\frac{x - x_i}{h}\right). \tag{12.7}$$

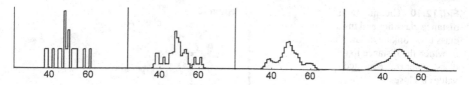

Fig. 12.9 Convolving the histogram of a feature distribution with Gaussian kernels with increasing variance produces an increasingly smoother estimate of the underlying distribution

In the case of the Gaussian kernel (see Fig. 12.9) this function is given by

$$K\left(\frac{x - x_i}{h}\right) = \frac{1}{\sqrt{2\pi}\,h} \exp\left(-\left(\frac{x - x_i}{h}\right)^2\right). \tag{12.8}$$

If it is known that features are uncorrelated (e.g., after carrying out PCA analysis and transforming the feature space[3]), the estimation of the likelihood function becomes much easier. In this case, $P(f|c_k) = \prod_{i=1}^{N} P(f_i|c_k)$ and the 1D likelihood functions can be computed separately for each feature.

Often, however, the likelihood function is constrained even more by assuming that it is a multivariate Gaussian distribution. Variation of feature values can often be assumed to be caused by a number of independent influences with appropriate properties so that we can make use of the Central Limit Theorem again. Assuming Gaussian distributions reduces necessary estimations to the computation of the expected value $\bar{\mathbf{f}}$ and the covariance matrix $\mathbf{\Sigma}$ of $\mathbf{f}$. The problem is further simplified if features are uncorrelated so that only their variances have to be estimated.

Computing the a priori probabilities $P(c_k)$ is usually easier. If it can be assumed that the samples in the training data set are representative for the population, the ratio of the number of samples of class c_k to the total number of samples estimates $P(c_k)$.

12.3   Classification Based on Distance to Training Samples

The number of training samples may not suffice for a good estimate of the feature likelihood function. On the other hand, in most regions of the feature space the difference between the most probable class assignment and its next competitor is very large. Estimation errors will not affect the classification result. Hence, several methods directly estimate the a posteriori probability using some simplifying assumptions.

Minimum distance classification requires univariate Gaussian feature likelihood functions with equal variances for each class. The a posteriori probability of a sample with feature vector $\mathbf{f}$ belonging to some class c_{opt} is maximized by selecting the

---

[3]It should be remembered that the PCA is based on an estimate of the covariance matrix. The reliability of this estimate depends on the dimensionality of feature space and the number of samples.

Fig. 12.10 The minimum distance classifier assigns a class to an unknown sample, of which the distance to the class center (the expected value) is closest

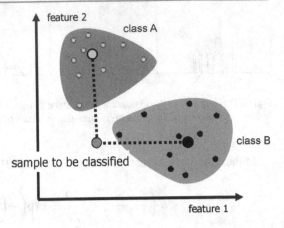

class with average feature vector $\bar{\mathbf{f}}_k$ to which it is the closest (see Fig. 12.10):

$$c_{\text{opt}} = \arg\min_{c_k} \|\mathbf{f} - \bar{\mathbf{f}}_k\|. \tag{12.9}$$

Computing the minimum distance classifier is slightly more costly than Bayesian decision-making as the computational cost increases linearly with the number of class centers. However, it does not require estimates of the likelihood function. The estimates for average values $\bar{\mathbf{f}}_k$ may be improved when newly classified samples are added to the training database.

Requiring univariate Gaussians with equal variances is rather restrictive, however, considering scatterplots of most distributions. A more accurate estimate for the a posteriori probability can be generated when the actual distribution of training samples is taken into account. To approximate the probability density function for some class c_k at a location $\mathbf{f}$ in feature space, the function is assumed to be locally constant in some vicinity f_δ around $\mathbf{f}$. Using f_δ as bin size, the normalized histogram serves as estimate for $P(c_k|\mathbf{f})$.

Samples may be distributed so sparsely that the size of f_δ needs to be large and constancy can no longer be assumed. Hence, classification schemes adapt neighborhood size according to local density of training samples.

The *nearest-neighborhood classifier* uses the smallest possible neighborhood size (see Fig. 12.11). The neighborhood around some sample $\mathbf{f}$ is the smallest hypersphere that contains the closest training sample to $\mathbf{f}$. If the class of the nearest sample is c_{near}, the estimate of $P(c_{\text{near}}|\mathbf{f})$ is 1 and $P(c|\mathbf{f}) = 0$ for all other classes c. Class c_{near} is assigned to the sample with features $\mathbf{f}$.

Using the nearest neighbor is a fairly rough estimate of the true probabilities and may deliver wrong results if the likelihood functions for the different classes have a complex shape. Hence, the adaptive neighborhood can be increased to include the first k samples. This is the *k-nearest-neighborhood (kNN) classifier* (see Fig. 12.12). Given that k_k of the k training samples belong to class c_k, the estimate of its probability is $P(c_k|\mathbf{f}) = k_k/k$. The kNN classifier is a voting mechanism where each of

Fig. 12.11 The Nearest
Neighborhood classifier
computes the closest
classified sample to a sample
with unknown class and
classifies the sample
accordingly

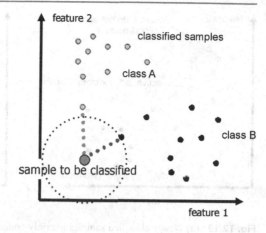

Fig. 12.12 The kNN
classifier classifies an
unknown sample according to
the class memberships of the
k nearest neighbors (shown
here for $k = 3$)

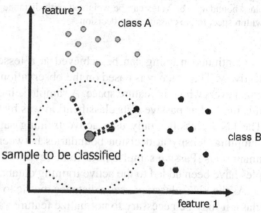

the k samples votes for a certain class. The class receiving the most votes is assigned
to the sample with feature vector **f**.

The quality of the estimate improves with the density of samples and the number k of voting samples. Better estimates let the classification error approach that of
Bayesian classification with known a priori probabilities and known feature likelihood functions.

Computing the result of a kNN classifier can be time-consuming. To find the
nearest neighbors to a given sample, distances to all samples in the training database
have to be computed. Many efficient schemes exist [e.g., the branch-and-bound
strategy in Jiang and Zhang (1993), the precomputation of a distance transform
in Warfield (1996), or the approximation in the wavelet domain in Hwang and
Wen (1998)], but the computational cost still increases with the size of the training
database. This can be critical if the accuracy of the computation is to be improved
by including classified samples into the database. The error rate may drop with time
as the average density of samples in feature space increases, but the computation
time increases. This is particularly disturbing when the user is not aware of the underlying reasons since the system seems to slow down with age.

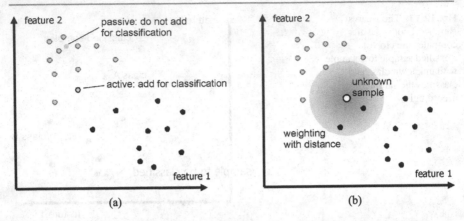

Fig. 12.13 (a) Newly classified samples are only added to the data base, if they are close to the class boundary. (b) Votes can be weighted with distance in order to account for their reliability with respect to the classification decision

Continued training can be achieved at a lesser cost if density is increased selectively. The strategy is based on the observation that accuracy does not need to be equal everywhere in feature space. A sample is included in the training database, but it is marked as passive if its classification was by unanimous vote (see Fig. 12.13a). The kNN classifier only uses active training samples. The strategy increases the sampling density at decision boundaries between classes where votes are seldom unanimous. Passive samples have to be reviewed from time to time after new samples have been added to the active training database.

As the kNN classifier uses a distance metric to compute the number of votes for a class, it may be necessary to normalize feature values with their standard deviation before computing nearest neighbors. However, if a high variance of a feature value indicates a higher importance of this feature, normalization should not be carried out.

Classification based on feature values may be unreliable if

- the data values are too small,
- the vote difference is too small, or
- the sample is too far away from any classified samples in the training data.

This reliability can be measured and if it is too low, a sample may be rejected. Votes can also be weighted with the distance to the sample, which automatically causes reliability to be low if a sample is too far away from any classified sample (see Fig. 12.13b).

12.4 Decision Boundaries

We already observed that estimates for a posteriori probabilities have to be most accurate at decision boundaries. In fact, the decision boundary alone, that is, the curve of equal a posteriori probability for at least two classes suffices if a method exists for determining on which side of such a boundary the feature vector of an unknown sample is located. Techniques for finding and applying decision boundaries will be discussed in this section. Most of the discussion will be based on a so-called *two-class problem* (i.e., the assignment of an unknown sample to one of two classes). Extensions to more than two classes will be discussed where appropriate.

All of the methods described below have in common that the search for a decision boundary is formulated as an optimization task that is usually solved iteratively. In general, the solution strategy does not guarantee that the global minimum (i.e., the optimal decision boundary) is found. This makes the use of decision boundaries sometimes inferior to the methods described in the previous section. The major advantages of decision boundaries are

- that their computation considers the need for increased accuracy at the boundary between two class regions,
- that the classification is faster requiring only constant computational cost once the decision boundary is defined.

12.4.1 Adaptive Decision Boundaries

If classes are well separated in feature space, linear *adaptive decision boundaries* may serve as classifier. A single linear decision boundary solves a two-class problem. It is represented by a linear equation in feature space

$$D(\mathbf{f}, \mathbf{w}, w_0) = \mathbf{w}^{\mathrm{T}}\mathbf{f} + w_0, \tag{12.10}$$

where $\mathbf{w} = (w_1, w_2, \ldots, w_N)$ and w_0 are weights determining the position of the hyperplane $D(\mathbf{f}, \mathbf{w}, w_0) = 0$ that separates the two classes. The constant w_0 is called the *bias* term. It is proportional to the distance of $\mathbf{f}$ to the hyperplane, if $D(\mathbf{f}, \mathbf{w}, w_0) \neq 0$. $D(\mathbf{f}, \mathbf{w}, w_0)$ is positive, if $\mathbf{f}$ is on the side of the hyperplane to which its normal points. Otherwise it is negative.

Classification into two classes requires weights to be found such that classified training samples are separated by the hyperplane. The iterative algorithm depicted in Fig. 12.14 will compute the hyperplane if it exists (i.e., if the classes are linearly separable; see Fig. 12.15 for an illustration).

Restricting the number of iterations irrespective of the current classification error is necessary because of several reasons.

- The samples may not be linearly separable. In this case, no hyperplane exists and the algorithm will only stop after the maximum number of iterations is reached.
- The correction factors c and k are set too high. The hyperplane oscillates around the correct solution because most correction steps are pushing the hyperplane too far in the opposite direction.
- The correction factors are set too low. The convergence to the solution is too slow and may not reach convergence after the maximum number of iterations.

Finding c and k is critical, and it is even more so the narrower the range of acceptable hyperplanes is (i.e., the closer the two classes are to each other).

initialize weights $w_0, \ldots, w_M$ with small random values
repeat until classification is perfect, average error is smaller than ε_{min} **or** maximum number of
steps is executed
       select sample **f** from training set and compute $D(\mathbf{f}, \mathbf{w}, w_0)$
      if class(**f**) $\neq$ sgn($D(\mathbf{f}, \mathbf{w}, w_0)$) **then**; with $c, k > 0$
            $w_i := w_i + c \cdot \text{class}(\mathbf{f}) \cdot f_i$
            $w_0 := w_0 + c \cdot \text{class}(\mathbf{f}) \cdot k$
      end_if
end_repeat

class(**f**) returns -1 if the sample belongs to the first and $+1$ if it belongs to the second class
sgn() is the signum function.

Fig. 12.14   Sketch of the loop for computing weights of a linear decision boundary

Fig. 12.15   If a selected
sample is not classified
correctly, the decision
boundary is moved towards
the incorrectly classified
sample

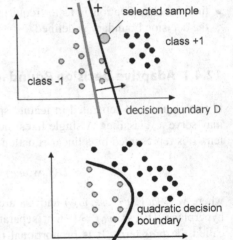

Fig. 12.16   A quadratic
decision boundary may
separate classes that are not
linearly separable

If classes are not linearly separable, they may be separated by a nonlinear
boundary. However, computing distances to a nonlinear boundary is much more
complex than computing the distance to the hyperplane. It gets simpler if the nonlinear boundary can be embedded in a higher-dimensional space in such a way
that the problem becomes linear. An example is a quadratic decision surface (see
Fig. 12.16) in two-dimensional feature space where the embedding is

$$D(\mathbf{f}, \mathbf{w}, w_0) = w_0 + w_1 u_1 + w_2 u_2 + w_3 u_3 + w_4 u_4 + w_5 u_5, \qquad (12.11)$$

with

$$u_1 = f_1, \quad u_2 = f_2, \quad u_3 = f_1 f_2, \quad u_4 = f_1^2, \quad u_5 = f_2^2. \qquad (12.12)$$

Similar embeddings can be created for other polynomial surfaces, but the dimensionality of feature space increases rapidly. Hence, embeddings are usually restricted to a low-dimensional feature space and polynomials of low order.

Decision boundaries can solve multiple class problems. A decision boundary D_{ij} needs to be trained for every pair of classes i and j. An unknown sample is inserted into all equations. It is classified as the one class that is not ruled out by any of the equations. The number of decision boundaries increases with the square of the number of classes. Furthermore, regions exist where all classes are ruled out. Samples in such a region are either classified as *undecided* or submitted to a second classifier (e.g., by computing the distance to the closest outruling class boundary).

12.4.2 The Multilayer Perceptron

Backpropagation neural networks deal with nonlinear decision boundaries and with multiple class problems more efficiently than the decision boundaries described above. They are also called *multilayer perceptrons* (MLP) as they consist of a sequence of perceptrons.

Perceptrons were introduced early in computer science (Rosenblatt 1958). They are a single layer neural network with all input nodes connected to a single output node. They model a linear decision boundary. Nevertheless, they introduce the concept of a neural network and will be described in more detail before continuing to the discussion of multilayer networks.

Any neural network can be represented by a graph with nodes—the cell body of the artificial neural network—and edges connecting the nodes—the dendrites. A great introduction into neural networks in general and their use for pattern recognition is Bishop (1995).

A neural network is hierarchical if it does not allow cycles in the graph. A hierarchical network is *layered* if nodes are organized in layers so that each node of a given layer is only connected to nodes of the previous layer—from which it receives input—and to nodes of the next layer—to which it gives input (see Fig. 12.17a). The input nodes of a perceptron are connected to a single output neuron.

Nodes "fire," that is, they give a signal through all their outgoing edges to nodes of the next layer based on input that they receive and based on a node-specific activation function f (see Fig. 12.17b).

To mimic the behavior of a nerve cell, this firing can be implemented as a threshold on the input. The input is produced by a gathering function g that integrates input received from other nodes. Input originates from firing nodes in the previous layer. The signal is weighted by edge-specific weights connecting the firing nodes with the receiving node. If we label nodes by layer l and their position k in the layer and if we assume a fully connected network, gathering is

$$g(n_{l,k}) = \sum_{i=0}^{K(l-1)} w_{l-1,i} f(n_{l-1,i}). \tag{12.13}$$

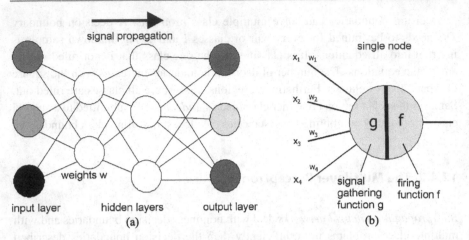

Fig. 12.17 (a) Structure of a layered neural network. (b) Nodes fire, if the gathered signal exceeds some threshold defined by the activation function

The number of nodes at layer $l - 1$ is $K(l - 1)$. The input from nodes $n_{l-1,0}$ is a constant representing the bias. Firing is

$$f(n_{l,k}) = \begin{cases} 1, & \text{if } g(n_{l,k}) > t, \\ 0, & \text{otherwise,} \end{cases} \tag{12.14}$$

where t is a threshold that determines when to fire. Node layers are counted from 1 to L with L being the output layer. The layer $L = 0$ receives input from the feature vector $\mathbf{f}$

$$g(n_{1,k}) = \sum_{i=0}^{K(0)} w_{0,i} f_i, \tag{12.15}$$

where f_i, $i = 1, K(0)$ is the ith feature of $\mathbf{f}$ with length $K(0)$ and $\mathbf{f}_0 = 1$ is the input bias.

It is now easy to see that, with firing threshold $t = 0$, a perceptron is a linear decision boundary. It is trained in the same fashion and solves the same kind of classification problems.

If a sequence of perceptrons is coupled, the capability of representing various decision boundaries increases dramatically (see Fig. 12.18). If the first layer feeds in several nodes and a second layer is added with a single node, the decision surface at the second layer is a convex, not necessarily closed polyhedron. Each of its bounding surfaces is determined by the output of one of the nodes in the previous layer. By increasing the number of nodes in the previous layer, the bounding polyhedron can approximate any convex surface with arbitrary precision. If several classes are to be separated, extra nodes per class representing their own decision boundary are created in the second layer.

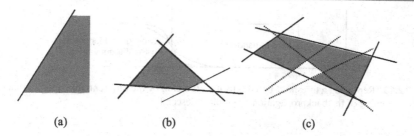

Fig. 12.18 (a) A single layer enables linear separation in feature space. (b) Adding nodes in an additional (hidden) layer, arbitrary convex decision boundaries can be represented. (c) With two hidden layers, convex figures can be combined to represent arbitrary concave decision boundaries

Arbitrary concave decision boundaries can be represented by adding a third layer. By addition and subtraction of the convex figures from the previous layer any decision boundary can be approximated with arbitrary precision, provided that the number of nodes in the first and second layers is arbitrarily large.

The middle layer of a three-layer perceptron is called the *hidden layer*. Although it can be shown that three layers suffice to approximate any decision boundary, multilayer perceptrons may contain more than one hidden layer. This accommodates different views on the data since each new layer adds a level of abstraction to the description of the decision boundary. The first layer separates space by hyperplanes, the second layer combines hyperplanes to convex figures, the third combines these to convex or concave figures, the fourth combines concave figures, and so on. Increasing the number of nodes within a layer adds capabilities to describe details of the decision boundary at the current level of abstraction. If a problem is known to be separable by a sequence of decisions, it is often advisable to choose a number of layers that corresponds to the number of hierarchy levels of this sequence.

Let us assume that the $K(L)$ nodes of the last layer L of a multilayer perceptron represent classes into which samples in feature space shall be sampled. These nodes could code the classification result in any convenient way. One could, for instance, use a binary code so that class membership to some class k would be a node pattern of the output nodes, which is the binary code of k. A simpler way would be that the desired output for a training sample belonging to class k is a vector $\mathbf{y}$ with $K(L)$ elements y_i such that $y_i = 1$ if $i = k$ and $y_i = 0$ otherwise. If the network is untrained, the output from an input feature vector $\mathbf{x}$ will differ from the desired pattern $\mathbf{y}$. The task is to find weights $w_{l,k}$ that minimize $\|\mathbf{y} - \mathbf{x}\|^2$ for all samples of the training data set.

Nothing has been said so far about the training of a multilayer perceptron. The simple algorithm for linear decision boundaries is not applicable. In turns out, however, that a generic method exists that computes a gradient descent on the weights for an arbitrary multilayer perceptron. It requires that the error function is differentiable. Hence, the thresholding in the activation function is replaced by the *sigmoid*

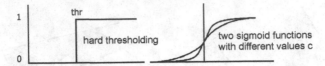

Fig. 12.19 Replacing a threshold-based activation function by the differentiable sigmoid function enables training of the backpropagation by gradient descend

function (see Fig. 12.19)

$$f(n_{l,k}) = \frac{1}{1 + \exp(c \cdot g(n_{l,k}))}. \tag{12.16}$$

It introduces fuzziness into the decision process. The function asymptotically approaches 0 for $f() \to -\infty$ and it approaches 1 for $f() \to \infty$. The rate of change is fastest at the origin. The steepness at the origin is controlled by c. The derivative of the sigmoid function is

$$f'(n_{l,k}) = f(n_{l,k})\big(1 - f(n_{l,k})\big). \tag{12.17}$$

It has been shown that the partial derivatives of the error function with respect to the weights can be computed by *backpropagating* the error from the output nodes into the network.[4] Iterative minimization starts with a feedforward step at each iteration n. It produces the output vector $\mathbf{x}^{(n)}$ using the current weights. Backpropagation then distributes the error correction, beginning at the output layer, back into the network. First, the derivative of the error $\|\mathbf{x}^{(n)} - \mathbf{y}\|$ with respect to the weights between the previous and last layers is computed. These weights are corrected accordingly and used to propagate the error into the previous layer. Error correction at this layer is again done by computing and applying partial derivatives of the error. The weight update of the current iteration terminates when the input layer is reached. For all but the last layer, the computation of the derivative requires the computation of derivatives in the higher layers. A sketch of the algorithm is depicted in Fig. 12.20.

The *learning rate* λ controls the speed with which learning converges. Large values for λ accelerate learning, but the probability of oscillation around a solution increases as well. Since gradient descent may become stuck in a local minimum, starting with a good guess for the weights improves the chances of convergence to a satisfactory solution. In the absence of such knowledge, random values for the weights should be chosen to avoid unwanted bias.

---

[4]The proof of this is a bit lengthy and will not be shown here. For a detailed treatment of backpropagation networks see Bishop (1995). The reasons why backpropagation produces a gradient descent are, briefly, the following: At each node, the gathering function sums up weighted results from the previous node and the derivative of a sum of functions is the sum of its derivatives. Fortunately, for computing the derivative of some weights, all previous weights can be treated as constants in the derivation. Applying the activation function to the sum is the application of a function to another function so that the chain rule applies to its derivative.

Initialize all weights $w_{l,k}^{(0)}$ to small random numbers
choose a positive constant λ (the learning rate)
for all samples **do**
    set $f_{0,1}, \ldots, f_{0,K(0)}$ to feature values of selected sample
    compute output vector $x_1, \ldots, x_{K(L)}$ at layer L with weights $w_{l,k}^{(n)}$
    compute partial derivatives at L: $\delta_{L,k}^{(n)} = x_k^{(n)}(1 - x_k^{(n)})(x_k^{(n)} - y_k)$
    for all layers $l = L - 1, \ldots, 1$ **do**

$$\delta_{L,k}^{(n)} = f_{l,k}^{(n)}\left(1 - f_{l,k}^{(n)}\right) \sum_{i=1}^{K(l)} \delta_{l,i}^{(n)} w_{l,i}^{(n)}$$

    end_for
    set $w_{l,k}^{(n+1)} = w_{l,k}^{(n)} - \lambda \cdot \delta_{l,k}^{(n)} f_{l,k}^{(n)}$ for all l, k
until weight change is insignificant

Fig. 12.20 Sketch of the backpropagation algorithm that realizes a gradient descent on the weights in the network

Convergence may be slow, especially if the network consists of many layers. Error distribution at every layer spreads the error more and more uniformly. Adding a *momentum* term to the correction may improve convergence speed:

$$w_{l,k}^{(n+1)} = w_{l,k}^{(n)} - \lambda \cdot \delta_{l,k}^{(n)} f_{l,k}^{(n)} + \alpha\left[w_{l,k}^{(n)} - w_{l,k}^{(n-1)}\right]. \qquad (12.18)$$

The momentum term $[w_{l,k}^{(n)} - w_{l,k}^{(n-1)}]$ weighted by α pushes the result toward the direction of change from the previous iteration.

There are three kinds of failures that may happen when a backpropagation network is trained.

- The data are not separable because the number of layers and nodes is too small for an appropriate approximation of the decision boundary.
- A local minimum may be found that does not optimally classify the data. The reason could be
  - an inadequate network topology (relation of the number of layers to the number of nodes in the layers),
  - a learning rate that is too high or too low,
  - an initialization that is too far from the global optimum.
- The decision boundary overadapts to the training data (see Fig. 12.21). It perfectly separates training samples but fails to separate the test data. The reasons for this are
  - too many nodes and layers so that the network does not properly generalize,
  - too many iterations in the optimization so that the boundaries approximate the training samples too closely.

Iterative optimization is stopped based on the average error on the test data set. The test error usually starts to increase while the training error still decreases which signifies loss of generalization (see Fig. 12.22).

Fig. 12.21 If training is carried out for a prolonged time, the large number of degrees of freedom of a backpropagation may cause the system to over-adapt to the training data

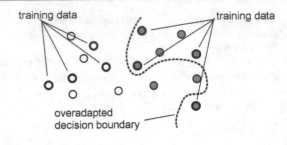

Fig. 12.22 The criterion for stopping the learning should be chosen based on the classification error on the test data

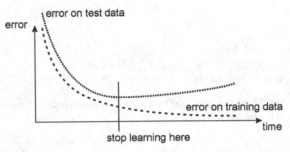

To find just the right number of nodes and layers for a proper generalization, an initial network may be repeatedly changed by removing nodes. Convergence of an optimally generalizing network can be further improved when edges are removed that carry very low weights. These edges mostly contribute noise to the classification result.

12.4.3 Support Vector Machines

More than one boundary may separate the samples of a classification problem. *Support vector machines* (SVM) are able to select among several possibilities the one boundary that maximizes the distance to the samples (see Fig. 12.23 for the principle). An introduction to SVMs is Steinwart and Christmann (2008), a detailed in-depth view by two of the important contributors in the field is Schölkopf and Smola (2002).

Maximizing sample distances from the decision boundary is a useful property considering that training data only sample the true distribution. It reduces the chance of misclassification.

Linear support vector machines solve a two-class problem. Consider the classification problem for linear decision boundaries in (12.10). The classifier can be rewritten such that

$$D(\mathbf{f}, \mathbf{w}, w_0) \cdot d > 0, \quad d = \text{class}(\mathbf{f}) \in \{-1, 1\}. \tag{12.19}$$

This can be reformulated as

$$d \cdot \left(\mathbf{w}^\mathrm{T}\mathbf{f} + w_0\right) \geq 1, \tag{12.20}$$

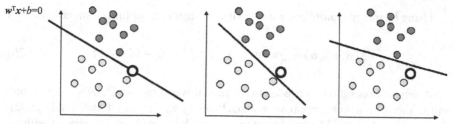

Fig. 12.23 Different, perfect separations of the training data lead to different classifications of unknown samples

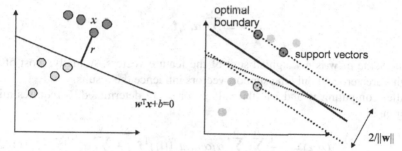

Fig. 12.24 Support vector machines maximize the distance from the decision boundary. The samples that define the course of the decision boundary are the support vectors

since weights for strictly separable sample distributions can always be properly scaled to make the minimum greater than one. The distance r of some sample $\mathbf{f}$ from the hyperplane is

$$r = \frac{\mathbf{w}^{\mathrm{T}}\mathbf{f} + w_0}{\|\mathbf{w}\|}. \tag{12.21}$$

The minimum distance for all samples $\mathbf{f}_i$ is then

$$\mu_L = \min_i \left(\frac{|\mathbf{w}^{\mathrm{T}}\mathbf{f}_i + w_0|}{\|\mathbf{w}\|} \right). \tag{12.22}$$

The training task is to find a hyperplane that maximizes μ_L. Given such a hyperplane, some samples $\mathbf{f}_b$ will have exactly this distance μ_L to the hyperplane, that is,

$$r_s = \begin{cases} \frac{1}{\|\mathbf{w}_s\|}, & \text{if } d_b = +1, \\ \frac{-1}{\|\mathbf{w}_s\|}, & \text{if } d_b = -1. \end{cases} \tag{12.23}$$

These vectors $\mathbf{f}_b$ are called the *support vectors* (see Fig. 12.24). Hence, no samples are in a corridor of width $2/\|\mathbf{w}\|$ implying that $\frac{\|\mathbf{w}\|}{2} = \frac{1}{2}\mathbf{w}^{\mathrm{T}}\mathbf{w}$ subject to the constraint

$$(\mathbf{w}^{\mathrm{T}}\mathbf{f}_i + w_0)d_i \geq 1 \quad \Rightarrow \quad (\mathbf{w}^{\mathrm{T}}\mathbf{f}_i + w_0)d_i - 1 \geq 0 \tag{12.24}$$

has to be minimized for finding the optimal decision boundary.

Using Lagrange multipliers $\boldsymbol{\alpha}$ for solving a constrained optimization task delivers

$$J(\mathbf{w}, w_0, \boldsymbol{\alpha}) = \frac{1}{2} \mathbf{w}^\mathrm{T} \mathbf{w} - \sum_{i=1}^{N} \alpha_i \left(d_i \left[\mathbf{w}^\mathrm{T} \mathbf{f}_i + w_0 \right] - 1 \right). \tag{12.25}$$

A series of operations is needed to arrive at this expression. Details can be found in the literature about support vector machines (e.g., Schölkopf and Smola 2002). The goal is to find a saddle point for $J(\mathbf{w}, w_0, a)$. It is done by minimizing J with respect to $\mathbf{w}$ and w_0 keeping α fixed, hence, computing partial derivatives with respect to $\mathbf{w}$ and w_0 and setting them to 0. Equating the derivatives of $\mathbf{w}$ to zero delivers

$$\mathbf{w} = \sum_{i=1}^{N} \alpha_i d_i \mathbf{f}_i. \tag{12.26}$$

The value of $\mathbf{w}$ is a weighted sum of the feature vectors. Actually, most of the weights are zero and only the support vectors influence the results.

After computing $\mathbf{w}$ and w_0, the values for $\boldsymbol{\alpha}$ are determined. It requires minimization of

$$Q(\alpha) = -\frac{1}{2} \sum_{i=1}^{N} \sum_{j=1}^{N} \alpha_i \alpha_j d_i d_j \left((\mathbf{f}_i)^\mathrm{T} \mathbf{f}_j \right) + \sum_{i=1}^{N} \alpha_i \tag{12.27}$$

subject to the constraint that $\sum_{i=1}^{N} \alpha_i d_i = 0$ (resulting from minimization for w_0) and $\alpha_i \geq 0$. This can be done using methods of linear algebra on constrained optimization.

The result is then inserted into (12.26) for delivering $\mathbf{w}$. The bias term w_0 is computed by choosing a support vector $\mathbf{f}_b$ and computing

$$\mathbf{w}^\mathrm{T} \mathbf{f}_s + w_0 = 1 \quad \Leftrightarrow \quad w_0 = 1 - \mathbf{w}^\mathrm{T} \mathbf{f}_s. \tag{12.28}$$

Although this sounds difficult, it is nothing but the application of standard linear algebra techniques. Linear support vector machines have the advantage over linear decision boundaries that they assert an optimal quality of the solution. This is probably the reason why they are popular, especially if few training samples exist (as it is often the case in medical image analysis).

Nonlinear decision boundaries can be computed similarly to the strategy discussed earlier by embedding the nonlinear space in a higher-dimensional linear space. However, the beauty of using support vector machines lies in (12.27) for computing the Lagrange multipliers. If the original feature space is mapped on some higher-dimensional space $\Phi(\mathbf{f}) = \mathbf{u}$, the new equation to be optimized becomes

$$Q(\alpha) = -\frac{1}{2} \sum_{i=1}^{N} \sum_{j=1}^{N} \alpha_i \alpha_j d_i d_j \left((\mathbf{u}_i)^\mathrm{T} \mathbf{u}_j \right) + \sum_{i=1}^{N} \alpha_i$$

$$= -\frac{1}{2} \sum_{i=1}^{N} \sum_{j=1}^{N} \alpha_i \alpha_j d_i d_j \left(\Phi(\mathbf{f}_i)^\mathrm{T} \Phi(\mathbf{f}_j) \right) + \sum_{i=1}^{N} \alpha_i. \tag{12.29}$$

In other words, just the dot product $\Phi(\mathbf{f}_i)^T\Phi(\mathbf{f}_j)$ has to be generated instead of spanning the space itself. If a simple function $K(\mathbf{f}_i, \mathbf{f}_j) = \Phi(\mathbf{f}_i)^T\Phi(\mathbf{f}_j)$ exists, it replaces the dot product in (12.29). This function is called a *kernel function*. It enables to find a nonlinear decision boundary by embedding $\mathbf{f}$ in a higher-dimensional space without actually carrying out the optimization in this space. This is sometimes called the *kernel trick*.

A number of such kernel functions exist and are used for nonlinear support vector machines. A polynomial surface with degree d is optimized using

$$K_{\leq d}(x, y) = \Phi_{\leq d}(\mathbf{x}) \bullet \Phi_{\leq d}(\mathbf{y}) = \left(1 + \mathbf{x}^T\mathbf{y}\right)^d. \tag{12.30}$$

Hence, the quadratic would be given by

$$\begin{aligned}
K_{\leq 2}\big((x_1 \quad x_2), (y_1 \quad y_2)\big) &= \left(1 + \mathbf{x}^T\mathbf{y}\right)^2 \\
&= (1 + x_1 y_1 + x_2 y_2)^2 \\
&= 1 + x_1 y_1 + x_2 y_2 + x_1^2 y_1^2 \\
&\quad + 2x_1 x_2 y_1 y_2 + x_2^2 y_2^2.
\end{aligned} \tag{12.31}$$

The dot product does not even have to be defined in Euclidean metrics. The following kernel (also known as *radial base functions* with variance σ^2)

$$K_\sigma(x, y) = \Phi_\sigma(\mathbf{x}) \bullet \Phi_\sigma(\mathbf{y}) = \exp\left(-\frac{\|\mathbf{x} - \mathbf{y}\|^2}{2\sigma^2}\right) \tag{12.32}$$

uses the angle between support vectors as metrics. Samples are classified according to their similarity to the support vectors. Results are somewhat similar to that of the discriminant functions discussed in the next section and to the association networks used for clustering, discussed in Sect. 7.2.3.

Originally, classification by support vector machines requires that training data sets are separable. Otherwise, no decision boundary exists that can be optimized. If some of the data are distorted so that features overlap in feature space, *slack variables* ξ_i can be introduced that make the problem separable again and therefore solvable.

Slack variables push the feature locations away from the boundary. This is done by modifying (12.24) to

$$\left(\mathbf{w}^T\mathbf{f}_i + w_0\right)d_i \geq 1 - \xi_i. \tag{12.33}$$

It was shown by Cortes and Vapnik (1995) that the introduction of slack variables adds an extra term to (12.25) but does not change the kernel property of (12.27).

12.5 Classification by Association

Adaptive linear discriminant functions bear similarities to the minimum distance classifier in that their classification criterion is based on the correspondence to a model feature vector given by weights $w_{k,0}, \ldots, w_{k,N}$ for a class k. Discriminant

Fig. 12.25 Adaptive
discriminant functions can be
thought of as vectors in a
feature space, where an
additional feature f_0 has been
added to represent the bias
term. Classification is then by
association to the most
similar discriminant function

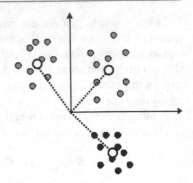

initialize weights $w_0, \ldots, w_M$ with small random values
repeat
      select sample **f** from training set
      compute all $D_k(\mathbf{f})$
      if the sample of class C_i is erroneously classified as C_j **then**
            for all features $m = 1, \ldots, M$ **do**
$$w_{i,m} := w_{i,m} + c \cdot f_{i,m}$$
$$w_{i,0} := w_{i,0} + c \cdot k$$
$$w_{j,m} := w_{j,m} - c \cdot f_{i,m}$$
$$w_{j,0} := w_{j,0} - c \cdot k; \quad \text{with } c, k > 0$$
          end_for
    end_if
until classification is perfect   **or** average error $< e_{\min}$
                                 or steps > max_steps

Fig. 12.26 Sketch of the algorithm to compute weights from training features for adaptive discriminant functions

functions have to be defined for each class

$$D_k(\mathbf{f}) = w_{k,0} + w_{k,1} f_1 + w_{k,2} f_2 + \cdots + w_{k,N} f_N. \tag{12.34}$$

The classification of an unknown sample with feature vector **f** happens by inserting **f** in each of the **K** discriminant functions and selecting the class k for which $D_k(\mathbf{f})$ is maximal (see Fig. 12.25).

Training of a set of discriminant functions is similar to the training of decision boundaries. Discriminant functions are evaluated for classified training samples. If the incorrect class is assigned to a training sample, its corresponding discriminant function is changed to deliver smaller values and the discriminant function of the true class is changed to deliver higher values. A sketch of the algorithm is depicted in Fig. 12.26.

The similarity to the minimum distance classifier is due to the fact that computing the discriminant function is similar to measuring a non-Euclidean distance between features **f** and the weight vector $\mathbf{w}_k = (w_{k,1} w_{k,2}, \ldots, w_{k,N})$ since

$$D_k(\mathbf{f}) = (\mathbf{w}_k)^{\mathrm{T}} \mathbf{f} + w_{k,0} = \|\mathbf{w}_k\| \cdot \|\mathbf{f}\| \cdot \cos(\angle \mathbf{w}_k, \mathbf{f}) + w_{k,0}, \tag{12.35}$$

with $\cos(\angle \mathbf{w}_k, \mathbf{f})$ being the distance measure. The bias can be integrated into the feature vector and the weight vector by setting $\mathbf{f}' = (1 f_1 f_2, \ldots, f_N)$ and $\mathbf{w}'_k = (w_{k,0}, w_{k,1}, w_{k,2}, \ldots, w_{k,N})$.

The discriminant functions can be turned into a distance classifier if the feature vectors and initial weights are normalized by letting $\mathbf{f}_{\text{norm}} = \mathbf{f}'/\|\mathbf{f}'\|$ and $\mathbf{w}_{k,\text{norm}} = \mathbf{w}'_k/\|\mathbf{w}'_k\|$. In this case, weights need to be normalized after each update. The trained classifier then decides based on the angle between $\mathbf{w}_{k,\text{norm}}$ and $\mathbf{f}_{\text{norm}}$.

The result is similar to a decision on distance between $\mathbf{f}$ and a class center of the minimum distance classifier presented earlier, except that the discriminant vector $\mathbf{w}_{k,\text{norm}}$ is trained based on a sample distribution. It also bears similarities to a support vector machine using radial base functions as explained in the previous section.

A discriminant function may also be used in a different way. If some order with respect to class membership can be assumed to be reflected in feature values of its samples (e.g., classes that represent stages of some process), a single function may suffice to discriminate between classes.

The approach is simple. Given V samples with N features, where the true class of a sample $\mathbf{f}_i = (f_{i1}, f_{i2}, \ldots, f_{iN})$ is represented by some number d_i, a function is searched that minimizes the distance $(D(\mathbf{f}_i) - d_i)^2$ for all samples

$$\mathbf{w}_{\text{opt}} = \arg\min_{\mathbf{w}} E(\mathbf{w}, \mathbf{f}) = \arg\min_{\mathbf{w}} \sum_{i=1}^{V} \left(D(\mathbf{f}_i, \mathbf{w}) - d_i\right)^2 \qquad (12.36)$$

with

$$D(\mathbf{f}_i, \mathbf{w}) = \mathbf{w}^T \mathbf{f}_i + w_0. \qquad (12.37)$$

Since the function is quadratic and nonnegative, parameters can be computed directly without requiring an iterative method and the result is guaranteed to be the global minimum. The desired weights w_i are those for which the partial derivative of the error function E is 0. The classifier is called *minimum square error discriminant function*.

It may seem that, if a single linear discriminant function solves the classification problem, it should be the eigenvector with maximal eigenvalue of a PCA. This is not necessarily the case because the PCA does not maximize class separability. However, if PCA indicates that reduction of a high-dimensional feature space to one or two dimensions covers most of the variance in the samples, it makes sense to investigate whether a minimum square error discriminant function can be applied.

12.6 Clustering Techniques

Clustering is sometimes called *class detection* since it analyzes sample distribution in feature space. Cluster members may be inspected after clustering and this may help to detect classes. Many different clustering techniques exist (Jain and Dubes

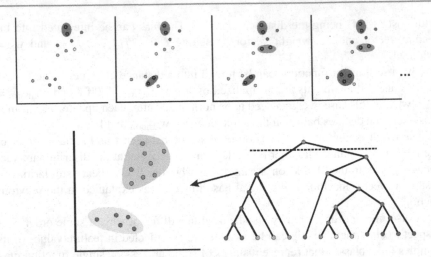

Fig. 12.27 Agglomerative clustering initially treats each sample as its own cluster. It then merges always the two closest clusters until all clusters are merged. The merging process is represented in a tree structure. The user then selects the desired number of clusters

1988; Xu and Wunsch 2005), of which some popular techniques for medical data will be described in the following sections.

The clustering of data is carried out in a top-down or a bottom-up fashion on un-classified samples. Examples of top-down clustering schemes have been presented in Sect. 7.2. The k-means clustering described in Sect. 7.2.1 can also be applied to high-dimensional sparse feature spaces, while mean-shift clustering (Sect. 7.2.2) gets very slow with increased dimension of feature space.

In this chapter, we will describe two further clustering techniques that are partic-ularly suitable if the number of samples is comparatively low.

If clustering is applied for class detection it is sometimes called *unsupervised classification* and the process is called *unsupervised training*, as it does not require assignment or checking the class membership of samples.

12.6.1 Agglomerative Clustering

Bottom-up clustering is also called *agglomerative clustering*. Initially, every sample is its own cluster. The pairs of closest clusters are then merged until the expected number of clusters is reached. If this is unknown, agglomeration continues until a single cluster is generated. Merging is documented by a binary tree with leaves being the initial clusters (see Fig. 12.27). A parent node is created from two nodes in the tree if their corresponding clusters are merged.

Storing the history of agglomeration in the tree enables later analysis of generated clusters. Some classes may fall into more than one cluster. Going up and down in the agglomeration tree and selecting and inspecting members of clusters helps to understand the true distribution of class members in clusters.

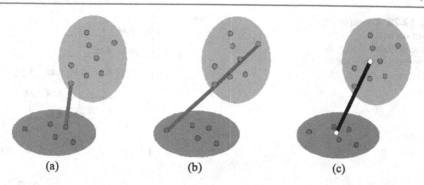

Fig. 12.28 Different kinds of distance measures between clusters: (**a**) single linkage, (**b**) complete linkage, (**c**) average linkage

Agglomerative clustering requires that the distance $d(C_1, C_2)$ between two clusters C_1 and C_2 can be computed. Different measures have been used (see Fig. 12.28).

- *Single linkage* defines the distance between two classes by the distance between its closest members.
- *Complete linkage* defines the distance by that of its furthest members.
- *Average linkage* defines the distance by the distance between centroids of two clusters.

Agglomerative clustering does not always delivers as good results as $d(M(C_1, C_2), C_3) \neq d(C_1, M(C_2, C_3))$, where $M()$ indicates the merging of two clusters. Hence, final clustering depends on the early decisions.

12.6.2 Fuzzy *c*-Means Clustering

Since clustering for class detection is provisional, it may be appropriate to model membership in a fuzzy way. Again, several different algorithms exist (see, e.g., Baraldi and Blonda 1999 for a survey) of which we present the base method.

A sample may belong to different clusters with different degrees of membership. The method is known as *fuzzy c-means clustering*. The degree of membership is given by the partition matrix **U**, where each entry u_{ij} determines the degree of membership of a sample i of N samples with feature vector $\mathbf{f}_i$ to cluster j of C clusters (see Fig. 12.29). The membership degree is normalized to a range of $[0, 1]$ so that the following two conditions must hold for the values u_{ij} in the partition matrix.

- Total membership for each sample to clusters 1 to C: $\sum_{j=1}^{C} u_{ij} = 1$.
- No empty clusters: $0 < \frac{1}{N} \sum_{i=1}^{N} u_{ij} < N$.

The objective is to create a good partitioning with compact clusters based on a compactness definition (see Fig. 12.30). Computing compactness requires a distance metric $d(\mathbf{f}_i, \mathbf{f}_j)$ to exist (e.g., the Euclidean distance). Compact clusters are created

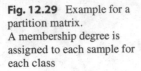

Fig. 12.29 Example for a partition matrix. A membership degree is assigned to each sample for each class

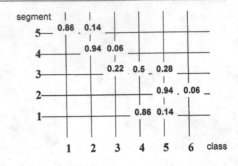

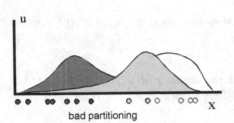 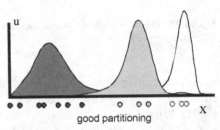

Fig. 12.30 The goal of fuzzy clustering is to find a partitioning with compact clusters

if the average distance between fuzzy members of a cluster is minimal:

$$\mathbf{U}_{\text{opt}} = \arg\min_{\mathbf{U}} \sum_{j=1}^{C} \frac{\sum_{k,l=1}^{N} u_{kj}^2 u_{lj}^2 d(\mathbf{f}_k, \mathbf{f}_l)}{2 \sum_{i=1}^{N} u_{ij}^2}. \quad (12.38)$$

Computing a fuzzy clustering is particularly simple if compactness is defined by the distance of a sample to its cluster center. A cluster center $\mathbf{c}_j$ for a given partition matrix $\mathbf{U}$ is the weighted sum of sample locations in features space. The weighting $w(u_{ij})$ is a function of the membership degree u_{ij} of a sample i to a cluster j:

$$\mathbf{c}_j = \frac{1}{\sum_{i=1}^{N} f(u_{ij})} \sum_{i=1}^{N} w(u_{ij})\mathbf{f}_i. \quad (12.39)$$

The iterative process starts with an initial partition matrix that could be generated, for example, from smoothing a hard partitioning by a Gaussian kernel. The objective is to find $\mathbf{U}_{\text{opt}}$ such that the sum of weighted distances $u_{ij}\|\mathbf{f}_i - \mathbf{c}_j\|$ between features $\mathbf{f}_i$ and cluster centers $\mathbf{c}_j$ is minimal. The function to be minimized is now

$$\mathbf{U}_{\text{opt}} = \arg\min_{\mathbf{U}} \sum_{i=1}^{N} \sum_{j=1}^{C} u_{ij}^m \|\mathbf{f}_i - \mathbf{c}_j\|^2, \quad 2 \le m < \infty. \quad (12.40)$$

The parameter m controls the fuzziness of the distribution. With m approaching infinity, the algorithm turns into hard clustering.

The matrix $\mathbf{U}_{\text{opt}}$ can be found by gradient descent in the space of the u_{ij}. The step for updating u_{ij} at iteration n is

$$u_{ij}^{(n+1)} = \frac{1}{\sum_{k=1}^{C}\left(\frac{\|\mathbf{f}_i - \mathbf{c}_i^{(n)}\|}{\|\mathbf{f}_i - \mathbf{c}_k^{(n)}\|}\right)^{\frac{2}{m-1}}}, \tag{12.41}$$

where $\mathbf{c}_j^{(n)}$ is a cluster center at iteration (n) defined by weighted clustering

$$\mathbf{c}_j^{(n)} = \frac{1}{\sum_{i=1}^{N}(u_{ij}^{(n)})^m}\sum_{i=1}^{N}(u_{ij}^{(n)})^m \mathbf{f}_i. \tag{12.42}$$

Optimization terminates if the change between partition matrices of subsequent iterations falls below some threshold. A matrix norm such as the maximum norm on matrices may be used to compute the stopping criterion:

$$\|\mathbf{U}^{(n)} - \mathbf{U}^{(n+1)}\| < \varepsilon \quad \text{with} \quad \|\mathbf{U}^{(n)} - \mathbf{U}^{(n+1)}\| = \max_{ij}\|u_{ij}^{(n)} - u_{ij}^{(n+1)}\|. \tag{12.43}$$

Fuzzy c-mean clustering is often intended to lead to a (fuzzy) classification of the samples. Hence, the number of clusters usually corresponds to the number of classes to be differentiated. Using gradient descent for optimization requires the initial partition matrix to be close to the final result.

12.7 Bagging and Boosting

Classification based on training from examples can be difficult if the decision boundary between classes is complex. The number of training samples may be insufficient to generate an appropriate classifier. *Bagging* and *boosting* are two techniques to arrive at a good classifier nonetheless by applying a kind of divide-and-conquer strategy. Instead of training a strong classifier that correctly classifies all samples, a set of weak classifiers is searched where each sample in the training set is classified by the majority of the classifiers. The advantage of combining weak classifiers lies in the fact that the absolute accuracy that is requested from the strong classifier is replaced by a relative accuracy of a combination of weak classifiers. A comparison of the performance of bagging and boosting algorithms can be found in Bauer and Kohavi (1999).

The main difference between bagging and boosting is that bagging generates a voting scheme, where each classifier votes for a class and the class with the majority of votes wins, while boosting generates a sequence of classifiers, where each classifier learns from the previous classifier and votes are weighted according to classifier quality. Both methods have in common that a given classification algorithm (e.g., kNN classification) is trained on a number of subsets of the training data producing the different classifiers.

Input: training set S of labeled pairs (s_i, l_i), $i = 1, N$, classification scheme CS,
              number of trials T
Output: combined classifier C^*

$S' = S$
initialize weights $w(s_i) = 1.0, i = 1, N$
for $i = 1, T$ **do begin**   ; create weak classifiers
    $\varepsilon_i = 1.0$
    $k = 0$
    while $\varepsilon_i > 0.5$ and $k < 25$ **do begin**   ; classifiers must have a minimum quality
                                    ; try up to 25 times to achieve this
$$C_i = \text{computeClassifier}(S', CS)$$
$$\varepsilon_i = \frac{1}{N} \sum_{s_j \in S': C_i(s_j) \neq l_j} w(s_j)$$
$$k = k + 1$$
    endwhile
    $\beta_i = \varepsilon_i / (1.0 - \varepsilon_i)$
    for $j = 1, N$ **do begin**   ; error-based sample weighting
        if $C_i(x_j) = l_j$ **then** $w(x_j) = w(x_j)/(2\varepsilon_i)$
              else $w(x_j) = w(x_j)/(2(1.0 - \varepsilon_i))$
    endfor
endfor
$$C^*(x) = \arg\max_{l \in L} \sum_{i: C_i(x)=l} \log \frac{1}{\beta_i}$$; final classifier

Fig. 12.31 Sketch of the AdaBoost algorithm (adapted from Freund and Schapire 1996 and Bauer and Kohavi 1999)

Bagging (*bootstrap aggregating*), presented by Breiman (1996), repeatedly selects subsets S_i from the training set and trains a classifier C_i based on this subset. The final classifier tries then all classifiers C_i on the unknown sample and assigns the class to it that receives the most votes.

Boosting was introduced by Schapire (1990) and was extended to AdaBoost (*Adaptive Boosting*) in Freund and Schapire (1996). AdaBoost, used in the context of medical image analysis (e.g., by Pujol et al. 2003; Ochs et al. 2007; and Takemura et al. 2010), trains each classifier on the complete training data. A sketch of the algorithm is depicted in Fig. 12.31.

Different classifiers are generated by weighting the samples based on the training error after a classifier has been trained. The weighted sample set is the submitted to the next classifier and weighted again. Samples receive higher weights for the next classifier if they were not classified correctly by the current classifier. Hence, the next classifier will be trained to remove errors not corrected sufficiently by all previous classifiers. The final classifier combines then, as in the case of bagging, the weak classifiers and decides by majority vote. However, different to bagging, classifier votes are weighted by their error rate.

While bagging may be carried out in parallel, AdaBoost is inherently sequential since its classifiers learn from their predecessors. Other boosting algorithms exist that define the search for the final classifier as an optimization task that can be solved in parallel. An example is LPBoosting (Demiriz et al. 2002) that defines boosting for linear decision boundaries as a linear programming task and that has been used to analyze cortical thickness from MRI for autism diagnosis (Singh et al. 2008).

12.8   Multiple Instance Learning

Although the scenario of multiple instance learning (MIL) is attractive and it is being investigated by many groups, it has currently few applications in analysis tasks in medical imaging such as Computer Aided Diagnosis, see Fung et al. (2006), Bi and Liang (2007). Hence, it will be briefly described.

The first application domain for MIL was drug design (Dietterich et al. 1997; Maron and Lozano-Péres 1997). It was investigated whether certain molecules bind or not. Molecules may have different spatial configurations. The binding ability depends not only on the molecule but also on the configuration. Hence, when observing relevant features of a molecule by some imaging technique, they may vary to a great extent for the same kind of molecule.

Each of the observations is treated as an instance of the same type of molecule that belongs to one of two classes ("binding" or "not binding"). Assigning this class membership to the molecule type to create a training set would result in distribution functions that overlap to a large extent as it is not part of the model that only some of the instances of a binding molecule may actually bind. The problem is represented better if all the instances of a molecule are treated as a bag of samples that is either labeled "binding" or "not binding." The former is known to contain at least one binding instance while the latter does not contain any binding instance. The task is to extract a decision boundary from a set of training bags that separates instances of the one class from those of the other class.

The problem can be put in a more abstract form. Two types of bags B exist in MIL: Positive bags $B = 1$ contain at least one sample s with $class(s) = 1$ and negative bags $B = -1$ contain only samples s with $class(s) = -1$. Having positive and negative bags is actually the key to solve the MIL problem. An optimal decision boundary will separate all samples from negative bags from positive samples such that at least one member of all positive bags is separated from the negative bags.

Since the positive samples in positive bags are unknown, different strategies can be and are used to arrive at a solution under various a priori assumptions (see Fig. 12.32). A decision boundary enclosing as many positive samples and as few negative samples as possible is searched when positive bags are assumed to be largely made up of positive samples. A nonoverfitting decision boundary enclosing no negative samples but as many positive samples as possible is searched if negative samples are reliable. A decision boundary enclosing dense clusters of positive samples is searched when it is assumed that only few feature value combinations constitute the unknown positive range (which is the case in searching for binding configurations).

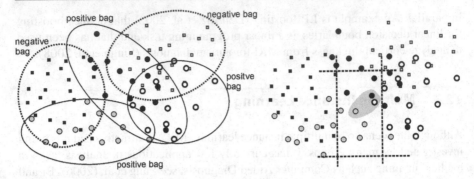

Fig. 12.32 In multiple instance learning, positive bags (*circles*) contain at least one positive instance, while negative bags (*squares*) contain only negative instances. Finding a decision boundary requires additional assumptions. Examples are to find the rectangle (*dashed lines*) that encloses the most instance of positive bags without containing instances from negative bags or the smallest region that contains at least one instance of each positive bag (*gray region*)

12.9 Concluding Remarks

Classification in sparse feature space mostly attempts to create a decision criterion without estimating likelihood functions. The strategy is successful when suitable features cluster well. Hence, errors in computing class membership will only result from samples close to the decision boundary.

Since the reliability and speed of most classification methods increase with the decreasing dimensionality of feature space, feature reduction should precede classification. This can be carried out with and without considering the distribution of classified samples in feature space.

A classification technique should be chosen based on knowledge about distribution characteristics in feature space. Simple techniques such as linear decision boundaries or linear support vector machines generalize well and are less dependent on initialization. Methods allowing for complex decision boundaries help to deal with data that are difficult to classify. They may, however, have the tendency to overadapt to training data.

12.10 Exercises

- Why is it difficult to derive a likelihood function from a sparsely populated feature space? Why does it help when features are independent of each other?
- When is it a disadvantage to use PCA for feature reduction? Please explain how training data can be used to arrive at a better feature reduction. Does this have limitations? What are they?
- How can independent component analysis be used for classification? What conditions must be met so that independent components can be found?

- Develop a situation where a kNN classifier would be preferred over a linear decision boundary. Discuss the attributes of this classification problem that lead to the preference.
- How can a kNN classifier "learn" from confirmed results? What is a potential disadvantage of this? And how can this be dealt with?
- What is the assumption under which a minimum distance classifier delivers the correct Bayesian decision (i.e., delivers the same result than that from evaluating the a posteriori probability)?
- Why is it useful to reject samples from classification by a kNN classifier? Which samples are rejected?
- How is classification by linear decision boundary related to classification based on the Bayesian theorem?
- How can the linear decision boundary approach be extended to nonlinear boundaries? What are the limitations of this approach?
- What kind of decision boundaries can be generated by a backpropagation network with two layers (hence, without a hidden layer) if the number of node per layer is not limited?
- Why is it necessary to use the sigmoid function as the activation function instead of thresholding? What effect does this have on classification?
- What is the optimization goal when training a support vector machine? What are the support vectors?
- What is meant by the "kernel trick"? How does it extend the capabilities of a support vector machine?
- How can a support vector machine be made to simulate an association network?
- How can an SVM be extended to deal with overlapping training samples?
- Which strategy should be followed if the number of clusters is not known for agglomerative clustering? How can clusters then be identified?
- How is fuzziness encoded in fuzzy clustering? What is the goal of finding an optimal fuzzy clustering?
- What is the advantage of using bagging instead of a single trained classifier? In what kind of distribution in feature space does bagging do particularly well?
- What is the main difference between bagging and boosting? Why should this be advantageous for using boosting?

References

Abdi H, Williams LJ (2010) Principal component analysis. Wiley Interdiscip Rev: Comput Stat 2(4):433–459

Baraldi A, Blonda P (1999) A survey of fuzzy clustering algorithms for pattern recognition. Part I+II. IEEE Trans Syst Man Cybern, Part B, Cybern 29(6):778–801

Bauer E, Kohavi R (1999) An empirical comparison of voting classification algorithms: bagging, boosting and variants. Mach Learn 36:105–142

Bi J, Liang J (2007) Multiple instance learning of pulmonary embolism detection with geodesic distance along vascular structure. In: IEEE conf computer vision and pattern recognition, CVPR'07, pp 1–8

Bishop CM (1995) Neural networks for pattern recognition. Oxford University Press, Oxford

Blanco Y, Zazo S (2003) New Gaussianity measures based on order statistics: application to ICA. Neurocomputing 51:303–320

Breiman L (1996) Bagging predictors. Mach Learn 24:123–140

Cortes C, Vapnik V (1995) Support vector networks. Mach Learn 20(3):273–297

Demiriz A, Bennett KP, Shawne-Taylor J (2002) Linear programming boosting via column generation. Mach Learn 46(1–3):225–254

Dietterich TG, Lathrop RH, Lozano-Péres T (1997) Solving the multiple-instance problem with axis-parallel rectangles. Artif Intell 89(1–2):31–71

Fisher RA (1936) The use of multiple measurements in taxonomic problems. Ann Eugen 7:179–188

Freund Y, Schapire RE (1996) Experiments with a new boosting algorithm. In: Machine learning: Proc of the 13th national conference, pp 148–156

Fung G, Dundar M, Krishnapuram B, Bharat Rao R (2006) Multiple instance learning for computer aided diagnosis. In: Proc 19th ann conf advances in neural information processing, pp 425–432

Hwang WJ, Wen KW (1998) Fast kNN classification algorithm based on partial distance search. Electron Lett 34(21):2062–2063

Hyvärinen A, Oja E (2000) Independent component analysis: algorithms and applications. Neural Netw 13(4–5):411–430

Hyvärinen A, Hurri J, Hoyer PO (2009) Independent component analysis. In: Natural image statistics. Computational imaging and vision, vol 39, 2nd edn, pp 151–175

Jain AK, Dubes RC (1988) Algorithms for clustering data. Prentice Hall, New York

Jiang Q, Zhang W (1993) An improved method for finding nearest neighbors. Pattern Recognit Lett 14:531–535

Maron O, Lozano-Péres T (1997) A framework for multiple instance learning. In: Proc conf on advances in neural information processing systems (NIPS), pp 570–576

Ochs RA, Goldin JG, Abtin F, Kim HJ, Brown K, Batra P, Roback D, McNitt-Gray MF, Brown MS (2007) Automated classification of lung bronchovascular anatomy in CT using AdaBoost. Med Image Anal 11(3):315–324

Pujol O, Rosales M, Radeva P, Nofrerias-Fernández E (2003) Intravascular ultrasound images vessel characterization using AdaBoost. In: Functional imaging and modeling of the heart. LNCS, vol 2674, pp 242–251

Rosenblatt F (1958) The perceptron: a probabilistic model for information storage and organization in the brain. Psychol Rev 65(6):386–408

Rosenblatt M (1956) Remarks on some non-parametric estimates of a density function. Ann Math Stat 27:832–837

Sarle WS (1994) Neural networks and statistical models. In: Proc. 19th ann SAS users group intl conf, pp 1–13

Schapire RL (1990) The strength of weak learnability. Mach Learn 5(2):197–227

Schölkopf B, Smola AJ (2002) Learning with kernels—support vector machines: regularization, optimization and beyond. MIT Press, Cambridge

Singh, Mukherjee L, Chung MK (2008) Cortical surface thickness as a classifier: boosting for autism classification. In: Medical image computing and computer-assisted intervention, MICCAI 2008. LNCS, vol 5241, pp 999–1007

Steinwart I, Christmann A (2008) Support vector machines. Springer, Berlin

Takemura A, Shimizu A, Hamamoto K (2010) Discrimination of breast tumors in ultrasonic images using an ensemble classifier based on the AdaBoost algorithm with feature selection. IEEE Trans Med Imaging 29(3):598–609

Warfield S (1996) Fast k-NN classification for multichannel image data. Pattern Recognit Lett 17(7):713–721

Xu R, Wunsch D II (2005) Survey of clustering algorithms. IEEE Trans Neural Netw 16(3):645–678

Validation

13

Abstract

Structures to be analyzed in medical images are usually inaccessible. The sufficiency and correctness of employed domain knowledge cannot be proven. Hence, validation of an analysis method estimates the correctness of results from tests on a limited number of samples. For carrying out the validation suitable samples need to be selected, comparison measures have to be chosen that reflect the quality of the result, and a norm is required against which the method is tested. These aspects are realized differently for a delineation task, a detection task, or a registration task. Requirements, means, and limitations of validation will be discussed in this chapter.

Concepts, notions and definitions introduced in this chapter

> Overlap and outlier measures for delineation tasks: oversegmentation and undersegmentation, Dice and Jacard coefficient, Hausdorff distance
> The ROC curve
> Success in detection: type I and type II errors, sensitivity and specificity, precision and recall rates
> Measuring registration errors
> Ground truth: manual delineation, hardware and software phantoms
> Training and test data
> Significance: t-test and Welsh test
> The p-value

An analysis method needs to be tested with respect to the quality with which results are achieved. Unfortunately, a direct way to prove the quality does not exist since the subjects of analysis are not accessible except by indirect means. It results in a number of characteristics of a validation procedure.

K.D. Toennies, *Guide to Medical Image Analysis*,
Advances in Computer Vision and Pattern Recognition,
DOI 10.1007/978-1-4471-2751-2_13, © Springer-Verlag London Limited 2012

- Validation is by statistical means because the quality of an analysis procedure is tested on a number of sample cases. The outcome is assumed to be representative for all cases.
- Validation is relative, as it gives information about the current method with respect to some other way to generate the analysis results.
- Validation is indirect by comparing features that a correct analysis method should produce instead of comparing analysis methodologies.

Even if validation shows success, the underlying assumptions of the validation must not be forgotten. Validation by statistical means, for instance, requires a representative set of data. It may be difficult to show to what extent a chosen set represents the totality of all data sets. A validation with respect to a reference method may be inconclusive if this method is inferior to other methods for the same analysis task. Finally, validation based on some criterion (e.g., the volume of a segment) may not reflect the attributes that are needed for the application of the method. Hence, the documentation of the validation scenario is an integral part of any validation. It gives a potential user of a method the chance to judge whether the validation is appropriate for his or her purpose.

For image-guided surgery that requires segmentation, registration, as well as object detection, Jannin et al. (2002) presented a number of characteristics that should be addressed and documented.

- *Accuracy* measures the deviation of results from the known ground truth.
- *Precision and reproducibility* measure the extent to which equal or similar input produces equal or similar results.
- *Robustness* characterizes the change of analysis quality if conditions deviate from assumptions made for analysis (e.g., when the noise level increases or if the object appearance deviates from prior assumptions).
- *Efficiency* describes the effort necessary to achieve an analysis result.
- *Fault detection* is the ability to detect potential false results during the application of an analysis method.

Except for the last, these attributes are also listed by Udupa et al. (2006) who subsumed precision and robustness under the same heading.

Accuracy is measured by computing a measure of the quality (Udupa et al. 2006 coined the phrase *figure of merit* = FOM for this), comparing analysis results with some ground truth. Useful measures of quality will be discussed in the next section followed by ways to generate ground truth data.

Quality measures are required for estimating reproducibility as well. However, ground truth is not necessarily required since only deviations of the results for the same or slightly deviating input shall be determined. High reproducibility does not differentiate between the correct or wrong results.

Robustness and reliability characterize reproducibility. They are similar in that both judge the dependencies of results on changes in the input. The difference is in the causes. A reliable method produces valid results within the range of expected input variation (e.g., acceptable variation of any initialization, expected variation of appearance of objects, etc.). A robust method is insensitive to variations outside of the expected range of variation (e.g., unexpected levels of noise, wrong parameterization, unexpected pathological variation, etc.). While reliability should be a given attribute of a method, robustness will always be limited. Data representing degrees of acceptable variation used for computing reliability should be extended to represent degrees of unacceptable variation (e.g., by adding unusual amounts of noise or by starting with an unacceptable initialization). Reliability and robustness estimates depend on representative data, a question that will be discussed in a separate section.

Efficiency describes the effort that is necessary to produce an analysis result. It seems to be easy to compute as it usually refers to the computational cost. However, most of the methods discussed in the previous chapters require some kind of interaction. Hence, Udupa et al. (2006) suggested including human operator time into the efficiency estimate. Even this may by insufficient as the kind of human interaction may influence other quality measures. For instance, expecting some difficult delineation from the human observer at irregular time intervals will lead to a different kind of operator fatigue than boredom from having to wait for giving some simple input. Its assessment requires setting up a user's study, which is often too expensive to be done. Still, as part of the validation, the kind of information requested through interaction, the kind of knowledge assumed from the human expert, and the occasions when interaction is requested should be documented.

Fault detection is a highly desirable feature. It requires a method to estimate the reliability of its own results. Fault detection can be realized by detecting faulty input, faulty intermediate results, or faulty output, each of which require a model of faultiness at the respective stage of processing. If the ranges of faulty behavior can be given, the validation of fault detection capabilities requires the corresponding ground truth data.

The documentation of the validation scenario builds on the description of the analysis method as mentioned in Chap. 1. Given the intended use of an analysis method and assumptions about the data, the description of a validation scenario should contain the following information.

- Description of the data on which the validation is to be carried out.
- Description and justification of what is assumed to be the ground truth.
- Criteria by which the quality is to be measured.
- Definition and justification of what constitutes a successful validation.

The results from validation are samples nonetheless. Hence, this chapter is concluded with a section on the computation of significance of a validation result.

13.1 Measures of Quality

Quality depends on the kind of analysis that has been carried out on the data. If an object is delineated, it will be a correspondence measure between the delineated object and some reference segmentation. If the task was object detection, it will be a ratio between the correct and incorrect decisions. If it has been a registration, it will be the deviation from the correct registration transformation. Since an analysis task may involve combinations of these methods, the kind of validation procedure will have to be selected based on the intended application.

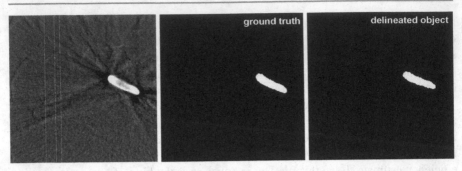

Fig. 13.1 Validation of a delineation requires a measure of comparison between some reference (the often so-called ground truth) and the delineated object

Let us illustrate this with an example. The delineation of an object boundary may be done by registering a shape model to the image data which is then deformed according to local image information. In this case, the quality of the desired result should be measured by the correspondence of the deformed model instance with the expected segmentation. The correctness of the registration transformation in itself plays only a minor role and will probably not be an interesting part of the validation for the user. However, since an incorrect registration will influence the performance of the subsequent model adaptation to the image data, measuring the registration error will tell something about the robustness of the method (the method may fail completely if the registration part fails). This may be helpful for a developer who wants to adapt this method.

In the following sections, measures for delineation tasks, object detection tasks, and image registration tasks will be listed separately, although the necessity for combining them should not be forgotten.

13.1.1 Quality for a Delineation Task

Measuring quality for a delineation task requires a measure of correspondence between the delineated structure f and some known, true reference delineation g (see Fig. 13.1). Generating ground truth will be discussed in detail in the next section. For now, let us assume that ground truth data exist. Hence, for an image consisting of voxels or pixels $\mathbf{v}$ a function g is known with

$$g(\mathbf{v}) = \begin{cases} 1, & \text{if } \mathbf{v} \text{ belongs to the delineated object,} \\ 0, & \text{otherwise.} \end{cases} \tag{13.1}$$

Correspondence can be measured in different ways.
- Volumetric measurements compute volume or area differences between f and g.
- Overlap measures compute the overlap between the object and background elements in f and g.

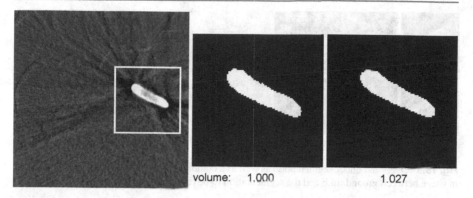

volume: 1,000   1.027

Fig. 13.2 The volume difference is the simplest FOM for comparing a delineation with the ground truth. It does, however, not account for shape differences

- Distance measurements compute the deviation between the boundaries of f and g.
- Outlier measures compute the maximum deviation between f and g.

It is easily seen that these measures capture different aspects of correspondence. A volumetric measurement only compares a property derived from the delineation. An overlap measure computes an element-wise correspondence. Distance measurements do the same with the corresponding boundary points. They may return substantially different results than an overlap measure since a large change of boundary detail does not necessarily result in an equally large change of volume.

Finally, outlier measurements capture singular deviations between f and g. Selecting a type of quality measure depends on the application. If a general quality shall be established (e.g., for promoting a method for other applications apart from that for which it has been developed) all types of quality measures should be used.

Volumetric measurements are easy to compute. They simply count the number of elements $|F|$ and $|G|$ with $F = \{\mathbf{v}|f(\mathbf{v}) = 1\}$ and $G = \{\mathbf{v}|g(\mathbf{v}) = 1\}$ weighted by the area or volume covered by each scene element (pixel or voxel) $\mathbf{v}$ (see Fig. 13.2). They are also the most unreliable measure since equal volume does not mean that the same object has been delineated. However, these or similar measures such as expected diameter or the size of a bounding box enclosing the object are sometimes the only way to get a quality measure at all when the exact delineation of the object is unknown.

Overlap measures compute the amount of oversegmentation, undersegmentation, or a combination of the two (see Fig. 13.3). *Oversegmentation* is simply the number of elements $\mathbf{v}$, for which $g(\mathbf{v}) = 0$ and $f(\mathbf{v}) = 1$, while *undersegmentation* is the opposite (i.e., $g(\mathbf{v}) = 1$ and $f(\mathbf{v}) = 0$). To make these numbers comparable for objects of different size the amounts are usually given as a percent oversegmentation or undersegmentation,

$$O = 100 \cdot \frac{|\{\mathbf{v}|g(\mathbf{v}) = 0 \wedge f(\mathbf{v}) = 1\}|}{|G|} \tag{13.2}$$

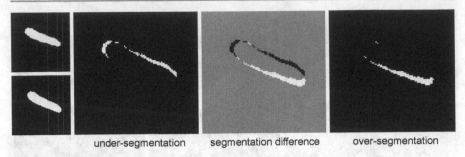

under-segmentation   segmentation difference   over-segmentation

Fig. 13.3 Over- and under-segmentation as well as a combination of the two represent differences in shape between ground truth and the segmentation to be tested

and

$$U = 100 \cdot \frac{|\{\mathbf{v}|g(\mathbf{v}) = 1 \wedge f(\mathbf{v}) = 0\}|}{|G|}. \tag{13.3}$$

It makes sense to evaluate the two measures separately when the criticality of oversegmentation is different than that of undersegmentation. However, for the compactness of presentation, results from the two measures may be combined. Two often-used quality measures are the *Dice coefficient* and the *Jaccard coefficient* (Crum et al. 2006). They are borrowed from statistics, where they are used to rate the similarity of data sets. The Dice coefficient (Dice 1945) is defined as

$$d = \frac{2|F \cap G|}{|F| + |G|}, \tag{13.4}$$

where $F \cap G$ is the set of all elements $\mathbf{v}$ with $f(\mathbf{v}) = 1$ and $g(\mathbf{v}) = 1$. The coefficient is 1 if the correspondence is perfect and smaller than 1 otherwise. The Dice coefficient was found to agree well with the perceived variability of results of a segmentation in Zou et al. (2004).

The Jaccard coefficient (Jaccard 1912) is given by

$$j = \frac{|F \cap G|}{|F \cup G|}, \tag{13.5}$$

where $F \cup G$ is the set of all elements $\mathbf{v}$ with $f(\mathbf{v}) = 1$ or $g(\mathbf{v}) = 1$. Again, this coefficient is 1 if the correspondence is perfect and decreases otherwise. The Jaccard coefficient is also known as the *Tanimoto coefficient* on sets.

Outliers cannot be measured by the criteria listed above, although they may be sometimes critical. An example would be a task where organ boundaries are to be delineated as part of access planning in minimally invasive surgery. In such a case, the maximum deviation of the delineated boundary from the true boundary is an important quality. It can be measured by the *Hausdorff distance* between the two data sets F and G (used, e.g., in Chalana and Kim 1997; Gerig et al. 2001; see Fig. 13.4). The Hausdorff distance h is the maximum of all minimal distances d

Fig. 13.4 The Hausdorff distance is the maximum of all shortest distances between points of one set to the other set

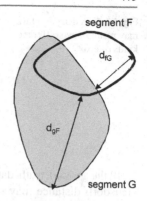

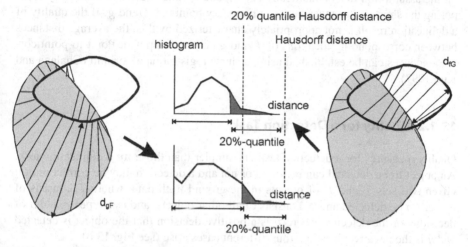

Fig. 13.5 The quantile Hausdorff distance for some quantile is computed from a quantile of a histogram of distances from F to G and from G to F

between points in F and points in G:

$$h = \max\left(\inf_{f \in F} d(f, G), \inf_{g \in G} d(g, F) \right). \tag{13.6}$$

It describes the largest distance of all smallest distances of points in one of the data sets to all points of the other data set. Since this measure is very sensitive to artefacts, a modified version of the Hausdorff distance is sometimes used that averages distances of the largest outliers. The *quantile Hausdorff distance* for the quantile h^q computes histograms of distances $d(f, G)$ and $d(g, F)$. For each of the histograms thresholds $t_q(d(f, G))$ and $t_q(d(g, F))$ are computed so that $q\%$ of all distances are smaller than t_q. The quantile Hausdorff distance is then (see Fig. 13.5)

$$h^q = \max\big(t_q\big(d(f, G)\big), t_q\big(d(g, F)\big)\big). \tag{13.7}$$

Fig. 13.6 A detection task may result in two different kinds of error

	object present	object not present
object found	True Positive	False Positive Type I Error
object not found	False Negative Type II Error	True Negative

If the ground truth data consist of the boundaries of delineated segments the Hausdorff distance may still be computed. Using the Hausdorff distance is based on the assumption that semantically corresponding points are determined by computing the shortest distances between boundary points of f and g. If the quality of a delineation result is not appropriately characterized by this, the average distances between corresponding locations of f and g can be computed. Point-to-point correspondences can be established using a shape registration algorithm (Chalana and Kim 1997).

13.1.2 Quality for a Detection Task

Quality measures for a detection task are simpler than those for a delineation task. An object to be detected can be found or not and a detection may be correct or not. Given two sets T and F of objects in the ground truth data, where T consists of objects to be detected and F consists of all other objects, and two types p and n of decisions of the detector, where p is a positive decision that the object is detected and n is the negative decision, four different cases arise (see Fig. 13.6).

- *True positive* detections TP are those belonging to T, which have been rightly detected by a positive decision p.
- *True negative* detections TN are those belonging to F, which are rightly resulted in a negative decision n.
- *False positive* results FP are those that do belong to F but resulted in a positive decision p.
- *False negative* results FN are those belonging to T but were classified as n.

A good detection method would produce as many TP and TN as possible. However, since false positive results (e.g., a tumor is detected while no tumor is present) and false negative results (e.g., a tumor is overlooked) may have wildly different consequences, the two types of errors are measured separately. The former is called a *type-I error* and the latter is a *type-II error*. Since the absolute numbers of FP or FN detections do not carry much information, they are normalized with the number of cases tested. This is expressed by the *sensitivity* and *specificity* of a method. Sensitivity Sv is defined as

$$Sv = \frac{TP}{T} = \frac{TP}{TP + FN}. \tag{13.8}$$

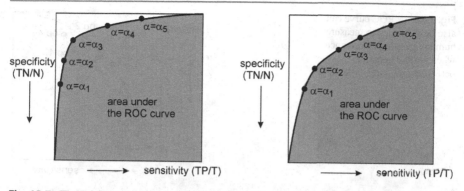

Fig. 13.7 The ROC curve rates sensitivity vs. specificity for different parameter settings of a detection method. The method described by the *curve on the right* is inferior to the method described by the *curve on the left*, since specificity decreases faster with increased sensitivity

It represents the rate of positive detections with respect to all elements of T. Sensitivity tells how likely it is to miss a detection by the analysis method (in the information retrieval community it is also called *recall rate*). The specificity Sp is defined as

$$Sp = \frac{TN}{N} = \frac{TN}{TN + FP}. \tag{13.9}$$

It represents the rate of negative decisions with respect to all elements of N. Specificity tells how likely it is that the detection method produces a false alarm. In the information retrieval community this is replaced by a different measure, called *precision rate Pr* of the retrieval

$$Pr = \frac{TP}{TP + FP}. \tag{13.10}$$

It reflects a different view at the detection task as it measures the amount of "noise" (the false positives), which is generated by the detection algorithm.

Often, a detection task can be parameterized to be more specific or more sensitive. Hence, this tradeoff itself is an important characteristic for evaluating a method (Popovic et al. 2007). A simple example would be a threshold classification where decreasing the threshold would increase the number of positive detections. This would increase the sensitivity since more elements of T would be included in TP, but it also decreases the specificity since more elements of F would falsely be classified as belonging to T. The tradeoff is specific to the detection method and independent of the threshold. Since it measures the performance of a parametrizable detector, it is also used as a quality measure for determining its performance. It is called the *receiver operator characteristic* (*ROC*) and measures the ratio of sensitivity versus specificity for each parameter setting α (see Fig. 13.7):

$$ROC(\alpha) = \big(Sv(\alpha), 1 - Sp(\alpha)\big). \tag{13.11}$$

Fig. 13.8 A ROC curve can
also be generated to measure
human operator performance
when several operators
performed the same task

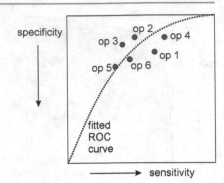

A curve can be drawn in a graph with axes Sv and Sp where different parameterizations α produce curve locations. This *ROC curve* represents the performance of the detector independent of the parameterization α. Hence, it is a way to compare two different, parametrizable detectors. An ideal ROC curve would produce a sensitivity and specificity of 100% irrespective of the value of α. Since the diagram is normalized with Sv and $1 - Sp$ ranging from 0 to 1, the area under this ROC curve would be 1.0. The worst result would be an ROC curve, where an increase of Sv would cause an equal increase of $1 - Sv$. This would mean that increasing the number of correct answers would increase the number of false answers in the same fashion. In this case, the ROC curve would be a diagonal and the area under the curve would be 0.5. Computing the *area under the ROC curve* allows comparing two different, parameterizable detectors.

Sometimes, the ROC curve cannot be generated for the ground truth. This would be the case when the ground truth is provided by human operator decision (it will be difficult to expect from an operator to be gradually more stringent in his or her decisions). A ROC curve can be estimated if several different, independent detection tasks were solved on the same data with the same detection system (e.g., by asking several human operators to solve the same detection task). Each of the solutions provides one point in the ROC diagram. Fitting a curve through these points gives an estimate of the ROC curve for this detector class (see Fig. 13.8).

Sensitivity, specificity, and the ROC curve have been used to measure the quality of a delineation task as well. In this case, the sets of T, F, p, and n are sets of pixels or voxels inside and outside the delineated object in the ground truth data and the data coming from the delineation method.

13.1.3 Quality for a Registration Task

The purpose of registration is to find a transformation that maps an n-dimensional image onto another m-dimensional image. If dimensions n and m are different, the transformation includes a projection step of the scene with higher dimension onto a space with dimensions of the scene with lower dimension.

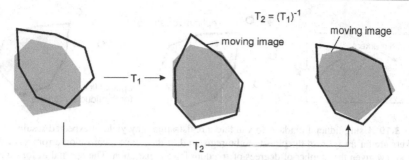

Fig. 13.9 If the still and the moving image are exchanged for registration, the resulting transformations should be the inverse of each other

   The quality of a registration task is measured by direct or indirect measurement of the difference between true and computed registration transformation. A direct comparison requires the true transformation parameters to be known (which is sometimes possible when phantom data are used for providing the ground truth). The average deviation of transformation parameters plus the detection of outliers is then the appropriate means to describe how well the registration method succeeded. For nonrigid registration, this transformation is given by a vector field defining local displacements. Differences in the true and the computed vector field are then used as a quality measure. For rigid transformations, differences in global rotation and translation are used as a quality measure. Since rotation and translation represent different kinds of transformation they should be measured separately.

   If the true transformation is unknown, an indirect way to compute a quality measure is to exchange moving and still images (see Fig. 13.9). The transformation should be the inverse and any deviations are taken as inaccuracies in the computation of the registration transformation. This way of validation should be used with care, however. It implicitly assumes that criteria to find a registration transformation from image A to image B are independent to that of finding a registration from B to A. If this is not the case, the quality measure does not tell much about the inherent quality of the registration method.

   If the data sets to be registered are of the same kind (e.g., when comparing images of the same patient using the same imaging device over time), the second image can be generated from the first image by transforming and resampling the data. This transformation is then compared with that of the registration transformation. Again, this has to be used with care since neither deviation between the two images to be registered nor resampling artefacts are considered.

   An indirect way, which is often used for computing the validity of a registration transformation, is to compute deviations of point locations after registration. If a number of point pairs are known that represent semantically equivalent locations in the two images, applying the registration transformation to these point locations in one image should map them exactly on locations of their counterparts in the other image. The point pairs are called *fiducial markers*. Of course, the point pair correspondence must not have been used for computing the registration transformation.

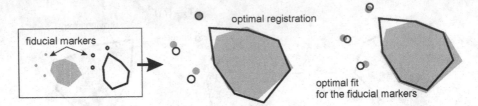

Fig. 13.10 Using fiducial markers to validate a registration may yield unexpected results, if the markers are far away from the objects to be registered, if they have localization errors, or if they are too few given the number of degrees of freedom for a registration. The optimal fit for fiducial markers does then not automatically mean that the registration itself is optimal

Using fiducial markers has the advantage that it evaluates a property that is usually the reason for computing the registration transformation in the first place. One has to be aware, however, that the quality of this mapping is evaluated only at the locations of the fiducial markers (see Fig. 13.10). This may become a problem if markers are placed in locations that are very different from those where a high accuracy is required (e.g., when only using skin surface markers to test a registration of brain images), or if the registration transformation has many degrees of freedom and only few marker positions are used (e.g., when evaluating a nonrigid registration transformation with few markers).

13.2   The Ground Truth

All measures to estimate the quality of an analysis procedure require a comparison of the analysis result with the true information. The truth is difficult to come by since the reason for producing images in the first place was to gather information about the human body that cannot be accessed otherwise.

Ground truth is the true analysis result of data to which the analysis method is applied. The data can be real or artificial. As we will see below, each of the strategies is tainted (i.e., it is never completely sure whether the selected data really represent the ground truth). An interesting suggestion to deal with this problem came from the validation committee within the ITK consortium (Yoo et al. 2000). They suggested a blind test. Independent observers evaluate analysis results of different data experts (which also could be different established computer analysis methods) with respect to a new method. The new method would be judged as accurate when no significant difference can be found. For automated analysis, the observers will be replaced by an automatic scoring system. Under the assumption that data experts produce unbiased variations of an unknown ground truth (an assumption that also gave rise to the STAPLE procedure, see Sect. 13.2.1 below), the method is able to rate a new method correctly even if the exact ground truth is unknown.

13.2.1 Ground Truth from Real Data

Ground truth from real data results from applying the currently established best method to it. This is often difficult to determine, however. If an established method exists at all, it may well be a different method for different kinds of image data, for different image acquisition protocols, and for different analysis questions. Hence, even if such a standard exists (e.g., to use active surfaces for liver segmentation in CT or to use mutual information and spline-based nonrigid registration for registering MR brain images), the developer will need to show that the conditions under which this standard is applied are comparable to the ones under which this is an established standard.

Another problem is that the implementation of the established state-of-the-art method is not always available. This is changing because many researchers make their code available and many of the state-of-the-art methods for segmentation and registration have been included into the freely available ITK package (www.itk.org, see Chap. 1).

If a currently best method does not exist, analysis by a human expert is an option to produce ground truth data. It requires some effort on the developer's side and a lot more effort on the data expert's side. The developer needs to provide an appropriate interactive interface for analyzing the data. The required effort from the expert's side is much higher. First, the expert has to carry out the analysis interactively on several data sets. In fact, the more data sets are analyzed, the easier it will be to differentiate between significant and insignificant results. Significance will increase further if the expert analyses the data several times. *Intraobserver variability* can be estimated that describes variation of judgment by the same individual. A high variability may indicate that the knowledge on which decisions are based is either not very clear, not sufficient, or cannot be applied easily. This is a reason to provide a good user interface since intraobserver variability should not rate the quality of the input component.

Different experts may have different opinions about the content in the data. Hence, *interobserver variability* should be measured as well by asking several experts to analyze the data. A good result for the automatic analysis method would be one that is close to a result on which experts agree and within the range of variation among experts. This requires a definition of what is meant by agreement among experts. It can be done using a voting system where each expert has a vote (Warfield et al. 1995). Agreement can be reached by majority vote, by requiring total agreement, or by something in between. The situation is less than ideal since each of the choices for defining agreement makes assumptions about the expertise of the voters without having the chance to validate these assumptions.

STAPLE (simultaneous truth and performance level estimation; Warfield et al. 2004) is an elegant way to solve this problem for delineation and object detection tasks. The ground truth is assumed to be a set of labeled voxels and the input is a labeling from different experts (or segmentation algorithms) whose reliability is unknown. STAPLE defines the problem probabilistically and treats expert segmentations as samples that deviate in an unknown fashion from the ground truth. It reconstructs the most likely ground truth data given the samples. This, in turn, defines the reliability of each sample. Hence, STAPLE is an application of a maximum likelihood (ML) algorithm to the sample results.

The STAPLE method for a two-label-segmentation (e.g., foreground vs. background) presumes that a number of R segmentations exist that assign a binary label to each of N scene elements. It estimates the true segmentation $\mathbf{t} = (t_1, \ldots, t_N)$ from the R segmentations $\mathbf{d}_j$, $j = 1, R$ and $\mathbf{d}_j = (d_{j,1}, \ldots, d_{j,N})$. It further estimates sensitivity $\mathbf{p} = (p_1, \ldots, p_R)$ and specificity $\mathbf{q} = (q_1, \ldots, q_R)$ for each of the R segmentations. The sensitivity and specificity of STAPLE relates to the number of classified voxels or pixels. If one of the R segmentations is new and shall be tested against the other segmentations, the sensitivity and specificity of the new method can be used to rate it against the other methods. Other quality measures such as the Dice coefficient can be computed based on $\mathbf{t}$.

Given an initial estimate of the sensitivities and specificities and an estimate for the a priori probability $P(t_i)$ of t_i being a foreground element, Warfield et al. (2004) showed how to use an EM algorithm for optimizing $\mathbf{p}$, $\mathbf{q}$, and $\mathbf{t}$. The E-step computes the current expected probability $w_i^{(k)}$ of an element i to have the label $t_i = 1$ by

$$a_i^{(k)} = P(t_i = 1) \prod_{j \in \{j \mid d_{i,j}=1\}} p_j^{(k)} \prod_{j \in \{j \mid d_{i,j}=0\}} \left(1 - p_j^{(k)}\right), \tag{13.12}$$

$$b_i^{(k)} = \left(1 - P(t_i = 1)\right) \prod_{j \in \{j \mid d_{i,j}=0\}} q_j^{(k)} \prod_{j \in \{j \mid d_{i,j}=1\}} \left(1 - q_j^{(k)}\right), \tag{13.13}$$

$$w_i^{(k)} = \frac{a_i^{(k)}}{\left(a_i^{(k)} + b_i^{(k)}\right)}. \tag{13.14}$$

The terms in the products in (13.12) and (13.13) represent the conditional probabilities of each segmentation j to arrive at a decision $d_{i,j}$ given that the true segmentation is either $d_i = 1$ or $t_j = 0$, and the current estimates of sensitivity and specificity. Together with the a priori probability $P(t_i = 1)$ and $P(t_i = 0) = 1 - P(t_i = 1)$, these are the right-hand sides of the Bayesian Theorem for computing the a posteriori probability for $t_i = 1$ or $t_i = 0$, respectively, given the decisions $\mathbf{d}_j$ and the current estimates for $\mathbf{p}$ and $\mathbf{q}$.

Computing the $w_i^{(k)}$ requires that the different segmentations are independent of each other since otherwise computing conditional probabilities by multiplying probabilities from each segmentation j is not permissible. A priori probabilities for segmentations where the result at some site i is independent of all other sites are the ratio of foreground elements to all scene elements. This assumes that segmentations j are also unbiased.

If a priori assumptions include information of spatial dependencies between scene elements this can be represented by a Markov random field (see Sect. 14.1). Optimization for the general case can be slow (e.g., simulated annealing) or may require a good initial estimate (ICM or graph cuts). However, as shown in Chap. 9, the graph cut solution is an efficient way to find the exact optimum if the number of labels is two.

Given the result of the E-step, the M-step of the EM algorithm updates sensitivity and specificity values by

$$p_j^{(k+1)} = \frac{\sum_{\{i|d_{i,j}=1\}} w_i^{(k)}}{\sum_{i=1}^{N} w_i^{(k)}}, \tag{13.15}$$

$$q_j^{(k+1)} = \frac{\sum_{\{i|d_{i,j}=0\}} (1 - w_i^{(k)})}{\sum_{i=1}^{N} (1 - w_i^{(k)})}. \tag{13.16}$$

The initial values for **p** and **q** use existing information about the performance of the segmentation methods to be tested. In the absence of such information, Warfield et al. (2004) suggested starting the system with very high values $p_j, q_j < 1$.

The STAPLE procedure can be extended to process multilabel segmentations, however, at the cost that the optimization of a spatially correlated segmentation via an MRF prior will become either slow or suboptimal.

If the comparison is carried out with the currently best method the burden of detecting the truth has been passed to the validation of this method (be it an automatic method or expert analysis). This is even true when elaborate reliability checks such as STAPLE are applied since they still rely on some basic assumptions (in this case, unbiased observers and a good initial estimate).

13.2.2 Ground Truth from Phantoms

Phantoms will exhibit varying degrees of realism. The more realistic a phantom is, the less accessible is the information represented by the phantom. Selecting the appropriate phantom is always a compromise. Based on the degree of realism, phantoms fall into four groups.

- Cadaver phantoms (human or animal).
- Artificial hardware phantoms constructed of material that is known to produce a similar image signal as real data.
- Software phantoms representing the imaged measurement distribution.
- Software phantoms representing the reconstructed image.

In their survey on image segmentation methods in medical imaging, Pham et al. (2000) classified phantoms of the first two kinds as *physical phantoms* and the latter two as *computational phantoms*. The main difference is that a physical phantom is imaged by the same imaging device as the patient data, while for the computational phantoms influences from imaging have to be simulated.

A cadaver or an animal specimen has similar properties as real patient data. Since image acquisition is equal to that generating patient data, the following attributes of the imaging procedure are represented by the phantom:

- material properties,
- measurement properties,
- influences from image reconstruction, and
- shape properties of the imaged object.

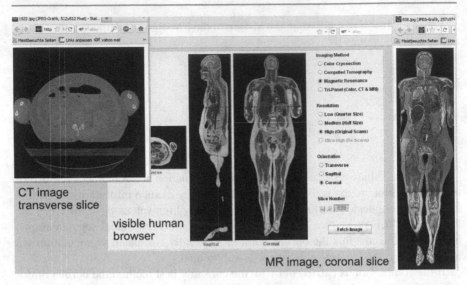

Fig. 13.11 CT and MRI slices and the imaged cytographic slices from the Visible Human Project (created using a browser of from the visible human page of the University of Michigan at http://vhp.med.umich.edu/)

To make the phantom data useful for validation analysis the results have to be generated in the phantom. That means the following.

- For a detection task the number and locations of the objects to be detected have to be specified.
- For a registration task fiducial markers have to be implanted that are visible in the images, or that the phantom is fixed to a reference frame from which the transformation parameters can be deduced.

Using a real phantom for a delineation task requires the object to be delineated in the phantom in a way that makes it visible in the images. If only indirect quality measures such as the volume of an organ are needed for validation, real phantoms can be used and the volume is measured afterward (requiring separation of the anatomic object from the rest of the phantom). Otherwise, delineation information has to be supplied from some other source. An example for this is the visible human project (http://www.nlm.nih.gov/research/visible/visible_human.html) where a male and a female cadaver were imaged by CT and MRI and specimen slices were then photographed (see Fig. 13.11). The information has been used to delineate anatomical structures in the images (Toh et al. 1996; Spitzer et al. 1996).

Some problems may arise when using such a phantom for validation.

- Attributes of the image phantom may still vary in an unknown fashion from that of the real data.
- Anatomical variability (normal as well as pathological) is not captured by the phantom.

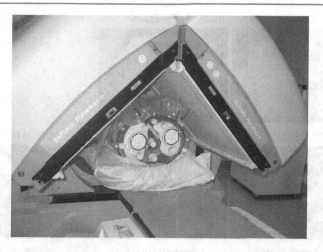

Fig. 13.12 Example of an artificial phantom. The picture shows a hardware phantom for the simulation of SPECT images of the heart. The phantom consists of several bottles of photon-emitting fluids that have a similar characteristic than the organs that are simulated. The shape of the bottles resemble (at the spatial resolution of SPECT imaging) the shape of the organs (with kind permission of Anna Celler, Department of Radiology, University of British Columbia, Vancouver)

Artificial hardware phantoms capture all but the material properties. Material properties are simulated by selecting material that produces a similar signal as the tissues to be imaged (see Fig. 13.12). Since the artificial structure is built on purpose, aspects for validation (the extent of an object, specific landmarks, delineation of object boundaries) are usually known and accessible. Simple hardware phantoms just capture the local properties to be measured by the imaging system (e.g., containers of some fluid that emit photons to test nuclear imaging systems). They are still appropriate to validate analysis methods if knowledge about the appearance and shape of the objects or features of interest as well as information about spatial relationships to surrounding tissues has not been used for the analysis. More realistic phantoms exist (e.g., for simulating imaging of vascular structures). Phantoms are usually single instances so that anatomical variation cannot be modeled. However, they are well suited to compare the quality of different methods applied to the same data such as the comparison of different image reconstruction algorithms (see Fig. 13.13).

Software phantoms representing the measured image signal are the next level of abstraction. The phantom consists of a 3D distribution of the signal to be measured by the image acquisition system (e.g., x-ray absorption for an x-ray CT phantom). The 3D signal distribution may be generated from interpreted image material (e.g., the MRI BrainWeb phantom; Collins et al. 1998). Creating the phantom requires knowledge about the original material coefficients (e.g., T_1, T_2, and proton density for the BrainWeb phantom). This information is taken from experiments. It is often idealized (e.g., by assuming that the material is homogeneous within an organ). Noise and artefact models of image acquisition are required for simulating the measurement. The effects from image reconstruction and shape properties of objects in

Emission   Transmission

OSEM   OSEM AC   OSEM RR

OSEM AC+RR   OSEM AC+RR+SC   Evolution AC+RR

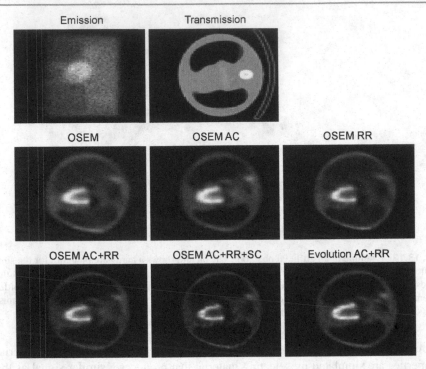

Fig. 13.13 Different reconstruction algorithms from data acquired from the phantom depicted in Fig. 13.12. The *top row* shows the measured emission and transmission data from the phantom, the *middle and the bottom rows* show reconstruction results using the OSEM algorithm (see Chap. 2) including various restoration techniques (AC: attenuation correction, RR: resolution recovery, SC: scatter correction) presented in Shcherbinin et al. (2008) compared to standard reconstruction technique of the GE evolution scanner (with kind permission of Anna Celler, Department of Radiology, University of British Columbia, Vancouver)

the image are part of the phantom. The advantage of a software phantom compared to a hardware phantom is that it easily allows the inclusion of known anatomical variation by creating several different shape phantoms. Also, the original properties of the objects to be represented are easily accessible. A number of software phantoms of this kind exist.

- The BrainWeb phantom, www.bic.mni.mcgill.ca/brainweb/ (Cocosco et al. 1997; Collins et al. 1998; Kwan et al. 1999) was created from a single subject. Although not representing interpatient variability, it gives a realistic representation of the typical appearance of brain structures (see Fig. 13.14). A simple user interface allows various parameterizations to produce different simulations of MRI images.
- The Field II ultrasound simulation program (see Fig. 13.15), to be found at server.electro.dtu.dk/personal/jaj/field/ (Jensen and Svendsen 1992; Jensen 1996, 2004), simulates the creation of ultrasound images from various input data. It is available as Matlab software.

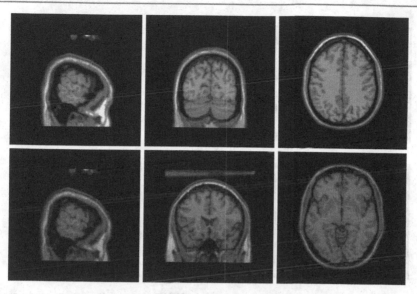

Fig. 13.14 Images generated from the BrainWeb software phantom (Collins et al. 1998) look very realistic. The simulation was done using the phantom that can be downloaded from www.bic.mni.mcgill.ca/brainweb/

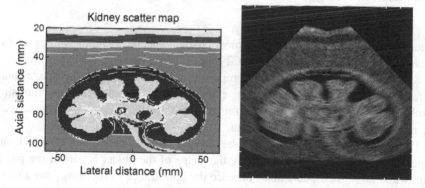

Fig. 13.15 Depiction of an ultrasound phantom and the simulated ultrasound image. The simulated image was created using the Field II ultrasound simulation program of Jensen (1992, 1996, 2004)

- The group of Segars et al., http://www.bme.unc.edu/~wsegars/index.html and http://dmip1.rad.jhmi.edu/xcat/, see Segars et al. (1999), Segars and Tsui (2009) developed several phantoms for CT and Nuclear Medicine such as the dynamic MCAT heart phantom simulating a moving heart, which is based on normal anatomy and the spline-based interpolation of dynamics, the NCAT phantom that has been extended to also include the upper airway tree and the lung lobes and to simulate normal and pathological variations (Garrity et al. 2003; Veress et al. 2006), and its extension, the XCAT. MCAT and XCAT are created from parame-

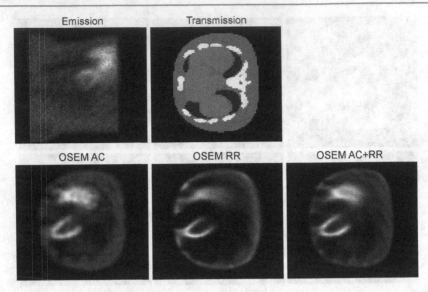

Fig. 13.16 Emission and transmission image of the NCAT phantom. Projections can be reconstructed to simulate CT, SPECT or PET imaging. In this case, different reconstruction algorithms for SPECT images are compared integrating attenuation correction (AC) and resolution recovery (RR) in the OSEM reconstruction algorithm (see Shcherbinin et al. 2008 for details; with kind permission of Anna Celler, Vancouver General Hospital)

terizable geometric primitives that model patient-specific anatomic variation. The phantoms are used to validate SPECT and PET data (see Fig. 13.16).

Since material and measurement properties are often idealized, the images may differ from the images of real objects even though they look realistic. Promising results on phantom data can then be misleading since they seem not to agree with the perceived performance on real data.

The highest level of abstraction is the use of a software phantom that models the appearance of an imaged object. Only the shape of the object is part of the phantom, while all other aspects that influence the appearance in the image need to be simulated. The shape information either stems from the interpreted images (e.g., the MNI brain atlas of Collins et al. 1998 to represent variation of the human brain anatomy) or—in an even more abstract fashion—it reflects just those shape properties that are assumed to be important for the analysis task. Artefacts from material, measurement, or reconstruction are simulated. Observed distortions in the image are modeled by the simulation model. The following are examples for artifacts that are modeled.

- Detector and measurement noise are usually combined as zero-mean Gaussian noise.
- Partial volume effects and the effects from the detector point spread function are modeled by smoothing the data.
- Variation in signal strength is modeled by including artificial shading.

The artefact model may be approximate, even if the images look similar to the true images.

In summary, the phantoms listed above produce ground truth only to the extent to which influences on the image generation have correctly been accounted for. Choosing a phantom is a compromise between the realism of the images generated and accessibility to the ground truth. Ideally, the phantom itself would be validated (i.e., to what extent the phantom data reflects the reality would be investigated). Since this is usually not done, using a phantom for validating an analysis procedure should include information as to what influences on the image content were simulated, on what information the simulated properties were based, and on what kind of information the analysis procedure relies. This gives others the chance to decide on the validity of arguments for their own purposes.

13.3 Representativeness of Data

Validation will be based on statistical arguments (such as "in 99.2% of all cases, volume deviated by less than 5% from the ground truth"). Hence, besides trusting ground truth and the appropriateness of the quality measures, representativeness is another issue for validation. Using representative data means that all data properties potentially influencing the performance of the analysis method are reflected in the test data. A couple of strategies strengthen the argument of representativeness.
- Separation between test and training data.
- Identification of sources of variation.
- Identification of outliers.
- Investigation of robustness with respect to parameter variation.

13.3.1 Separation Between Training and Test Data

The separation between training data and test data is self-evident if classification is the goal of the analysis. However, other analysis tasks include training as well, for instance, when optimal parameters have to be determined. Parameters are anything that need to be fixed prior to carrying out the analysis. This could be a stopping criterion for an iterative algorithm or a threshold for a decision component. As in classification, it is not acceptable to validate a parameter-dependent segmentation on ground truth data that have been used to compute the optimal parameter value.

Often, the set of data that can be used for training and testing is very small. Separating it into two even smaller subsets would reduce the significance of the results further. A work-around is to use the *leaving-one-out technique* (also called *jackknife technique*, see Fig. 13.17 for an example). A data set of N elements, for which the ground truth is known, is separated in a training set of $N - 1$ elements and a test set consisting of just one element. Parameter estimation is done on the training set and the quality is then measured on the single test element. This is done for all N subsets of $(N - 1)$-element training sets and 1-element test sets. The overall quality is then computed by combining the N different test results.

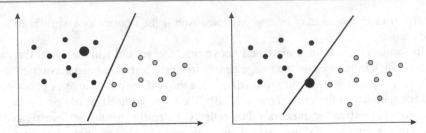

Fig. 13.17 Leaving-One-Out technique for a classification task. Repeatedly, a sample is left out from training and the resulting decision boundary is tested on this sample. The test is to be carried out using every sample as left-out sample

13.3.2 Identification of Sources of Variation and Outlier Detection

Representativeness means that the typical sources of variation in the data are covered by the ground truth data. To test the behavior in extreme cases outliers should be identified. If data consist of patient data that have been analyzed by the current best method or by a human expert, sources of variation and outliers can be found with the help of an expert. The expert will be able to tell whether the images reflect the "usual appearance" of the objects to be analyzed, but it will require some discussion between the data expert and method expert nonetheless. The reason is that analysis methodology will act differently for different sources of variation. A detection method that mainly relies on the detection of objects in the vicinity of other objects will be insensitive to object variations, but very sensitive to variations in the appearance of neighboring objects. A data expert will only perceive this as important if it is a criterion for the expert's decision as well.

Another source of misunderstanding regarding variation and outliers is the difference of the task for the expert and for a computer method. The expert often analyses single cases with the correct output expected for this case while the computer-assisted analysis method has to work in general for all potential cases. The expert judges the single case using additional information from anamnesis and other diagnostic imaging or nonimaging information. The notions of "usual" or "outlier" may be based on all this information and not on the image alone. To prevent this kind of misunderstanding, it should be made very clear that the discussion is about the appearance of an object in the image.

The discussion is usually easier for the engineer or computer scientist when phantoms are the ground truth. The phantom is generated with keeping variation with respect to appearance in the image in mind. Furthermore, if variable phantoms have been created, the different sources of variation (noise, artifacts, patient-specific changes in shape and appearance) have been identified and the ranges of normal and abnormal variation have been defined. It may be difficult to establish whether all sources of variation are covered, however. This is true for technical as well as for anatomical sources of variation. For variation of technical parameters or models it cannot often be proven that the model captures exactly the reality (e.g., when assuming a certain kind of noise) and it is left to the developer to decide whether the model still produces a good validation scenario. For anatomical variation, certain simple parameters (e.g., size or length-to-breadth ratio) are often measured, but it cannot be guaranteed that these parameters reflect everything that is necessary for producing a representative set of phantoms. Furthermore, pathological variations are often not captured at all.

Given the remarks above, it seems that estimating normal and extraordinary variation is impossible. This is fortunately untrue since some sources of variation can be captured with some accuracy. Using this information is preferable to using the argumentation above for just choosing arbitrary data for validation. Disclosing assumptions about sources of variation helps others to rate the validity of these arguments.

Outliers can also be detected based on their very nature. If they are so different from the rest of the cases, computable properties used as a priori knowledge for the analysis method will exist that are different for these data sets as well. Hence, it will be possible to predict the property of an outlier from nonoutlier data. This can be used in *cross-validation*.

Given N data sets, cross-validation computes predictions of these properties from all subsets of $N - 1$ elements and applies this prediction to the remaining data set. The $N - 1$ elements would be a sufficiently high number to generate an estimate of a likelihood function. If the property value of the left out Nth element has a low probability according to this likelihood function, the element is probably an outlier and should be removed. Outlier removal continues until no further outliers can be found, or if the data set becomes too small. In the latter case, the outliers actually characterize the data. There are a number of reasons for this.

- The properties used as a priori knowledge are inappropriate for the analysis method because the parameter settings have to be adapted for every single case.
- The data fall into several classes for which separate methods need to be found.
- The acquisition of ground truth data failed as the data are apparently not representative for the totality of all data (if it were representative, outliers would not occur this often).

13.3.3 Robustness with Respect to Parameter Variation

Given the argumentation above, it can be assumed that a developer or user will never be completely sure that test data were representative. Any parameterization from a training stage will have been generated from (slightly) nonrepresentative data. Hence, parameters would be preferred where small changes do not cause a large change in the analysis result. It simply means that the main power of the analysis is in the method and combination of submethods rather than in the parameterization.

Finding parameters and testing the method with respect to changes of parameter values can be costly because every possible combination of parameters needs to be tested. It may become unfeasible if the number of parameters is large. Hence, it is worthwhile to try to detect parameters that are most likely independent of each other. Doing this by simply testing would be unfeasible again. However, if the analysis

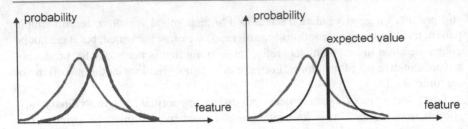

Fig. 13.18 The purpose of the student-t test is to determine how likely two distributions of observations belong to the same observation. It is often tested by estimating how likely the expected value of one of the two distributions belongs to the other distribution

methodology has been developed with exact documentation about information that is exploited for the analysis and about ways how this is used for carrying out the analysis, it is usually possible to hypothesize which parameters may be independent.

This is especially the case when the method is organized as a sequence of processes where each process has its own set of parameters and produces a well-defined intermediate result. If the intermediate results can be predicted for the ground truth data, parameters can be optimized and tested for each process independently. Even if subsequent processes are able to correct erroneous intermediate results, the optimal result for each step can be defined independent of the other steps.

13.4 Significance of Results

The results of an analysis may be satisfactory, but there is always the question whether the number of samples was sufficiently high for having a predictive value for the universe. Given a data set $S = \{s_1, \ldots, s_N\}$ reflecting the ground truth represented by a quality value $q_G(s)$ and test results $q_T(s)$, the question is how likely they describe the same entity except for some error $E(q_G - q_T)$. Given ground truth, an established method T_e, and a new method T_n, the question is whether T_n really produces better results.

The *significance* of a test result can be computed by estimating the probability that it arose by chance. This percentage is the p-value that is used to describe the significance of the outcome of an experiment. The statement "the results are significant with $p < 0.01$" simply means that the probability that the results arose by chance is less than 1%.

Intuitively, significance depends on the number of samples and on the amount of similarity or dissimilarity between the two populations (ground truth vs. test or method A vs. method B). Significance can be tested by the *student-t-test* (also called t-test). It computes the probability whether quality measurements q_{new} from a new method can be the result of some natural fluctuation of measurements q_{old} that were computed with an earlier method (see Fig. 13.18).

To formulate this as a problem of computing probabilities several aspects have to be specified. First, a *null hypothesis* is formulated. A null hypothesis assumes that nothing has happened. In our case, this means that the new method produces the same kind of results as the old method. A probability has to be computed that they have been drawn from the same probability distribution.

The new method is significantly different if this is not likely. It is significantly better if it is significantly different and the results are better. If the probability characteristics of quality measures of both the new and the old methods were known this would be easy. One could simply compute the probability with which the expected value of the distribution of the new method is a value from the distribution of quality measures of the old measure.

Probability distributions are usually unknown and can only be estimated from the sample results from q_{new} and q_{old}. The reliability of this computation depends on the number of samples for these estimates. This is captured by the student-t test. Many different variants of this t-test exist and the interested reader is referred to Aron et al. (2004) for further details. Here, we will present two versions that are often appropriate for computing the significance of the performance of an analysis method compared to the performance of some previous method. They are called the unpaired and paired t-test. It will be presented for normal distributed data where the mean and variance are unknown.

Let us assume that we have samples $X_1, X_2, \ldots, X_N$ (e.g., some quality measure with respect to ground truth) with mean μ and variance σ^2. The average of the samples is

$$\bar{X}_N = (X_1 + \cdots + X_N)/N. \tag{13.17}$$

The estimated variance of the samples is then

$$S_N^2 = \frac{1}{N-1} \sum_{i=1}^{N} (X_i - \bar{X}_N)^2. \tag{13.18}$$

The following parameter is then normal-distributed with zero mean and normalized variance

$$Z = \frac{\bar{X}_N - \mu}{\sigma/\sqrt{N}}. \tag{13.19}$$

Now let us assume that we have an unknown sample w. How likely is it that this sample is the mean of a distribution from which we have the N samples X_i? For this, a *confidence interval* is computed. It is

$$\int_{-a}^{a} Z(w)\,dw = p \tag{13.20}$$

and defines an interval $[-a, a]$ so that the probability for w is p. For example, the 90% confidence interval

$$\int_{-a}^{a} Z(w)\,dw = 0.90 \tag{13.21}$$

defines an interval bounded by $[-a, a]$ for which the probability is 90% that w belongs to Z. In other words, if w is outside the interval, the probability is only 10% that w belongs to Z. If we restrict a to be positive (e.g., if our value of w represents a change in quality and we are only interested in positive changes), then the same a characterizes a 95% confidence interval.

To compute the confidence interval from the samples Z, w is transformed into the normalized normal distribution

$$P(-a < w < a) = p$$

$$\Leftrightarrow \quad P\left(-a < \frac{\bar{X}_N - \mu}{\sigma/\sqrt{N}} < a\right) = p \tag{13.22}$$

$$\Leftrightarrow \quad P\left(\bar{X}_N - a\frac{\sigma}{\sqrt{N}} < \mu < \bar{X}_N + a\frac{\sigma}{\sqrt{N}}\right) = p.$$

This allows us to compute the value for a given the standard deviation σ. Since σ is unknown, the distribution is replaced by the estimate from the samples (this is the *t-distribution*)

$$P(-a < w < a) = p$$

$$\Leftrightarrow \quad P\left(-a < \frac{\bar{X}_N - \mu}{S_N/\sqrt{N}} < a\right) = p \tag{13.23}$$

$$\Leftrightarrow \quad P\left(\bar{X}_N - a\frac{S_N}{\sqrt{N}} < \mu < \bar{X}_N + a\frac{S_N}{\sqrt{N}}\right) = p.$$

Hence, $\bar{X}_N \pm a\frac{S_N}{\sqrt{N}}$ is the confidence interval with probability p that w is in Z. The values for a are tabulated and tables and Excel sheets exist for given probabilities p. When computing the t-test, one-sided and two-sided tests have to be differentiated. A one-sided t-test assumes an interval $[-\infty, a]$ and w is outside the interval if $w > a$. Hence, the 90% confidence interval of a two-sided t-test results in the same value of a as the 95% confidence interval of the one-sided t-test.

In the t-test above, pairings between results from the old method and those from the new method were not considered. This allows a comparison between methods even if the samples were generated from different data sets, as long as they can be assumed to be equally representative for the problem. However, since this cannot always be shown (or even made plausible), tests are often carried out on the same data set. Pairs of results $(X_1, Y_1), \ldots, (X_N, Y_N)$ exist where X is the quality of the old method and Y the result of the new method.

A *paired t-test* accounts for this using the mechanism above, but now with the following distribution function

$$t = \frac{\bar{P}_D - \mu}{S_D/\sqrt{N}}, \tag{13.24}$$

$$\bar{P}_D = \frac{1}{N} \sum_{i=1}^{N} (X_i - Y_i), \tag{13.25}$$

$$S_D = \frac{1}{N-1} \sum_{i=1}^{N} [(X_i - Y_i) - \bar{P}_D]^2. \tag{13.26}$$

The difference between the results of the old and new methods is taken as the sample value. The null hypothesis would be $\mu = 0$.

Since the t-test essentially tests the probability of the expected value of a distribution to be a value of the distribution of the null hypothesis, it implicitly assumes that the variances of the two distributions are equal. If this cannot be assured, the *Welch test* (Welch 1947) is a variant that should be applied. The difference between the t-test and the Welch test is that the t-distribution is now generated from the two different sample distributions X_1 and X_2 by normalizing them with the estimated variances s_1 and s_2 from both distributions, leading to

$$t = \frac{\bar{X}_1 - \bar{X}_2}{\sqrt{\frac{s_1^2}{N_1} + \frac{s_2^2}{N_2}}}. \tag{13.27}$$

This is then used in the same way for computing significance s the unpaired t-test for the student-t distribution.

13.5 Concluding Remarks

Validation of an analysis method is a necessary prerequisite for introducing any new analysis method to the scientific community since it cannot be verified that domain knowledge is sufficient and correct for solving the analysis problem. Validation is difficult because sufficiency and correctness have to be corroborated from results on representative test data. An acceptable validation needs to show to what extent tests are estimates for such a generalization. Furthermore, that quality measures and comparison data really support the argumentation has to be made plausible.

Validation is often a hen-and-egg problem. Hence, a detailed description of the validation scenario and a well-founded justification as to why which measures were selected is mandatory. Even though this is still not a formal verification, it enables the reader and potential future user of a method to investigate the validity of the arguments used for setting up the validation scenario.

13.6 Exercises

• Why is it necessary to document the validation scenario and not just the results from validation?

- What are the major components of a validation scenario and what should be documented?
- Describe a situation where volume computation would be an appropriate criterion for measuring the quality of a delineation task. When should it not be used?
- Under what conditions does it make sense to differentiate between oversegmentation and undersegmentation?
- What information about delineation quality is revealed by the Hausdorff distance? Please describe a scenario where this measure is important to rate a delineation method.
- What information is captured by sensitivity and specificity? For what reason is specificity needed to rate a detection method? Give an example.
- Imagine a registration method that has been developed to register preoperative and postoperative CT scans. What are the options to be used as ground truth? Discuss the advantages and disadvantages of the different options.
- What needs to be made sure when selecting test data for ground truth?
- Why is it necessary to carry out manual segmentation several times by different people and by the same person if it shall be used for ground truth? How is the information that is gained from these multiple segmentations used for rating the performance of an algorithm?
- What is the difference between hardware phantoms and software phantoms? What are the advantages of using a software phantom?
- Which kinds of influences from image acquisition be represented in a software phantom?
- What are the limitations when representing anatomic variations by a software phantom?
- What is meant by robustness with respect to parameter variation? Why is it important that a method is robust with respect to parameter variation?
- Give an example from segmentation where it is necessary to differentiate between training and test data.
- What is the basic idea of STAPLE? What advantage does this have when validating a method?
- What is the meaning of "p-value"?
- Assume that the results of a method A on data AT and the results of method B on data BT have been generated. It can be assumed that AT and BT are samples from the same distribution of test data. What would be an appropriate null hypothesis for a t-test?

References

Aron A, Aron EN, Coups E (2004) Statistics for the behavioral and social sciences: a brief course. Prentice Hall, New York

Chalana V, Kim Y (1997) A methodology for evaluation of boundary detection algorithms on medical images. IEEE Trans Med Imaging 16(5):642–652

Cocosco CA, Kollokian V, Kwan RKS, Pike GB, Evans AC (1997) BrainWeb: online interface to a 3d MRI simulated brain database. NeuroImage 5:452

Collins D, Zijdenbos A, Kollokian V, Sled J, Kabani N, Holmes C, Evans A (1998) Design and construction of a realistic digital brain phantom. IEEE Trans Med Imaging 17(3):463–468

Crum WR, Camara O, Hill DLG (2006) Generalized overlap measures for evaluation and validation in medical image analysis. IEEE Trans Med Imaging 25(11):1451–1461

Dice LR (1945) Measures of the amount of ecologic association between species. Ecology 26(3):297–302

Garrity JM, Segars WP, Knisley SB, Tsui BMW (2003) Development of a dynamic model for the lung lobes and airway tree in the NCAT phantom. IEEE Trans Nucl Sci 50(3):378–383

Gerig G, Jomier M, Chakos M (2001) Valmed: a new validation tool for assessing and improving 3D object segmentation. In: Proc 4th intl conf medical image computing and computer-assisted intervention (MICCAI 2001). LNCS, vol 2208, pp 516–523

Jaccard P (1912) The distribution of flora in the alpine zone. New Phytol 11:37–50

Jensen JA (1996) Field: a program for simulating ultrasound systems. In: 10th Nordic-Baltic conf biomedical imaging, medical & biological engineering & computing, vol 34(Suppl 1(part 1)), pp 351–353

Jensen JA, Svendsen NB (1992) Calculation of pressure fields from arbitrarily shaped, apodized, and excited ultrasound transducers. IEEE Trans Ultrason Ferroelectr Freq Control 39(2):262–267

Jensen JA (2004) Simulation of advanced ultrasound systems using field II. IEEE Int Symp Biomed Imaging: Nano Macro I:636–639

Jannin P, Fitzpatrick JM, Hawkes DJ, Pennec X, Shahidi R, Vannier MW (2002) Validation of medical image processing in image-guided therapy. IEEE Trans Med Imaging 21(12):1445–1449

Kwan RKS, Evans AC, Pike GB (1999) MRI simulation-based evaluation of image-processing and classification methods. IEEE Trans Med Imaging 18(11):1085–1097

Pham DL, Xu C, Prince JL (2000) Current methods in medical image segmentation. Annu Rev Biomed Eng 2:315–337

Popovic A, de la Fuente M, Engelhardt M, Radermacher K (2007) Statistical validation metric for accuracy assessment in medical image segmentation. Int J Comput Assisted Radiol Surg 2(3–4):169–181

Segars WP, Lalush DS, Tsui BMW (1999) A realistic spline-based dynamic heart phantom. IEEE Trans Nucl Sci 46(3):503–506

Segars WP, Tsui BMW (2009) MCAT to XCAT: evolution of 4-d computerized phantoms for imaging research. Proc IEEE 97:1954–1968

Shcherbinin S, Celler A, Belhocine T, Vanderwerf A, Driedger A (2008) Accuracy of quantitative reconstructions in SPECT/CT imaging. Phys Med Biol 53(17):4595–4604

Spitzer V, Ackerman MJ, Scherzinger AL, Whitlock D (1996) The visible human male: a technical report. J Am Med Inform Assoc 3(2):118–130

Toh MY, Falk RB, Main JS (1996) Interactive brain atlas with the visible human project data: development methods and techniques. RadioGraphics 16:1201–1206

Udupa JK, LeBlanc VR, Zhuge Y, Imielinska C, Schmidt H, Currie LM, Hirsch BE, Woodburn J (2006) A framework for evaluating image segmentation algorithms. Comput Med Imaging Graph 30:75–87

Veress AI, Segars WP, Weiss JA, Tsui BMW, Gullberg GT (2006) Normal and pathological NCAT image and phantom data based on physiologically realistic left ventricle finite-element models. IEEE Trans Med Imaging 25(12):1604–1616

Warfield SK, Dengler J, Zaers J, Guttmann CR, Wells WM III, Ettinger GJ, Hiller J, Kikinis R (1995) Automatic identification of grey matter structures from MRI to improve the segmentation of white matter lesions. J Image Guid Surg 1(6):326–338

Warfield SK, Zou KH, Wells WM III (2004) Simultaneous truth and performance level estimation (STAPLE): an algorithm for the validation of image segmentation. IEEE Trans Med Imaging 23(7):903–921

Welch BL (1947) The generalization of "Student's" problem when several different population variances are involved. Biometrika 34(1–2):28–35

Yoo TS, Ackerman MJ, Vannier MW (2000) Toward a common validation methodology for segmentation and registration algorithms. In: Medical image computing and computer-assisted intervention—MICCAI 2000. LNCS, vol 1935, pp 217–225

Zou KH, Warfield SK, Bharatha A, Tempany CMC, Kaus MR, Haker SJ, Wells WM III, Jolesz FA, Kikinis R (2004) Statistical validation of image segmentation quality based on a spatial overlap index. Acad Radiol 11(2):178–189

Appendix

14

Abstract

The Appendix contains a detailed discussion of selected mathematical aspects that are necessary for many of the methods presented in this book. In its three sections Markov random fields and their optimization, a derivation of the solution of a variational problem for a function of a single variable and a description of the principal component analysis including a solution that is robust with respect to outliers in the sample are presented.

Concepts, notions and definitions introduced in this chapter

> Markov random fields, neighborhood systems, simulated annealing, mean-field annealing, iterated conditional modes
> Variational calculus, Euler–Lagrange equation
> Principal component analysis, robust PCA, outliers and outlyingness

14.1 Optimization of Markov Random Fields

14.1.1 Markov Random Fields

If a vector $\mathbf{g}$ is an observation of a random process with mean $\mathbf{f}$, the relation between $\mathbf{g}$ and $\mathbf{f}$ is given by the likelihood function $p(\mathbf{g}|\mathbf{f})$ of observing $\mathbf{g}$, if the mean were $\mathbf{f}$. A priori knowledge about the nature of $\mathbf{f}$ is given by the a priori probability $P(\mathbf{f})$ of observing $\mathbf{f}$. If the random process is assumed to be an artefact of the observation (which is the case when noise is distorting a deterministic $\mathbf{f}$), restoration aims to recover the expected value $\mathbf{f}$ given the observation $\mathbf{g}$. This is expressed by the Bayesian theorem

$$P(\mathbf{f}|\mathbf{g}) = \frac{1}{P(\mathbf{g})} p(\mathbf{g}|\mathbf{f}) \cdot P(\mathbf{f}), \qquad (14.1)$$

where $P(\mathbf{g})$ is the a priori probability of $\mathbf{g}$ and acts as a normalizing factor.

K.D. Toennies, *Guide to Medical Image Analysis*,
Advances in Computer Vision and Pattern Recognition,
DOI 10.1007/978-1-4471-2751-2_14, © Springer-Verlag London Limited 2012

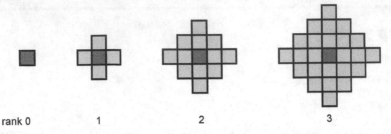

rank 0   1   2   3

Fig. 14.1 Neighbor sizes on a regular grid can be differentiated by the distance to the furthest pixel, which is indicated by the rank

If **f** and **g** represent images, the a priori knowledge about **f** is often related to local homogeneity (e.g., when predicting that it is likely that neighboring pixels have the same gray value). Hence, neighborhood has to be defined among elements of **f**. The probability $p(\mathbf{f})$ must take this neighborhood information into account. It can be expressed by defining the probability as a *Markov random field* (*MRF*). The following is an overview about Markov random fields in their use for restoration and segmentation. Further details and a detailed discussion of other types of MRFs can be found in Li (2009). Details on the optimization of MRFs are also found in the chapter on stochastic optimization in Duda et al. (2001).

A set of random variables $\mathbf{f} = \{f_1, f_2, \ldots, f_i, \ldots, f_k, \ldots,\}$ is an MRF if the conditional probability of an element f_i only depends on the probabilities of elements f_k in some neighborhood of i. Neighborhood can be arbitrary but must be finite. Variables and the neighborhood system constitute a graph with f_i being the nodes and neighboring nodes being connected by an edge.

For regular lattices representing images, neighborhood systems can be ranked by the distance of neighboring elements to the center. A neighborhood of rank 1 of a 2D image would comprise the 4-neighbors, a rank-2 neighborhood would include the 8-neighbors plus pixels in the x- and y-directions that are two pixels away, and so on (see Fig. 14.1).

For a given neighborhood system, dependencies between nodes are defined by clique potentials. A *clique* in a graph is a collection of nodes that is fully connected (every node is connected to every other node, see Fig. 14.2 for rank-1 cliques). The potential V determines the dependency between members of a clique.

The Hammersley–Clifford-Theorem states that for random variables ω, possessing MRF quality, the probability distribution is a Gibbs distribution depending on clique potentials

$$P(\mathbf{f} = \omega) = \frac{1}{\sum_\omega \exp(-U(\omega))} \exp(-U(\omega))$$

$$= \frac{1}{\sum_\omega \exp(-U(\omega))} \exp\left(-\sum_{c \in C} V_c(\omega)\right), \qquad (14.2)$$

clique size   1   2   3

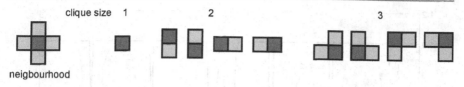

neigbourhood

Fig. 14.2 In a neighborhood of rank 1 several 1st, 2nd, and 3rd order cliques exist

where the potential $U(\omega)$ is the sum of all clique potentials $V_c(\omega)$ of cliques $c \in C$ for a given neighborhood system. The normalization factor sums potentials over all possible configurations. If we assume that the likelihood function $p(\mathbf{f}|\mathbf{g})$ is a Gaussian with mean vector $\mathbf{f}$

$$p(\mathbf{g}|\mathbf{f}) = \frac{1}{Z} \exp\left(-\frac{1}{2}(\mathbf{f}-\mathbf{g})\,\Sigma\,(\mathbf{f}-\mathbf{g})^T\right), \qquad (14.3)$$

this is the energy U for a clique of size 1. It can be integrated into the a priori probability term so that the probability to maximize is

$$p(\mathbf{f}|\mathbf{g}) = \frac{1}{P(\mathbf{g})} p(\mathbf{g}|\mathbf{f}) \cdot P(\mathbf{f}) = \frac{1}{\sum_{\omega} \exp(-U(\omega))} \exp\left(-\sum_{c \in C} V_c(\omega)\right). \quad (14.4)$$

For maximizing $p(\mathbf{f}|\mathbf{g})$ using a maximum likelihood approach, it is necessary to proceed from some configuration $\omega^{(n)}$ to the next configuration $\omega^{(n+1)}$ so that the a posteriori probability of the configuration increases. It requires computation of the normalizing constant in (14.4), which is called the *partition function*. This is unfeasible, however, since it sums over all possible configurations and increases exponentially with the number of nodes.

The partition function can be neglected if $U(\omega)$ is fixed. Given an appropriate definition of the potentials V, maximizing (14.4) then means minimizing

$$e = \sum_{c \in C} V_c(\omega). \qquad (14.5)$$

Optimization is still not simple since elements of $\mathbf{f}$ and $\mathbf{g}$ are dependent on each other through the covariance matrix Σ and the neighborhood dependencies contained in the definition of the clique potentials. Optimization is further complicated by the fact that the landscape produced by the energy function has many local maxima. Finding the global maximum cannot be done by a simple gradient ascent.

Several methods have been presented to find an optimal $\mathbf{f}$ based on (14.5) of which some of the established methods will be discussed in the following sections.

14.1.2   Simulated Annealing

Optimization for solving a restoration task by *simulated annealing* was presented by Geman and Geman (1984). It is a stochastic optimization technique that iterates

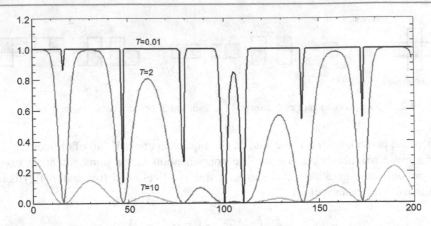

Fig. 14.3 The energy function is rather flat at high temperatures T. With decreasing temperature the minima get more pronounced

through configurations of **f**. The term of the method refers to the simulation of an annealing process of heated metal that—starting from an arbitrary configuration—takes its energy-minimal configuration during the cooling process. Locally and globally minimal configurations are the local maxima of a parameterized Gibbs distribution where a temperature parameter T represents the actual state of cooling. Equation (14.2) now reads

$$
\begin{aligned}
P(\mathbf{f} = \omega) &= \frac{1}{\sum_\omega \exp(-U(T, \omega))} \exp\left(-\frac{U(\omega)}{T}\right) \\
&= \frac{1}{\sum_\omega \exp(-U(T, \omega))} \exp\left(-\frac{\sum_{c \in C} V_c(\omega)}{T}\right).
\end{aligned}
\tag{14.6}
$$

If the temperature is very high, the distribution function is rather flat (see Fig. 14.3). Moving through the configuration space by iterative maximization is easy since the energy differences between configurations are small. Determining the global maximum is difficult, however, since moving away from the maximum is just as easy.

The maxima get more pronounced with decreasing temperatures. Finding a local maximum becomes simpler, while moving out of a local maximum becomes less likely. When the temperature approaches $T = 0$, only the local maxima have nonzero probability.

The annealing process is simulated by gradually decreasing the temperature. At each temperature level the process is allowed to search for the optimal configuration for some time. The search is stochastic. Randomly chosen new configurations are accepted unconditionally if the total energy decreases. The probability of accepting an energy increase depends on the current temperature and the ratio between energy before and after selecting the new configuration. Since the temperature remains constant while iterating through the configurations, the partition function is

```
set temperature T = T0
set initial configuration ωcur
while T > ε do
   while sites have not been polled several times do
      select site i randomly from all sites
      compute perturbed version ωnew of the current estimate ωcur
         by selecting new site label Lnew(i) ≠ L(i)
      compute change of potential between ΔU = U(ωcur) − U(ωnew)
      if ΔU > 0 then
         ωcur = ωnew
      else
         if exp(−ΔU/T) > random(0, 1) then ωcur = ωnew
   end_while
   reduce T according to cooling schedule
end_while
```

Fig. 14.4   Sketch of the annealing algorithm

constant as well and cancels out when computing the ratio. Hence, it does not need to be computed. A sketch of the algorithm can be found in Fig. 14.4.

Geman and Geman (1984) showed that the algorithm produces the optimal solution regardless of the initial configuration if the following annealing schedule is applied

$$T^{(n)} \geq \frac{m \cdot \Delta}{\ln(t+1)}, \tag{14.7}$$

where m is the number of sites and Δ is the energy difference between the configuration with highest energy and the one with lowest energy. Since m is usually large and Δ (if it is known at all) is large as well, the procedure converges very slowly. Hence, approximate schedules are often used such as (Geman and Geman 1984)

$$T^{(n)} = \frac{C}{\ln(t+1)}, \tag{14.8}$$

where the parameter C is chosen based on domain knowledge, or (Kirkpatrick et al. 1983)

$$T^{(n)} = \kappa T^{(t-1)}, \tag{14.9}$$

with parameter κ chosen based on domain knowledge. The selection of C or κ depends on knowledge as to how close the initial configuration is to the optimal result.

14.1.3   Mean Field Annealing

Mean field annealing (Peterson and Soderberg 1989; Zhang 1992) uses a different approach to deal with the fact that computing the partition function is unreasonable.

Instead of iterating through configurations by single state changes it tracks the mean field

$$\langle \omega \rangle_T = \sum_\omega \omega_i P_T (\omega) = \sum_\omega \omega_i \frac{1}{\sum_\omega \exp(-U(T,\omega))} \exp\left(-\frac{U(\omega)}{T}\right). \quad (14.10)$$

The mean approaches the optimal solution when the temperature reaches 0. The advantage of this approach is that the mean reaches the optimal solution much faster than by going through stochastic changes at single sites.

For computing the a posteriori probability the mean from neighboring sites is used to estimate the a priori probability. Equation (14.6) is replaced by

$$P(\mathbf{f} = \omega) \approx \prod_i \frac{1}{\sum_\omega \exp(-U^{MF}(T,\omega))} \exp\left(-\frac{U^{MF}(\omega_i)}{T}\right), \quad (14.11)$$

where U^{MF} is the mean field local energy from neighboring sites. It is assumed to be known.

Since the energy from interaction with neighboring sites is only an estimate based on the current configuration, mean field annealing has to be iterated in a similar fashion as simulated annealing. However, since the U^{MF} estimates are constant for the current iteration, all sites can be updated simultaneously.

Estimates from the mean interaction with neighboring sites are converging faster to the true means than updates from stochastic interaction. Hence, the temperature can be lowered faster than in simulated annealing. There is a heuristic component involved, however, since minima in the mean field are only equal to those in the original energy function if the temperature is zero.

14.1.4 Iterative Conditional Modes

Optimization is much faster using a strategy suggested by Besag (1986) which is called *iterative conditional modes* (ICM). ICM is a greedy strategy that only accepts improvements of the overall potential of a configuration. Hence, it requires a good initial guess for $\mathbf{f}$. As such, ICM is similar to simulated annealing with $T = 0$. The initial guess is readily available if a maximum likelihood estimate is generated from the distorted image without considering neighborhood dependencies of the MRF.

Optimal values for $\mathbf{f}$ are found by changing pixel values at one site f_i at a time. Given an image $\mathbf{f}^{(n)}$ at iteration n, the next image at iteration $(n+1)$ is created by maximizing

$$P\left(f_i^{(n+1)} \mid f_{S-i}^{(n)}, \mathbf{g}\right) = p\left(\mathbf{f}|\mathbf{g}\right) \cdot P\left(f_i \mid f_{\text{Nbs}}\right)$$

$$= p\left(f_i|g_i\right) \cdot P\left(f_i \mid f_{\text{Nbs}}\right)$$

$$= \exp\left(-\frac{(f_i - g_i)^2}{2\sigma^2} - \beta \sum_{k=0}^{K-1} u_{ik}\right), \quad (14.12)$$

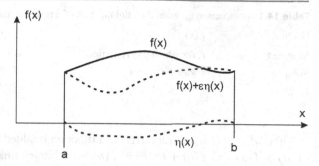

Fig. 14.5 The goal of variational calculus is to find a function $f(x)$ that minimizes a functional of F. Such function is found when any variation by an added test function $\varepsilon\eta(x)$ increases the value of the functional

where $f_{S-i}^{(k)}$ includes all pixels except f_i. Maximizing the probability means minimizing the sum of clique potentials

$$f_i^{(n+1)} = -\arg\min_{f_i}\left[\frac{(f_i^{(n)} - g_i)^2}{2\sigma^2} + \beta\sum_{k=0}^{K-1} u_{ik}^{(n)}\right]. \qquad (14.13)$$

If the neighborhood influence is 0, it turns into a maximum likelihood estimator.

ICM computation can be parallelized if pixels are grouped into sets of nonadjacent pixels.

14.2 Variational Calculus

The goal of variational calculus is to find a minimizing function for a functional (i.e., a function F of a function f). The strategy is similar to the minimization of a function $f(x)$. While for the latter a value x is searched, where $f(x + \Delta x) > f(x)$ for arbitrary changes Δx, in variational calculus a function $f(x)$ is searched of which arbitrarily small changes $\varepsilon \cdot \eta(x)$ cause an increase of the value of the functional F (see Fig. 14.5). The functional is a function of f and its derivatives. How such test functions are applied to solve a general variational problem can be found in textbooks on the calculus of variations (e.g., Weinstock 1974 or Gelfand and Fomin 2003).

The derivation of the solution for the simple variational problem of the kind

$$E(x) = \int_a^b F\left(f(x), f'(x), x\right) dx, \qquad (14.14)$$

where $f(x)$ is twice differentiable on the interval $[a, b]$, will be presented here. It covers the variational problems for the methods presented in this book. The strategy in comparison to minimizing a function is depicted in Table 14.1.

To find a function $f(x)$ that minimizes (14.14), small variations $f(x) + \varepsilon \cdot \eta(x)$ are introduced. The function $\eta(x)$ is twice differentiable on $[a, b]$ with boundary conditions

$$\eta(a) = 0, \qquad \eta(b) = 0. \qquad (14.15)$$

Table 14.1 Comparison between the minimization of a function and that of a functional

Given	$f(x)$	$F(f(x), f'(x), x)$
Searched	x, for which $f()$ is minimal	$f(x)$, for which $\int F()$ is minimal
Solution	x with $f'(x) = 0$	$f(x)$ with $\frac{dE}{df} = \frac{d}{dx}\frac{\partial F}{\partial f'} - \frac{\partial F}{\partial f} = 0$
Iteration	$x^{(n+1)} = x^{(n)} - f'(x^{(n)})$	$f^{(n+1)}(x) = f^{(n)}(x) - dE/df$

Otherwise $\eta(x)$ is arbitrary. Hence, a function is added to $f(x)$ such that $f(a) + \varepsilon\eta(a) = f(a)$ and $f(b) + \varepsilon\eta(b) = f(b)$ for arbitrary functions $\eta(x)$ and arbitrary values ε. The value of ε is now taken as variation parameter

$$J_{f(x)}(\varepsilon) = \int_a^b F\big(f(x) + \varepsilon\eta(x), \, f'(x) + \varepsilon\eta'(x), \, x\big)\, dx. \qquad (14.16)$$

If $f(x)$ is a minimum, any $\varepsilon \neq 0$ will increase $J_{f(x)}(\varepsilon)$. Hence, a necessary condition for $f(x)$ that minimizes E is

$$\left.\frac{dJ_{f(x)}(\varepsilon)}{d\varepsilon}\right|_{\varepsilon=0} = \int_a^b \frac{d}{d\varepsilon}\big[F\big(f(x) + \varepsilon\eta(x), \, f'(x) + \varepsilon\eta(x), \, x\big)\big]\, dx = 0. \quad (14.17)$$

Applying the chain rule (and dropping the arguments for clarity) results in

$$\left.\frac{dJ_{f(x)}(\varepsilon)}{d\varepsilon}\right|_{\varepsilon=0} = \int_a^b \frac{dF}{df}\eta + \frac{dF}{df'}\eta'dx = 0. \qquad (14.18)$$

For using the Lagrangian symbolic of the solution, the following variable substitution is made

$$\delta(x) = \varepsilon\eta(x). \qquad (14.19)$$

Multiplying (14.18) with ε on both sides and making the substitution results in

$$\delta J = \varepsilon\left.\frac{dJ_{f(x)}(\varepsilon)}{d\varepsilon}\right|_{\varepsilon=0} = \int_a^b \frac{\partial F}{\partial f}\delta + \frac{\partial F}{\partial f'}\delta'\, dx = 0. \qquad (14.20)$$

The partial integration[1] of the second term in (14.18) delivers

$$\delta J = \left[\frac{\partial F}{\partial y}\delta\right]_a^b + \int_a^b\left[\frac{\partial F}{\partial f} - \frac{d}{dx}\left(\frac{\partial F}{\partial f'}\right)\right]\delta\, dx = 0. \qquad (14.21)$$

---

[1] Partial integration of an integral of the kind $\int_{a..b} f'g$ uses the multiplication rule from differentiation to arrive at $\int_{a..b} f'g = [fg]_{a..b} - \int_{a..b} fg'$. In the case above $f' := \delta'$ and $g := \partial F/\partial f'$.

The first term vanishes since the boundary conditions require $\delta(a) = \delta(b) = 0$ resulting in

$$\int_a^b \left[\frac{\partial F}{\partial f} - \frac{d}{dx} \left(\frac{\partial F}{\partial f'} \right) \right] \delta \, dx = 0 \tag{14.22}$$

for arbitrary functions δ. The fundamental lemma of calculus states that

$$\int_a^b f(x) \cdot \delta(x) \, dx = 0 \tag{14.23}$$

for a continuous function f and arbitrary, twice differentiable functions δ obeying the boundary conditions $\delta(a) = \delta(b) = 0$. This implies $f(x) = 0$ on $[a, b]$.

The sketch of the proof is as follows. Since δ is arbitrary, it can be selected as $r(x) \cdot f(x)$ with $r(x)$ positive on $]a, b[$, twice differentiable and $r(a) = r(b) = 0$ (e.g., $r(x) = (x - a)(x - b)$). It results in

$$\int_a^b [f(x)]^2 \cdot r(x) \, dx = 0. \tag{14.24}$$

Since $r > 0$ on $]a, b[$, it is easily seen that $f(x) = 0$ must hold on $]a, b[$ for (14.24) to hold. Since f is continuous, $f(x) = 0$ must hold on $[a, b]$ as well. Hence, (14.22) is only true if

$$\frac{\partial F}{\partial f} - \frac{d}{dx} \left(\frac{\partial F}{\partial f'} \right) = 0. \tag{14.25}$$

This condition is called the *Euler–Lagrange equation* giving rise to the iterative solution scheme listed in Table 14.1.

14.3   Principal Component Analysis

Principal component analysis (PCA) is a way for linear decorrelation in feature space (Abdi and Williams 2010). If many of the original features are correlated, the distribution of samples in feature space actually occupies a lower-dimensional sub-space. The PCA produces an orthogonal transformation in feature space such that all covariance values between features are zero. Coordinate axes after transformation are aligned or orthogonal to this subspace (see Fig. 14.6). Features corresponding to axes orthogonal to the subspace can be identified and removed.

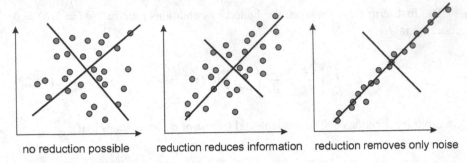

no reduction possible   reduction reduces information   reduction removes only noise

Fig. 14.6 PCA produces an axis system that decorrelates the data. It is oriented along the data distribution in feature space. Features of this new coordinate system may be removed if projection on the remaining axes produces only a small error

14.3.1 Computing the PCA

The covariance matrix $\mathbf{C}$ of the original feature space can be estimated from sample covariances

$$\mathbf{C} = \begin{pmatrix} c_{11} & c_{21} & & c_{N1} \\ c_{12} & & & \\ & & & \\ c_{1N} & & & c_{NN} \end{pmatrix},$$

(14.26)

$$c_{ij} \approx \frac{1}{K-1} \sum_{k=1}^{M} \left(f_{ik} - \bar{f}_i \right) \left(f_{jk} - \bar{f}_j \right), \quad \bar{f}_i \approx \frac{1}{K} \sum_{k=1}^{K} f_{ik},$$

where K is the number of samples available, and f_{ik} is the ith feature of the kth feature vector in the set of samples.

If features were (linearly) uncorrelated all off-diagonal elements should be zero. If features are uncorrelated and occupy only a lower-dimensional subspace that is aligned with features axes some of the variances in the diagonal should be zero as well. Any location of a sample in feature space can still be exactly represented if these features were removed.

Covariance between features usually exists. Hence, $\mathbf{C}$ will contain nonzero off-diagonal elements. The PCA will create a set of new features $\mathbf{f}'$ of which their elements are linear combinations of features of $\mathbf{f}$

$$f_j' = \sum_{i=1}^{N} f_i e_{ij}$$

(14.27)

so that the covariance matrix of the sample distribution $\mathbf{f}'$ no longer has nonzero off-diagonal elements. The beauty of the method is that a closed-form solution exists for computing weights e_{ij}, which we will describe below (see also Fig. 14.7).

Fig. 14.7 The PCA solves an Eigen problem for the covariance matrix **C**. The eigenvectors $\mathbf{e}_i$ are the axes of the new co-ordinate system and the eigenvalues λ_i are variances σ_i^2 along these axes (of which standard deviations σ_i are shown in this picture)

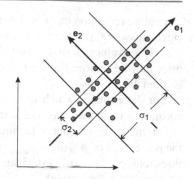

Given an estimate of **C**, a new orthogonal system of feature axes $f_1', \ldots, f_N'$ will be computed with covariance matrix **C'**

$$\mathbf{C}' = \begin{pmatrix} \sigma_1^2 & 0 & 0 \\ 0 & \sigma_2^2 & \\ & & \\ 0 & & \sigma_N^2 \end{pmatrix}, \tag{14.28}$$

with σ_i^2 being the variance of feature f_i. Computing eigenvalues λ_i and eigenvectors $\mathbf{e}_i = (e_{i1}\ e_{i2}\ \ldots\ e_{iN})$ for **C** with

$$\mathbf{C}\mathbf{e}_i = \lambda_i \mathbf{e}_i \quad \Rightarrow \quad \mathbf{C}\mathbf{E} = \mathbf{E}\mathbf{\Lambda} \quad \Leftrightarrow \quad \mathbf{E}^\mathrm{T}\mathbf{C}\mathbf{E} = \mathbf{\Lambda},$$

$$\mathbf{E} = \begin{pmatrix} \mathbf{e}_1 & \mathbf{e}_2 & \ldots & \mathbf{e}_N \end{pmatrix} = \begin{pmatrix} e_{11} & e_{21} & & e_{N1} \\ e_{12} & e_{22} & & \\ & & \ldots & \\ e_{1N} & & & e_{NN} \end{pmatrix} \tag{14.29}$$

produces the decomposition immediately because

$$\mathbf{\Lambda} = \mathbf{E}^\mathrm{T}\mathbf{C}\mathbf{E} \approx \mathbf{E}^\mathrm{T} \left[\frac{1}{K} \sum_{k=1}^{K} (\mathbf{f}_k - \bar{\mathbf{f}}) \times (\mathbf{f}_k - \bar{\mathbf{f}})^\mathrm{T} \right] \mathbf{E}$$

$$= \frac{1}{K} \sum_{k=1}^{K} [\mathbf{E}^\mathrm{T}(\mathbf{f}_k - \bar{\mathbf{f}})] \times [(\mathbf{f}_k - \bar{\mathbf{f}})^\mathrm{T}\mathbf{E}] = \frac{1}{K} \sum_{k=1}^{K} \mathbf{f}_k' \times (\mathbf{f}_k')^\mathrm{T}. \tag{14.30}$$

The matrix $\mathbf{\Lambda}$ is a diagonal matrix containing the eigenvalues of **C**. They correspond to the feature variances of the covariance matrix $\mathbf{C}' = \mathbf{\Lambda}$ in a transformed system where a new feature f_{ik}' is computed by projecting the feature vector $\mathbf{f}_k$ on the ith eigenvector

$$f_{ik}' = (\mathbf{e}_i)^\mathrm{T} (\mathbf{f}_k - \bar{\mathbf{f}}). \tag{14.31}$$

Feature reduction can now be carried out by investigating the variances (i.e., the eigenvalues of $\mathbf{C}$). A feature f_i' can be removed if its corresponding eigenvalue λ_i is zero. Eigenvalues close to zero indicate high linear correlation. Corresponding features may be removed as well since the uncorrelated contribution of those features is often due to noise.

For determining which features are to be removed, features $\mathbf{f}'$ are ordered according to their variance. The accumulated variance $\sigma^2_{\mathrm{accum}}(n) = \sum_{i=1}^{n} \sigma_i^2$ is used to determine the amount of feature reduction. A value of $n < N$ is chosen such that the percentage of $p_{\mathrm{var}}(n) = \sigma^2_{\mathrm{accum}}(n)/\sigma^2_{\mathrm{accum}}(N)$ of the total variance exceeds some threshold (e.g., $p_{\mathrm{var}}(n) > 0.95$ signifying that the first n features explain 95% of the variance in feature space).

14.3.2 Robust PCA

Principal component analysis is often applied when the number of samples is low and the dimension of the feature space is high. However, covariances in the matrix $\mathbf{C}$ are estimated from the samples. Its reliability depends on the size K of the sample set and the dimension of the feature vector. If the PCA is carried out, for instance, in 100-dimensional feature space using just 50 samples, the subspace spanned by the samples will be at most 50-dimensional. Covariance estimates can then be unreliable for two reasons (as has been already noted in Sect. 11.5).

- There is no redundant information about the variance. Hence, any influence from measurement noise in the feature values is interpreted as legal co-variance. This is unwanted when reduced features shall describe some class-specific variation.
- Any outlier in the feature values directly influences the variance estimates of the data (see Fig. 14.8). This is unwanted, as the low probability of measuring an outlier value is not reflected in the covariance estimation.

Several ways exist for a robust PCA that attempt to solve these issues (Wang and Karhunen 1996; Li et al. 2002; Skočaj et al. 2002; Hubert et al. 2005) by assuming that the number of degrees of freedom (i.e., the number of dimensions needed to characterize class attributes by features) is substantially lower than the number of samples. It is furthermore assumed that outliers can be detected by measuring some distance from nonoutlying feature vectors. The main characteristic of a covariance matrix, which is not influenced by outliers, is therefore a low but nonzero determinant. All of the methods work in an iterative fashion.

In the following, the robust PCA by Hubert et al. (2005) will be described which combines several strategies of previous attempts. The method is available as "robpca" in Matlab. It proceeds in three stages.

In the *first stage*, the dimension of the data is reduced to the subspace that is spanned by the samples. If the number of samples is n and the original dimension of the data is d, the subspace is $d_0 \le \min(n, d)$. In other words, if—which is often the case—the number of samples of n is lower than d, the dimension d_0 can be at most n (and may be lower if some of the samples are linear dependent on each other). The result of this stage is the largest subspace in which variances can be estimated from the sample data.

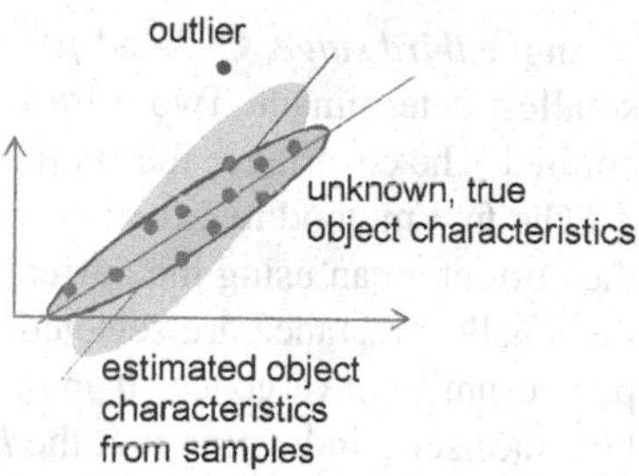

Fig. 14.8 Error in the PCA
due to an outlier in the
samples

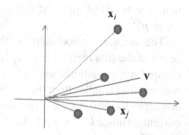

Fig. 14.9 The outlyingness
for some sample x_i is
computed by comparing a
distance measure to arbitrary
directions v with distances of
all other samples x_j to this
direction v

In the *second stage*, the h least outlying samples are searched. In Hubert et al.
(2005) it was shown that h must be larger than $[(n + d_0 + 1)/2]$ and low enough as to
not include any outliers. In the absence of knowledge about the number of outliers
and of d_0, the authors suggested selecting

$$h = \max\left(\alpha n, \frac{n + d_{max} + 1}{2}\right), \qquad (14.32)$$

where d_{max} is the maximum number of principal components that will be selected
as features and α is a control parameter with $\alpha =]0, 1]$.

Selecting α and d_{max} depends on domain knowledge about the data. Hence, it is
not advisable to use any default values from a given implementation. If d_{max} is too
small it may be that too much of the natural class-specific variance in the data is not
accounted for, and if it is set too high outliers may not be removed. The value of α
controls this behavior as well. A high value overrides a too conservatively chosen
maximum of dimensions, while a lower value will increase the robustness.

Given the number nonoutlying samples h, outlyingness will be computed for
each sample. This is essentially a distance measure between the sample in question
and all other samples. The main component of the measure (details can be found
in Hubert et al. 2005, see also Fig. 14.9) is a normalized sample distance to all
lines through pairs of other samples. Since distances are computed with respect to
other samples, they are independent of an external coordinate system. The outlyingness measure is a relative measure that rates this distance to the average normalized
distance of all samples for all possible directions. Only the h samples with lowest
outlyingness are kept for further processing. The first estimate of a robust covariance
matrix $\mathbf{C}^{(0)}$ and a robust mean $\boldsymbol{\mu}^{(0)}$ are computed from these h samples.

In the *third stage*, $\mathbf{C}^{(0)}$ and $\boldsymbol{\mu}^{(0)}$ are used for computing a covariance matrix with smallest determinant. Two different, nonoptimal methods for this computation are applied. The covariance matrix that has the lowest determinant of the two is chosen.

The first method iteratively computes Mahalanobis distances for each sample to the current mean using the current covariance matrix estimate. The h samples with the smallest distance are selected to compute the next estimate. The process is repeated until convergence. It may happen that during the process the determinant becomes zero, indicating that the h samples span a subspace of the d_0-dimensional space. In such a case d_0 is reduced to this subspace and the process is continued. The result of this first method is a covariance matrix $\mathbf{C}^{(1)}$ and the associated mean $\boldsymbol{\mu}^{(1)}$.

The second method starts with the number of dimensions $d_1 \leq d_0$ that is the result of the first method and repeatedly and randomly selects $(d_1 + 1)$ samples and computes a covariance and mean estimate from this subset. If the determinant is nonzero and smaller than the current estimate, the new covariance matrix and mean are kept. The results are estimates $\mathbf{C}^{(2)}$ and $\boldsymbol{\mu}^{(2)}$. If $\det(\mathbf{C}^{(2)}) < \det(\mathbf{C}^{(1)})$ then the current estimate $\mathbf{C}^{(3)}$ is set to $\mathbf{C}^{(2)}$. Otherwise $\mathbf{C}^{(1)}$ is selected as the current estimate $\mathbf{C}^{(3)}$. The means are selected accordingly.

The covariance matrix $\mathbf{C}^{(3)}$ is then used to compute distances between each sample and the estimated mean $\boldsymbol{\mu}^{(3)}$. Samples are weighted by the distances. The final covariance matrix is then computed from the weighted samples. In Hubert et al. (2005) a hard rejection (weights are 0 or 1) is applied depending on this distance, but soft weighting would be possible as well if domain knowledge indicates that outlier characterization by distance may not be reliable.

References

Abdi H, Williams LJ (2010) Principal component analysis. Wiley Interdiscip Rev: Comput Stat 2(4):433–459

Besag J (1986) On the statistical analysis of dirty pictures. J R Stat Soc B (Methodol) 48(3):259–302

Duda RO, Hart E, Stork DG (2001) Pattern classification, 2nd edn. Wiley Interscience, New York

Gelfand IM, Fomin SV (2003) Calculus of variations. Dover, New York

Geman S, Geman D (1984) Stochastic relaxation, Gibbs distributions, and the Bayesian restoration of images. IEEE Trans Pattern Anal Mach Intell 6(6):721–741

Hubert M, Rousseeuw PJ, Branden KV (2005) ROBPCA: a new approach to robust principal component analysis. Technometrics 47(1):64–79

Kirkpatrick S, Gelatt CD Jr, Vecchi MP (1983) Optimization by simulated annealing. Science 220(4598):671–680

Li Y, Xu LQ, Morphett J, Jacobs R (2002) An integrated algorithm of incremental and robust PCA. In: Proc IEEE intl conf image processing, ICIP 2003, vol I, pp 245–248.

Li SZ (2009) Markov random field modeling in image analysis, 3rd edn. Springer, Berlin

Peterson C, Soderberg B (1989) A new method for mapping optimization problems onto neural networks. Int J Neural Syst 1(1):3–22

Skočaj D, Bischof H, Leonardis A (2002) A robust PCA algorithm for building representations from panoramic images. In: Europ conf computer Vision—ECCV 2002. LNCS, vol 2353, pp 81–85

Wang L, Karhunen J (1996) A unified neural bigradient algorithm for robust PCA and MCA. Int J
    Neural Syst 7(1):53–67
Weinstock R (1974) Calculus of variations. Dover, New York
Zhang J (1992) The mean field theory in EM procedures for Markov random fields. IEEE Trans
    Signal Process 40(10):2570–2583

Index

0

0-level set, 272

α

α–β swap move, 244
α-expansion move, 244

A

A posteriori probability, 212
    direct estimation, 387
A priori probability, 213
    Bayesian image restoration, 141
    estimation, 219
AAM, *see* Active appearance model
Absolute connectivity, 251
Absorption edge, 28
Accuracy, 414
Active appearance model, 352
    combining shape and appearance, 353
Active contour, 262
    external energy, 263
    geodesic, 288
    internal energy, 263
    optimization, 264
    without edges, 291
Active geodesic regions, 293
Active shape model, 347
    alignment of landmarks, 350
    combination with FEM, 369
    decorrelation, 348
    landmark selection, 348
    modes of variation, 349
    segmentation, 351
    training, 348
AdaBoost, 408
Adaptive decision boundary, 391
    bias term, 391
    multiple class problem, 393
    nonlinear, 392
Adaptive linear discriminant function, 401
Advection force, 286

Agglomerative clustering, 404
Algebraic reconstruction technique, 67
Analysis software, 8
Anatomical landmark, 305
Anger camera, 65
Angiography, 33
Anisotropic diffusion filtering, 134
Annealing schedule, 447
Anterior commissura, 306, 326
Application entity, 94
ART, 67
Artificial hardware phantom, 429
ASM, *see* Active shape model
Assemblage, 362
Association cost, 248
Association network, 228
Atlas mapping, 325
Attenuation coefficient, 37
Attenuation correction, 70
Attenuation
    SPECT, 67
    ultrasound imaging, 62
    X-ray, 30
Average linkage, 405

B

Backpropagation, 396
Backpropagation network, *see* Multilayer
        perceptron
Bag of features, 165
Bagging, 407
Balloon model, 266
    inflation force, 266
Bayesian classifier, 386
Bayesian image restoration, 138
Bayesian theorem, 212, 443
Beam hardening, 27
Between-class scatter matrix, 383
Binomial filter, 128
Blackening curve, 32
Blob detection, 157

Blood oxygen level dependency, 56
BOLD imaging, 56
Boundary condition
    essential, 362
    natural, 362
Boxcar filter, 128
BrainWeb, 430
Bremsstrahlung, 26
Butterworth filter, 130

C

Canny edge operator, 149
CAT, *see* Computed tomography
Cathode ray tube, 26, 30
Central slice theorem, 38
Chemical shift, 54
Classification
    adaptive decision boundary, 391
    adaptive linear discriminant function, 401
    bagging, 407
    Bayesian classifier, 386
    Bayesian theorem, 212
    kNN classifier, 388
    minimum distance classifier, 387
    multilayer perceptron, 393
    nearest neighborhood classifier, 388
    support vector machine, 398
Clinical study, 5
Clinical workflow, 5
Clique, 444
Clique potential, 444
Clustering, 221, 403
    agglomerative, 404
    fuzzy c-means, 405
    interactive, 221
    k-means, 223
    mean shift, 225
    self-organizing map, 228
Competitive learning, 229
Complete linkage, 405
Composite object, 92
Composite service, 92
Composite SOP class, 93
Compton scatter, 28
Computational phantom, 427
Computed tomography, 35
Computer-aided detection, 6
Computer-aided diagnosis, 6
Computer-assisted surgery, 6
Confidence interval, 437
Contrast, 113
    GLCM, 116
    global, 113
    Michelson, 113
        resolution, 112
        rms, 114
        root-mean-square, 114
Contrast enhancement, 119
    linear, 119
    windowing, 119
    histogram equalization, 119
Convolution backprojection, 40
Corner detector, 155
    Harris, 155
    SUSAN, 157
Correlation coefficient, 309, 339
Correspondence criterion, 301
    anatomical and geometrical landmarks, 302
    image-based features, 307
Covariance, 339
Covariance matrix, 218, 452
Cross-validation, 435
CRT, 26
CT, 35
CT angiography, 43
CT artefacts
    metal artefact, 42
    motion, 42
    noise, 41
    partial volume effect, 41
    step-ladder-artefact, 42
    streak artefacts, 42
CTA, *see* CT angiography
Curvature from divergence, 287

D

Damping matrix, 363
Data dictionary, 98
Decision boundary, 390
Deformable curve, 263
Deformable model, 336
Deformable shape model, 353
Dermoscopy, 74
Deterministic sign change criterion, 308
Diagnosis support, 6
Dice coefficient, 418
DICOM, 91
    application entity, 94
    compression, 106
    conformance statement, 96
    connectivity, 96
    file format, 98
    service class, 92
    service class provider, 94
    service class user, 94
    tag elements, 98
    viewer, 105
DICOM message service element, 93

Difference of Gaussians, 158
Diffusion filtering, 133
Diffusion imaging, 58
Diffusion tensor, 134
Diffusion tensor imaging, 58
Digital mammography, 34
Digital subtraction angiography, 33
Digitally reconstructed radiograph, 319
DIMSE, see DICOM message service element
Discriminant function minimum square error,
    403
Display ACR recommendations, 103
Divergence, 287
DoG, see Difference of Gaussians
Domain knowledge, 7, 16
    in MRF, 139
    in segmentation, 172
    medial axis representation, 346
    representation, 183
    segmentation, 182
    training, 185
    variability, 184
Doppler imaging, 62
DRR, 319
DSA, 33
DSM, 353
DTI, 58
Dynamic level set, 274
    evolution, 275
    stopping criterion, 288
    upwind scheme, 284

E
Edge detection
    Canny, 149
    multi-resolution, 150
Edge enhancement, 123
Edge tracking, 148
    multi-resolution, 151
Edge-preserving smoothing
    Bayesian image restoration, 138
    diffusion filtering, 133
    median filter, 131
EEG, 76
Efficiency, 415
Elastic registration, 323
Elasticity, 263, 364
    modulus, 364
Elasticity matrix, 363
Electroencephalogram, 76
Electromagnetic wave, 24
Electron volt, 25
Element matrix, 361
    assemblage, 362

Endianity, 100
Entropy, 114
Essential boundary condition, 362
Euler–Lagrange equation, 451
    active contour, 264
    variational level sets, 290
Eulerian solution, 278
Evaluation, 7, 17
Expansion move, 244
    graph, 246
Expectation maximization algorithm, 216
Explicit model, 336
External energy, 263
Extrinsic marker, 304

F
F-factor, 25
False negative, 420
False positive, 420
Fast marching algorithm, 282
Fault detection, 415
FBP, see Filtered backprojection
Feature linear decorrelation, 380
Feature reduction, 380, 454
    by principal component analysis, 382
    interactive, 381
Feature similarity, 302
Feature space
    active shape model, 347
    classification, 380
    in registration, 301
Feature vector multi-dimensional, 217
FEM, see Finite element model
Fibre tracking (DTI), 58
FID, 47
Fiducial marker, 314, 423
Fiducial registration error, 314
Field II ultrasound simulation, 430
Field of view, 40
Figure of merit, 414
Filtered backprojection, 38
Finite element model, 360
    acceleration, 363
    combination with ASM, 369
    dynamic, 362
    external force, 365
    searching model instances, 370
    shape function, 360
    static, 361
    velocity, 363
Fisher's discriminant analysis, see Linear
                discriminant analysis
Flat panel detector, 32
Floyd-Fulkerson algorithm, 240

Fluorescence microscopy, 75
Fluoroscopy, 32
fMRI, *see* Functional MRI
Focal spot (CRT), 30
FOM, 414
Foreground segmentation, 172
FOV, 40
Free induction decay, 47
Free vibration mode, 367
Free-form deformation, 323
Functional MRI, 56
Fuzzy c-means clustering, 405
Fuzzy connectedness, 250
   connectivity, 251

G
Gabór filter, 127
Gamma camera, 65
   collimator, 65
Gamma ray, 25
Gantry
   CT, 38
   MRI, 50
Gaussian filter, 128
Gaussian mixture model, 215
   expectation maximization algorithm, 216
Gaussianity, 385
Generalized cylinder, 344
Generalized Hough transform, 340
Geodesic active contours, 288
Geometrical landmark, 306
Ghosting, 54
GHT, 340
Gibbs distribution, 444
Gist, 165
GLCM, *see* Grey-level co-occurrence matrix
Global contrast, 113
Gradient echo imaging, 53
Gradient histogram
   HOG, 164
   SIFT, 161
Gradient magnetic fields, 48
Gradient vector flow, 267
Graph cut, 236
   a priori knowledge, 240
   connecting extrusions, 247
   data cost, 243
   expansion move, 244
   initialization, 243
   interaction cost, 243
   MRF optimization, 242
   normalized, 247
   shape prior, 247, 372
   sink, 236

   source, 236
   swap move, 244
   weights, 237
Grey-level co-occurrence matrix, 115, 181
Ground truth, 424
   from human expert, 425
   from phantoms, 427
   from real data, 425
   STAPLE, 425
GVF, 267
Gyromagnetic constant, 46

H
Hamming filter, 39, 130
Hann filter, 130
Harris corner detector, 155
Harris matrix, 155
Hausdorff distance, 418
   quantile, 419
Head-hat registration, 317
Heaviside function, 291
Hessian matrix, 126
   determinant, 158
Hidden layer, 395
Hierarchical FEM, 370
Hierarchical segmentation, 173
Hierarchical watershed transform, 197
HIS, 85
Histogram, 114
Histogram equalization, 119
   adaptive, 120
Histogram of gradients, 164
Hit-or-miss operator, 345
HL7, 88
   reference information model, 89
HOG, *see* Histogram of gradients
Homogeneous diffusion filtering, 133
Hospital information system, 85
Hough transform
   accumulator cell, 153
   circles, 340
   generalized, 340
   straight lines, 152
Hounsfield unit, 41
HU, 41

I
ICA, 384
ICM, 448
ICP algorithm, 318
Ideal low pass filter, 129
IDL, 9
IFT, *see* Image foresting transform
Image foresting transform, 252

Image foresting transform *(cont.)*
    node load, 252
    path cost, 253
    watershed transform, 254
Image intensifier, 31
    pincushion distortion, 31
    S-distortion, 31
    vignetting, 31
Image-based features, 307
Implicit model, 336, 341
Incompatibility
    DICOM, 97
    HL7, 90
Independent component analysis, 384
Information object, 92
Information object description, 92
Inhomogeneous diffusion filtering, 134
Initialization graph cut, 243
Intelligent scissors, 203
Intensity gradient, 123, 148
    in speed functions, 288
Interaction
    confirmation, 186
    correction, 186
    feedback, 186
    guidance, 186
    guidelines, 186
    parameterization, 186
Interactive delineation, 189
Interactive graph cut, 242
Internal energy, 263
    elasticity, 263
    stiffness, 263
Interobserver variability, 425
Intraobserver variability, 425
Intrinsic landmark, 305
Inversion recovery sequence, 52
IOD, *see* Information object description
Ionizing radiation, 25
Ising model, 220
Iterative closest point algorithm, 318
Iterative conditional modes, 448
ITK, 11

J
Jaccard coefficient, 418
Jackknife technique, 433
Joint entropy, 310

K
K-means clustering, 223
    diversity criterion, 224
    itialization, 224

K-nearest-neighborhood classifier, 388
K-space imaging, 50
Kernel density estimator, 214, 386
Kernel function support vector machine, 401
Kernel trick, 401
KNN classifier, 388
    active and passive samples, 389
    sample normalization, 390
Kohonen network, 228
    clustering, 230
    neighborhood activation, 230
    training, 229
Kurtosis excess, 385

L
Lagrangian solution, 277
Laplace operator, 124
Laplacian of Gaussian, 125, 157
Larmor frequency, 46
LDA, *see* Linear discriminant analysis
Leaving-one-out technique, 433
Level (display), 41
Level set, 270
    evolution computation, 277
    evolution step size, 280
    evolution upwind scheme, 278
    function, 271
    interface, 272
    topologically constrained, 294
    variational, 290
Light box, 101
Light microscopy, 75
Likelihood function, 213
    estimation, 214
    partial volume effect, 215
Line of response, 72
Line pairs per millimeter, 112
Linear discriminant analysis, 382
Linear discriminant function, 401
Linear support vector machine, 398
Live wire, 203
    3D, 206
    cost function, 204
    noise, 205
    optimality criterion, 203
Local affinity, 250
Local shape context, 163
LoG, *see* Laplacian of Gaussian
Longitudinal relaxation, 47
Lpmm, 112

M
M-rep, 346
Magnetic resonance, 45

Magnetic resonance (*cont.*)
   diffusion imaging, 58
   longitudinal relaxation, 47
   perfusion imaging, 57
   T_2* effect, 48
   transverse relaxation time, 47
   proton density, 47
Magnetic resonance imaging, 44
   data acquisition times, 52
   echoplanar imaging (EPI), 53
   frequency encoding, 49
   RARE sequence, 53
   readout gradient, 49
   slice selection, 48
   techniques, 48
Magnetoencephalogram, 77
Mammography, 34
   digital, 34
MAP-EM, 70
Marginal probability, 213
Marker particle solution, 277
Marker-based watershed transform, 199
Markov random field, 138, 443
   graph cut optimization, 242
   neighborhood, 444
Marr-Hildreth filter, 126
Mass matrix, 363
Mass spring model, 354
   external force, 356
   internal force, 357
   node coordinate system, 358
Matching, 300
MatLab, 9
Maximally stable extremal regions, 161
Maximum a posteriori expectation
      maximization, 70
Maximum flow, 240
Maximum likelihood expectation
      maximization reconstruction, 68
MCAT heart phantom, 431
Mean field annealing, 447
Mean filter, 128
Mean shift clustering, 225
   mean shift, 226
   mode, 225
Mean square distance, 339
Mean transit time, 57
Medial axis, 343
   representation, 346
   scale space, 345
   transform, 344
Median filter, 131
   artefacts, 132

Medical workstation, 101
   software, 104
MEG, 77
MevisLab, 9
Mexican hat filter, 126
Microscopy, 75
MIL, 409
Mincut maxflow, 240
Minimum cost graph cut, 236
Minimum distance classifier, 387
Mixture of Gaussians, 215
MLEM, 68
MLP, *see* Multilayer perceptron
Model, 334
   explicit representation, 262
   implicit representation, 262
   instance, 334
Model-driven segmentation appearance model,
      352
Model-driven segmentation
   by active contours, 261
   shape model, 335
Modes of variation, 349
Modulation transfer function, 117
MR angiography, 54
   flow void, 54
   phase contrast, 54
   gadolinium-enhanced, 54
MR artefact
   chemical shift, 54
   ghosting, 54
   noise, 54
   partial volume effect, 54
   shading, 54
MRA, *see* MR angiography
MRF, *see* Markov random field
MRI, *see* Magnetic resocance imaging
MSER, 161
MTF, 117
Mulitlayer perceptron momentum term, 397
Multi-resolution edge detection, 150
Multi-resolution edge tracking, 151
Multi-resolution MRF, 221
Multilayer perceptron, 393
   for classification, 395
   learning rate, 396
   overadaptation, 397
Multilayer segmentation, 173
Multiple instance learning, 409
Mumford–Shah functional, 290
Mutual information, 310
mWST, 199

N

N-link, 236
Narrow band method, 285
Natural boundary condition, 362
NCAT phantom, 431
NCut algorithm, 250
Nearest neighborhood classifier, 388
Neighbor link, 236
Neighborhood similarity, 324
Newmark-β algorithm, 365
    computation, 367
Noise, 117
    reduction, 127
Non-rigid registration, 322
    initialization, 324
    smoothness constraint, 322
Nonlinear decision boundary, 392
    support vector machine, 400
Normalization, 300, 325
    ROI-based, 327
Normalized graph cut, 247
    approximation, 248
    association cost, 248
Normalized histogram, 115
Normalized object, 92
Normalized service, 92
Normalized SOP class, 93
Nuclear imaging, 64
Null hypothesis, 436

O

One-sided t-test, 438
OpenCV, 11
Ordered subset expectation maximization, 70
OSEM, 70
OSI, 88
OSL algorithm, 70
Otsu's method, 191
Outlier detection, 435
    paired landmarks, 316
    PCA, 454
    unpaired landmarks, 316
Outlyingness, 455
Over-segmentation, 173, 197
Overlap measure, 417
Oversegmentation, 417

P

p-value, 436
PACS, 87
Pair production, 29
Paired landmarks, 313
Paired t-test, 438
Partial volume effect, 41

Partition function, 445
Partitional clustering, 222
Parzen window, 214
Pattern intensity criterion, 321
PCA, *see* Principal component analysis
PDM, 347
Peak SNR, 117
Perceptron, 393
Perfusion imaging, 57
PET, *see* Positron emission tomography
PET artefacts, 73
Phantom, 427
Photoelectric absorption, 28
Photon, 24
Physical phantom, 427
Picture archiving and communication system,
    87
Pincushion distortion, 31
Point distribution model, 347
Poisson ratio, 364
Positron emission tomography, 72
Posterior commissura, 306, 326
Precision rate, 421
Primary landmarks, 348
Principal axis, 315
Principal component analysis, 382, 451
    feature reduction, 454
    for registration, 315
Probabilistic Talairach coordinates, 326
Procrustes distance, 304
Proton density, 47
Pull mode, 95
Push mode, 94
PVE, 41

Q

QoF, 335
Quadric, 342
Quality
    delineation task, 416
    detection task, 420
    registration task, 422
Quality of fit, 335
Quantile Hausdorff distance, 419
Quaternion, 314

R

Radiation
    characteristic, 26
    excitation, 26
    monochrome, 26
    polychrome, 26
Radiation absorbed dose, 25
Radiation exposure, 25

Radiology information system, 85
Radon transform, 36
RAG, 195
Raleigh damping, 363, 368
Raleigh scatter, 28
Random walk, 254
  algorithm, 257
  computation, 255
  for segmentation, 255
  probability function, 255
Recall rate, 421
Receiver operator characteristic, 421
Reference information model, 89
Region adjacency graph, 195
Region growing, 199
  homogeneity, 200
  leaking, 202
  seeded, 201
  symmetric, 201
  two pass, 200
Region merging, 195
Registration, 299
  components, 300
  digitally reconstructed radiograph, 319
  features, 302
  pattern intensity criterion, 321
  projection image, 319
  with quaternions, 314
  with segmentation, 328
Reinforcement learning, 229
Relative cerebral blood flow, 57
Relative cerebral blood volume, 57
Relative connectivity, 252
Relaxation labeling, 193
Reliability, 414
Representation, 334
Resolution enhancement, 120
Retina photography, 74
Rigid registration, 312
  from paired landmarks, 313
  in frequency domain, 317
RIS, 85
Robust PCA, 454
Robustness, 414, 435
ROC, 421
ROC curve, 422
  area under the ROC curve, 422
Rotation
  matrix, 313
  with quaternions, 314

S
S-distortion, 31
Saliency, 165

Scale space, 337
Scale-invariant feature transform, 159
Scintigraphy, 65
SCP, 94
SCU, 94
Secondary landmarks, 348
Seeded region growing, 201
Segmentation
  active contour, 262
  by classification, 212
  clustering, 221
  data knowledge, 175
  domain knowledge, 172, 182
  finite element model, 360
  fuzzy connectedness, 250
  Gaussian pyramid, 177
  geodesic active contours, 288
  graph cut, 242
  image foresting transform, 252
  influence from noise, 177
  interactive, 188
  interactive graph cut, 236
  kinds of interaction, 185
  level sets, 285
  live wire, 203
  mass spring model, 354
  normalized graph cut, 247
  random walks, 254
  region growing, 199
  region merging, 195
  shading, 177
  split and merge, 196
  texture, 179
  thresholding, 190
  variational level set, 290
  watershed transform, 197
  with active shape models, 351
  with shape prior, 371
Self-organizing map, 228
  clustering, 230
  neighborhood activation, 230
  training, 229
Sensitivity, 420
Service class provider, 94
Service class user, 94
Service object pair, 93
Shading, 54
Shadow groups, 99
Shape context, 163
Shape decomposition, 337
Shape descriptor, 343
Shape detection, 335
Shape deviation, 335
Shape distance, 372

Shape feature vector, 347
Shape function, 360
Shape hierarchy, 338
Shape matching
    dummy points, 164
    with local shape context, 164
Shape model, 334
Shape prior, 247, 371
Shape representation, 335
Shape-based interpolation, 121
SIFT, 159
    feature computation, 160
    key point generation, 159
    key point reduction, 159
    matching, 161
Sigmoid function, 396
Signal-to-noise ratio, 117
Signed distance function level sets, 273
Significance, 436
Simple point, 294
Simulated annealing, 142, 445
    optimal solution, 447
    schedules, 447
Single linkage, 405
Single photon emission computed tomography,
    71
Skeleton, *see* Medial axis
Slack variable, 401
Slice interpolation, 121
Smoothness constraint, 322
Snake, 262
SNR, 117
Sobel operator, 124
Software phantom, 429
SOM, *see* Self-organizing maps
Sonography, *see* Ultrasound imaging
SOP, 93
Spatial resolution, 112
Specificity, 421
Speckle artefact, 62
SPECT, 71
Speed function, 277, 285
    advection force, 286
    curvature, 286
    data knowledge, 288
    intensity gradient, 288
Speeded-up robust features, 161
Spin echo sequence, 51
Spin (of an atom), 44
Spin precession, 46
Spin-lattice-relaxation time, 47
Spin-spin-relaxation time, 47
Spiral scanner, 38
Split and merge, 196

Spring force, 357
STAPLE, 425
    sensitivity and specificity estimation, 426
Stationary level set, 274
    arrival time, 281
    evolution, 275
    upwind scheme, 281
Stereotaxic coordinate system, 325
Stiffness, 263
Stiffness matrix, 361
Stochastic sign change criterion, 308
Stopping criterion
    dynamic level set, 288
    stationary level set, 283
Stress matrix, 363
Student-t-test, 436
Superellipsoid, 342
    with free-form deformation, 343
Support vector, 399
Support vector machine, 398
    linear, 398
    nonlinear decision boundary, 400
    radial base functions, 401
    slack variables, 401
SURF, 161
SUSAN corner detector, 157
SVM, *see* Support vector machine
Swap move, 244
    graph, 245
Symmetric region growing, 201

T
T-distribution, 438
T-link, 236
T-snake, 268
    evolution, 269
T-surface, 269
T-test, 436
T_1-time, 47
T_2* effect, 48
T_2-time, 47
Talairach coordinates, 325
Tanimoto coefficient, 418
Template matching, 338
Terminal link, 236
Tertiary landmarks, 348
Texture, 179
    Haralick's features, 181
    Law's filter masks, 181
    spectral features, 181
Thinning algorithm, 345
Thresholding, 190
    connected component analysis, 190
    Otsu's method, 191

Thresholding (*cont.*)
    relaxation labeling, 193
    shading correction, 193
    using fuzzy memberships, 191
    Zack's algorithm, 191
Topologically constrained level sets, 294
Torsion force, 358
Transfer function, 119
Transverse relaxation, 47
Treatment planning, 6
True negative, 420
True positive, 420
Turbo spin echo sequence, 53
Two-sided t-test, 438

U

UID, 92
Ultrasound artefacts, 62
Ultrasound imaging, 60
    A-scan, 61
    B-scan, 61
Under-segmentation, 417
Unique identifier, 92
Upwind scheme, 278

V

Valence electron, 25
Validation, 413
    documentation, 414
    quality measures, 415
    robustness, 435
    sources of variation, 434
Variational calculus, 449
Variational level set, 290
    with shape prior, 372
Variational level sets
    active contours without regions, 292
    active geodesic regions, 293

Euler–Lagrange equation, 290
    geodesic active contour, 289
Vibration mode, 367
    object-specific symmetry, 369
Viewer software, 8
Vignetting, 31
Viscous fluid model, 323
Visible human, 428

W

Watershed transform, 197
    by image foresting transform, 254
    flooding, 197
    hierarchical, 197
    marker-based, 199
    over-segmentation, 197
Wave propagation, 273
Welch-test, 439
Window (display), 41
Within-class scatter matrix, 383
WST, *see* Watershed transform

X

X-ray, 24
    attenuation, 27
    contrast, 28
    generation, 25
    imaging, 29
    tube, 27
XCAT phantom, 431

Y

Young's modulus, 364

Z

Z message (HL7), 90
Zack's algorithm, 191